THE A to Z OF

COSMETIC AND PLASTIC SURGERY

THE A to Z OF

COSMETIC AND PLASTIC SURGERY

Carol Ann Rinzler

Foreword by
Robert T. Grant, M.D., M.Sc., F.A.C.S.
and by
Stanley Darrow, D.D.S., F.A.C.D., F.A.G.D.

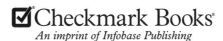
☑️Checkmark Books®
An imprint of Infobase Publishing

The A to Z of Cosmetic and Plastic Surgery

Checkmark Books
An imprint of Infobase Publishing
132 West 31st Street
New York NY 10001

ISBN-13: 978-0-8160-7908-7
ISBN-10: 0-8160-7908-0

The Library of Congress has cataloged the
hardcover edition of this work as follows:

Library of Congress Cataloging-in-Publication Data
Rinzler, Carol Ann.
The encyclopedia of cosmetic and plastic surgery / Carol Ann Rinzler; foreword by Robert T. Grant and by Stanley Darrow.
p. ; cm.
Includes bibliographical references and index.
ISBN-13: 978-0-8160-6285-0 (alk. paper)
ISBN-10: 0-8160-6285-4 (alk. paper)
1. Surgery, Plastic—Encyclopedias. I. Title.
[DNLM: 1. Reconstructive Surgical Procedures—Encyclopedias—English. 2. Cosmetic Techniques—Encyclopedias—English. 3. Surgery, Plastic—Encyclopedias—English. WO 13 R584e 2009]
RD118.R56 2009
617.9'5—dc22   2008016098

Checkmark Books are available at special discounts when purchased in bulk quantities for businesses, associations, institutions, or sales promotions. Please call our Special Sales Department in New York at (212) 967-8800 or (800) 322-8755.

You can find Facts On File on the World Wide Web at http://www.factsonfile.com

Text and cover design by Cathy Rincon

Printed in the United States of America

VB Hermitage 10 9 8 7 6 5 4 3 2 1

This book is printed on acid-free paper and contains 30 percent postconsumer recycled content.

CONTENTS

FOREWORD

Plastic and reconstructive surgery is a "quality-of-life" specialty. Plastic surgeons are devoted to improving the health, wellness, and life experience of their patients. We do not "save" lives in the sense that a cardiac surgeon helps repair the heart's blood supply after a heart attack or the breast surgeon fights a woman's cancer by removing part or all of her breast. It is in reconstructing the breast after an operation and restoring a women's sense of wholeness, or addressing a skin wound that will not heal after open heart surgery that plastic surgeons add tremendously to the patient's overall recovery and ability to enjoy life most completely. It can be hard to assess the value of the contributions of plastic surgery. Deaths from diseases treated by plastic surgeons and "traditional" complications, like bleeding and infection, while seen, are not as commonplace as after procedures in other specialties. How does one assess the success of the operation in plastic surgery? We talk of a quick return to work and baseline health for the patient after plastic surgery, an improvement in self-esteem that results from the procedure and enhancement of the patient's personal perspective on life and relationships as markers for successful outcomes from our procedures. How does one measure the improved social skills seen in people previously too shy to express themselves completely because of a body part that they were born with or that develops that is not in proportion to the rest of their frame, who blossoms after the face or body are put in better harmony by a plastic surgery procedure? It is in meeting or exceeding the patient's reasonable expectations of the result from the planned procedure that plastic surgeons excel.

Plastic surgery is also a specialty not restricted by anatomic boundaries. When you make an appointment to see an orthopedic surgeon, you are going to have a bone or joint problem addressed. Likewise, when you see a neurosurgeon, your likely ailment involves the brain, spinal cord, or peripheral nervous system. Since plastic surgery is defined by the kinds of procedures that are performed and the techniques the surgeon utilizes, every plastic surgeon's practice is unique, so if you have met one plastic surgeon, you have met one plastic surgeon! Plastic surgeons operate all over the body, on the surface, and in the deepest recesses of remote body cavities. They operate on newborns and elderly patients, patients with acute reconstructive needs, and patients who are having truly elective surgery. Plastic surgeons' clinical practices can vary widely from practitioner to practitioner. Some plastic surgeons specialize in surgery of the hand, others in pediatric facial and congenital anomalies like cleft lip and palate. Others can reconstruct a portion of the jawbone removed to treat a cancer by fashioning a new jaw out of the "spare parts" portion of one of the bones of the leg, the fibula. They then use microsurgery to reconnect the bone's blood supply to ensure it stays alive after it has been moved into its new position in the body. Joseph Murray, M.D., the surgeon who pioneered the first kidney transplant, is a plastic surgeon. All of the advances today in transplantation of solid organs such as livers, hearts, and kidneys, including the amazing advances with "composite" organ transplants (tissues made up of a variety of differing cell types like hands and faces) all owe their success to the work of plastic surgeons.

Finally, there is the cosmetic surgeon—the kind of plastic surgeon most lay people think is representative of the work done in the specialty. Not only mainstream American media, but most Americans themselves are fascinated not just with the lives and lifestyles of cosmetic surgery patients, but with those of the practitioners as well! It is no secret that as the American population ages, the "baby boomer" population is carrying to new levels the search to remain not only active but to look younger than their parents did at the same age. There has been dramatic growth in the past decade in both of the noninvasive techniques available—fillers that replace lost facial volume due to age as well as injectable toxins that erase the wrinkles that come over time. Laser and other light-based technologies also are now available to "rejuvenate" the face, hands, and chest, working to counter the deleterious cosmetic effects of a lifetime of sun exposure, poor dietary habits, and smoking. Men, too, have jumped on the cosmetic surgery bandwagon, accounting for as many as 15 to 20 percent of patients seeking cosmetic services in recent surveys. They also desire the vigorous look of youth at home and in their workplaces. The time-honored proverb may state that "appearance isn't everything," but survey after survey confirms that in today's culture and society people who are considered more youthful and pleasing in appearance get promoted faster and make more money than their older-appearing, less attractive peers.

Plastic surgeons are leading the way among medical professionals in building wellness relationships with their patients, partnering with them in defining lifestyle choices that make one beautiful both within and without.

But not all plastic surgery is performed by plastic surgeons. Because there is no traditional anatomic border to this specialty, other doctors have flocked to cosmetic surgery and medicine as a way to protect their own personal financial bottom line from the economic realities of the increasingly dysfunctional health care system. When a doctor puts self-interest ahead of the interests of his or her patients, trouble follows. Whether it is in the exploitation of the doctor-patient relationship for entertainment purposes on "reality TV" or the shameless promotion of new, untested, or unproven treatments for aging or for rejuvenation, doctors practicing cosmetic surgery and medicine fail their patients and their profession. "Newer" is not always necessarily better.

So where does this leave the patient? Bombarded by images daily in the media or online, how does one cut through the morass of information related to plastic surgery, yet not be overwhelmed and still feel in control of one's life and health? Referring to trusted sources of information is the best prescription for moving forward. The information contained in *The A to Z of Cosmetic and Plastic Surgery* is indeed comprehensive. Making reference to the topics reviewed in this volume is an outstanding way to familiarize oneself with the language, traditions, and techniques of the specialty of plastic and reconstructive surgery. After reading through the topics here, use the Internet and consult the Web sites of the American Society of Plastic Surgeons or the American Society for Aesthetic Plastic Surgery, as both contain additional resources designed specifically for the education of patients and providers. Finally, find a board-certified plastic surgeon who shares your same life perspective and goals for health and wellness.

Before you agree to undergo any procedure, your plastic surgeon should be seeking to explore the potential motivations for why you might be considering a certain procedure. The doctor should be asking questions such as "How long has this issue been bothering you?" or, "How do you see the potential for improvement from the procedure affecting your life?" Plastic surgeons know that the more specific they can frame the issue that bothers the patient, the higher the likelihood of a successful surgical outcome. Most accomplished plastic surgeons can deliver the desired enhancement in one's appearance if they feel the patient is a reasonable and realistic candidate. What no surgeon can do is say whether an enhanced post-operative body image will improve one's relationship with a spouse or make one more desirable to a potential employer. That part is up to you!

Remember that all procedures, even the less invasive ones like fillers and lasers, have risks and side effects, even in the most skilled hands. If it seems "too good to be true," well, it probably is. Medicine and surgery have made quantum leaps over past generations, but the basic components of human healing and frailty remain. Complete healing takes time, a commodity increasingly in short supply in today's hectic pace of work and home life. When surgery is truly elective, make sure you are in the best physical and mental health possible before proceeding. If there are unresolved health or wellness issues, there is no reason to move forward. Reschedule the planned procedure or return later for another consultation once your life and health are in better order. Having a complication or less than optimal outcome will not make you feel better about yourself at all! You are in control of when you want to consider scheduling a consultation or potential operation.

The elective nature of the aesthetic marketplace is a great advantage. Be sure to visit a number of plastic surgeons before undergoing any type of procedure to be sure you have found the best practitioner and feel confident with the choice and the advice received. You should like and trust your plastic surgeon and should never feel rushed or harried. By doing your "homework," through this book, online, and in person, you will have become empowered in harnessing those areas where traditional medical doctors can assist in improving how you look and feel.

Robert T. Grant, M.D., M.Sc, F.A.C.S.,
Plastic-Surgeon-in-Chief, New York Presbyterian
Hospital, the University Hospital of Columbia and
Cornell; Associate Clinical Professor of Surgery,
College of Physicians and Surgeons of Columbia
University; Adjunct Associate Professor of Clinical
Surgery (Plastic Surgery), Weill Medical College
of Cornell University

The dentist is a major figure in the enhancement of facial cosmetic improvement. He or she is not only concerned with the teeth but with all of the jaw apparatus. Without properly functioning jaw joints, muscles, and lips, facial expression may be compromised. Probably the most commonly addressed issue is the position of the teeth, which are visible, and their appearance, color, and shape. Missing teeth can be a functional and aesthetic problem.

Replacement of missing teeth has been a major concern of restorative dentists in recent years as well as far back in history as the earliest civilizations. Modern techniques for replacement have been enhanced and refined, giving the dentist many new and effective tools. This includes refinement and scientific validation of implant procedures, a process of giving a patient replacement teeth. Currently this system is in the hands of the trained general dentist or a team of surgical and restorative practitioners.

Other advances in dentistry provide for new and improved restoration of individual teeth after carious (affected by cavities) or traumatic injury. Newer materials and techniques are aimed at attaining maximum aesthetic results and longevity. The smile as a social and business asset helps create a first impression of great significance. In the forefront of an engaging smile is a pleasing presentation of the teeth. The aesthetic dentist is instrumental in creating the most natural shape and color of teeth, which should conform to the facial features of his or her patient. The teeth are not only framed by the face and lips but also by the gingival (gum) tissue displayed. Healthy pink gum tissue is pleasing to the observer. The periodontal specialist is sometimes needed to restore healthy-looking gingival tissue. Some of the more technically exacting procedures may involve grafting tissue from other areas of the mouth.

New techniques that allow doctors to change the shape and color of teeth include direct bonding, ceramic veneers, and enhanced-strength porcelain crowns. It should be noted that chalky white coloration or straight lines do not make for great aesthetics. Restorative dentists are trained to relate tooth form and shading to the facial contours and complexion of the patient. There are many simple and noninvasive procedures that can enhance the appearance of teeth. The aesthetic dentist will consider all aspects and choose procedures that will help the patient in line with financial limitations.

Pathological lesions in the oral cavity or externally on the face are not only aesthetically unpleasant but can be life threatening. Disclosure and biopsy aids are available for discovery of early cancer lesions. Other lesions are diagnosed or treated or may be referred to the required specialty areas.

Prevention of oral disease is in the hands of the patient at home and in regular visits to the dentist. Properly timed regular visits can forestall the breakdown of teeth and expensive and extensive restorative procedures later in life.

It should also be noted that certain habitual or dysfunctional jaw movements can change the shape of teeth by wear or by destruction of restorations. The dentist is the only health practitioner who has the knowledge and experience to treat such jaw dysfunction and associated joint and muscle pain. Pain can disfigure a smile as can physical aberrations.

The potential facial aesthetics patient should search for a skilled aesthetic dentist with whom he or she can relate and fully discuss needs and expectations. Just as dental correction offers an addition to surgical facial improvements, it may effectively be complemented by various forms of plastic surgery. This volume will supply much needed information relevant to all aspects of cosmetic improvement.

Stanley Darrow, D.D.S., F.A.C.D., F.A.G.D.
Former professor of operative dentistry at
New York University College of Dentistry and
currently attending dentist at Flushing Hospital
and Medical Center

INTRODUCTION
Changing Faces, Changing Bodies, Changing Lives

Throughout history, people have done interesting things to make themselves look better. Ancient Egyptians plucked their body hair. Africans stretched their necks and earlobes. Asians bound their feet. Western Europeans plastered their faces with fashionable but deadly lead-based powder. In modern America, people pass up these simple body alterations in favor of plastic surgery (from the Greek word *plastikos,* which means "to mold or to form").

According to the American Society of Plastic Surgeons (ASPS), the largest organization of board-certified plastic surgeons in the world, in 2006 Americans signed up for nearly 2 million cosmetic plastic surgeries such as face-lifts, "tummy tucks," liposuction, and implants for body parts from cheek to calf and everything in between. The five most popular were breast augmentation (329,000 procedures), followed by nose reshaping (307,000), liposuction (303,000), eyelid surgery (233,000), and tummy tightening abdominoplasty (146,000) and a list of other procedures ending with pectoral implants (403), surgery designed to make a man's chest look more manly.

In the same year, there were more than 9 million minimally invasive procedures recorded. These are cosmetic treatments that are not actually surgery but change one's appearance. The five most popular: Botox injections (4,000,000), chemical face peels (1,000,000), laser hair removal (887,000), skin-smoothing microdermabrasion (816,000), and "plumping" wrinkle fillers (778,285).

Not all plastic surgery is cosmetic or elective. Noting that physicians in India are reported to have been using skin grafts as early as 800 B.C.E., the American Society of Plastic Surgeons calls its discipline "one of the world's oldest healing arts." They would also be justified in calling it "an art born of war." As discussed in the entry titled "plastic surgery" on page 150, much of modern plastic surgery is reconstructive, procedures that evolved from techniques that were born on the battlefield as emergency measures to replant limbs, protect burned skin, and prevent death from catastrophic blood loss.

Today, these procedures have been refined so that the same skilled surgeons who performed cosmetic surgery also undertake lifesaving or life-changing reconstructive procedures. They may remove tumors, rebuild malformed hearts, correct devastating structural birth defects such as cleft lip and palate or a misaligned face, repair injuries, remove scars, and restore catastrophically burned skin. In 2006, more than 5,000,000 such surgeries were performed in the United States.

About This Book

The public's modern fascination with youth and cosmetic surgery, demonstrated by the popularity of such television attractions as the wily *Nip/Tuck* and the astonishing *Extreme Makeover* specials and the parade of celebrities showing off their new-and-improved bodies, has created a large market for books on cosmetic plastic surgery. A quick flip through the virtual pages of Amazon.com or BarnesandNoble.com, though, shows that virtually all the books currently available for lay readers focus tightly on elective cosmetic surgeries.

True, these books are informative; some are also entertaining. But as a group they may lack medical authority. For example, many mention "nose jobs," the lay term for plastic surgery to slim and shape the nose. But few list the term *rhinophyma*, a synonym for small fibrous tumors characteristic of the thickening of the skin on the nose due to rosacea that are sometimes removed with plastic surgery.

The emphasis on the cosmetic aspect of plastic surgery is fine for readers looking for a chatty guide to better appearance through surgery. However, students researching reconstructive surgery or a seriously curious layperson who wants to know how to heal the rosacea rhinophyma that turned early film comedian W. C. Fields's or former president Bill Clinton's noses red and bumpy needs something more complete.

The obvious answer is a medical text, but textbooks are written for medical students, which means lay readers need to know more than they know to find out what they don't know. Hence, *The A to Z of Cosmetic and Plastic Surgery.*

This book, like other Facts On File's Library of Health and Living volumes, is designed to help the lay reader bridge the gap between *lightweight* and *technical* while also serving as an accessible source of current information for various medical professionals who appreciate a clear, direct encyclopedia-style presentation. The elastic A to Z format accommodates a wealth of information such as

- Individual entries for health conditions such as cleft lip and/or palate that may require plastic surgery or conditions such as roughened facial skin that can be treated with a noninvasive, nonsurgical procedure. Each medical condition entry begins with a brief description of the condition, followed by a section listing Symptoms and Diagnostic Path, one listing Treatment Options and Outlook, and, finally, an overview of the Risk Factors and Preventive Measures relevant to the condition.

- Individual entries for specific cosmetic and surgical procedures such as abdominoplasty and nonsurgical treatments such as acupuncture. Each entry starts with a brief introduction identifying the condition for which the surgery/procedure is prescribed. Next is a section describing the Procedure, one listing the surgical Risks and Complications, and, finally, a concluding section on postsurgical Outlook and Lifestyle Modifications.

- Individual entries to describe the structure and function of organs and body systems such as the immune system and the circulatory system and why they are relevant to cosmetic and plastic surgery procedures.

- A glossary of the medical and technical terms from *abscess* to *zone* commonly used when describing human anatomy, medical conditions, and cosmetic and plastic surgeries.

- A bibliography listing the sources—books, periodicals, pamphlets, Internet sites—reviewed while writing this book.

- An appendix, Web Sites for the cosmetic and plastic surgery patient, which includes the Internet sites for medical associations for plastic surgeons and physicians in related disciplines; general medical information; technical information; and medical and surgical language; plus a list of Web addresses for the state and District of Columbia medical societies, giving access to information about the surgeon one may choose to do a procedure.

Clearly, this guide to the procedures and practices plastic surgeons use to enhance or repair the human body is a valuable first step not only for researchers but for potential patients as well. Taking the next steps—deciding whether plastic surgery is the right choice and whether the surgeon under consideration is the right person for the job—requires the reader to ask some serious questions.

Looking before You Leap into Plastic Surgery

Reconstructive surgery is rarely an elective procedure. The defects and injuries it repairs are crippling at best and life-threatening at worst.

Cosmetic surgeries, on the other hand, are elective. That is not to say that they are minor or that their effects are trivial. Appearance is important to one's self-esteem, and the variety of procedures created by modern cosmetic plastic surgery can, indeed, change lives.

However, there are pitfalls along the way. For some patients, the desire to look better escalates to an obsession that leads to multiple unnecessary surgeries. Others are so determined to have surgery that they ignore doctors who say their health may make the surgery too risky and seek out someone who will wield the knife. The best-known example of the former may be singer Michael Jackson. One sad example of the latter is Donda West, mother of rap star Kanye West. Turned down by a reputable surgeon, Ms. West found another who was willing to proceed, and she died due to complications from cosmetic surgery in 2007.

To avoid these problems and help ensure a successful experience, the American Society of Plastic Surgeons recommends the all prospective plastic surgery patients ask—and answer—some basic questions about their forthcoming surgical experience.

Questions to Ask the Doctor

1. Are you certified by the American Board of Plastic Surgeons?
2. Are you a member of the American Society of Plastic Surgeons?
3. How many procedures of this type have you done?
4. Do you have hospital privileges (the right to admit patients to or perform surgery in a specific hospital)?
5. What specific risks are associated with this surgery?
6. How long will my recovery take? What limits will I face in my daily life (including work)?
7. How much will this procedure cost? Is it covered by insurance, or will we set up a payment schedule?

Questions to Ask about the Surgical Site

1. Is the hospital where this procedure will occur accredited by the Joint Commission on the Accreditation of Healthcare Organizations?
2. If the procedure will be done at a freestanding outpatient facility, is the facility accredited by the Accreditation Association for Ambulatory Health Care, Inc. or the American Association for Accreditation of Ambulatory Surgery Facilities?
3. Is the facility associated with a nearby hospital in case an emergency arises?
4. Is the person providing anesthesia for this procedure a board-certified physician (anesthesiologist) or a certified registered nurse anesthetist?
5. If the doctor performs procedures in his or her office, is there lifesaving equipment available in case of emergency?

Questions to Ask Yourself

1. Do I have a health condition that would rule out the surgery I am considering or make it more complicated than expected?
2. Can I comply with any medical regimens or tasks required to make my surgery successful?

When deciding to have elective surgery, one has the chance to elect. That is, to choose to have the surgery and to choose, at will, the surgeon. To do this well and safely, it is essential to get complete answers to all the questions listed above before proceeding.

Carol Ann Rinzler
March 2008

ACKNOWLEDGMENTS

In writing this book, I owe a debt of gratitude to Robert T. Grant, M.D., and Stanley Darrow, D.D.S., who were kind enough to read and comment on the manuscript. I would also like to thank Keith B. Raskin, M.D., and his office manager, Teresa B. Hallinan, in whose presence one experiences the true spirit of medicine.

As always, I appreciate the editorial guidance of James Chambers of Facts On File and the support of my agent, Phyllis Westberg.

Finally, this book is dedicated to my husband, Perry Luntz, a fellow writer whose encouragement has never wavered and whose vision remains true.

ENTRIES A–Z

Abbe flap   See SKIN FLAP.

abdominal zipper   See SURGICAL ZIPPER.

abdominoplasty   This cosmetic surgery, some-times called a "tummy tuck," reshapes and slims the area of the body between the chest and the pelvis to give the patient a trimmer body. This surgery may be done by removing a fat deposit that does not respond to diet; or by cutting away excess skin left after extreme weight loss; or by reducing sagging due to pregnancy or natural age-related loss of skin elasticity; or by tightening muscles stretched by multiple pregnancies; or by repairing a pregnancy-related separation of muscle from the abdominal wall.

Procedure

The common types of abdominoplasty are *traditional abdominoplasty* (also known as complete abdomi-noplasty or full abdominoplasty), *fleur-de-lis (lys) abdominoplasty, endoscopically assisted abdominoplasty, high-lateral-tension abdominoplasty, partial abdomino-plasty* (miniabdominoplasty or mini-tummy tuck), and *dermolipectomy.* Another procedure, *circumfer-ential abdominoplasty* (midbody lift), is used in cases where extreme weight loss has left excess skin around the entire midsection of the body.

All forms of abdominoplasty are considered major surgery, most often performed under general anesthesic and usually in a hospital setting. Some patients may be released within hours after a partial abdominoplasty, but most abdominoplasty patients spend a day or two in the hospital.

Traditional abdominoplasty is surgery to remove a large amount of excess skin and fat. The surgeon makes one long incision from hip to hip, just above the pubic bone, then lifts the skin up and away from the underlying tissues. She next removes excess fatty tissue; repairs the rectus abdominus muscle separation and sutures it into a tighter position, bringing the edges of the incision together and removing excess skin to make a smooth closure. If necessary, she repositions the navel and closes the incision with sutures or surgical staples. The procedure for a *partial abdominoplasty* is similar to that for a traditional abdominoplasty, but the incision is shorter; less skin and fatty tissue are removed; and the navel is not likely to be repositioned.

Fleur-de-lis abdominoplasty is also surgery to remove large amounts of excess skin and fat. The procedure is named for the shape of the two-part, T-shape vertical and horizontal incision in the center of the abdomen, which resembles the flower of Lyons (*fleur-de-lis [lys]* in French), a heraldic device used by French kings. As with a full abdomino-plasty, the surgeon lifts the skin; removes excess fat; tightens the muscle; brings the edges of the incision together; repositions the navel (if necessary); and closes the incision.

Endoscopically assisted abdominoplasty is a procedure used to tighten the abdominal muscles without removing much skin or fat. The surgeon makes several small incisions across the abdomen; inserts an endoscope (see ENDOSCOPY) (a flexible tube with a light that enables the surgeon to see under the skin) through one incision and a second instrument to lift the skin away from the muscle through another incision; stitches and tightens the muscle; and closes the incisions.

High-lateral-tension abdominoplasty surgery flattens the abdomen by tightening abdominal muscles and removing excess tissue, including rolls of skin left after massive weight loss. The surgery, distinguished by an incision that extends around the body into the flank area, may be combined with LIPOSUCTION of the upper thigh to provide a smoother line down the body.

Miniabdominoplasty is a procedure most often used when the abdominal fat is found only in the area under the navel. The surgeon makes a short incision just above the pubic region, lifts the abdominal skin up toward the belly button, trims away excess skin, tightens muscles if required, and sutures the skin in place under the navel. *Dermolipectomy* is similar to miniabdominoplasty, except that it may remove more skin but does not involve tightening the abdominal muscles; the procedure is used for patients whose abdominal skin is looser than those for whom the miniabdominoplasty is sufficient.

Circumferential abdominoplasty removes excess skin from the stomach, thighs, and buttocks in a single procedure. The surgeon makes an incision across the abdomen in the area of the navel, frees and lifts the skin toward the middle of the abdomen, cuts away excess tissue, repositions the navel if necessary, and closes the incision. She next turns the patient over on the operating table, makes an incision across the lower back at a point corresponding to the incision on the abdomen, and repeats the procedure. Note: Several months after this surgery, the patient may undergo additional procedures to trim excess skin from under the upper arms, breast area, thigh, neck, and face.

Note: Before closing the incision(s) after abdominoplasty, the surgeon may insert a drain to allow blood and other liquids to flow out of the wound rather than pool under the skin.

Risks and Complications

Common side effects include pain, tenderness, loss of sensation at the site of the incision, and/or swelling of the abdomen, the labia (women), and the scrotum (men) for up to six weeks after surgery.

Possible complications include continued bleeding that may cause a hematoma (pooling of clotted blood under the skin) that may become infected, or a seroma (pool of fluid under the skin that may require surgical drainage), or blood loss severe enough to require a transfusion. As the wound heals, the stitches may fail to dissolve properly.

The navel may be off-center or otherwise oddly positioned due to contraction of the various scars, and the blood supply to the newly positioned navel or to the abdominal wall may fail to develop properly (more commonly in people with vascular problems), leading to tissue death requiring a skin graft. The death of fat cells/fatty tissue under the skin may cause infection requiring further surgery. The incision may separate, creating a thicker-than-normal scar requiring surgery to reduce it. As with all major surgery, there is a risk of life-threatening blood clots in legs and lungs, as well as a reaction to the anesthetic. Because circumferential abdominoplasty is a more complex procedure than other forms of abdominoplasty, it carries a higher risk of possible complications.

Outlook and Lifestyle Modifications

This surgery is most effective for healthy adults. It is not a substitute for proper diet and exercise to achieve weight reduction. It is not recommended for people who are extremely obese or for those who plan to lose more weight or for women who plan to become pregnant again, because the abdominal muscles may separate from the abdominal wall during future pregnancies.

ABO system   See BLOOD TYPE.

absorbable suture   See SUTURE.

absorbent foam   Also known as an alginate dressing, a highly absorbent bandage containing alginates, material derived from compounds in the cell walls of algae. Types of algae used for this include the *Macrocystis pyrifera* from California and Mexico, and *Ascophyllum nodosum* and *Laminaria hyperborea* from Ireland, Norway, and Scotland, and *Laminaria japonica* from China and Japan. Some alginates dissolve in cold water to produce a thick sticky solution, calcium alginate. This is insoluble in water and is used to produce fibers to be woven into a gauze dressing that provides a network on which a scab can form over a wound, particularly a burn. The bandage is easily and painlessly removed by moistening it with a saline (saltwater solution); removing the bandage does not damage the tissue underneath.

The dressing is designed for wounds with a heavy discharge; for example, after plastic surgery to repair a deep skin ulcer. The foam not only provides a cushion around the wound, it also draws exudate (liquid seeping from the wound) into the center of the dressing, away from the skin. As a result, the area around the wound stays drier. The dryness promotes healing by reducing the risk of maceration (tissue damage due to constant moisture) and infection.

Another type of absorbent dressing is collagen dressing, a flexible wound covering made from a porous membrane of purified bovine (cow) collagen (connective tissue) attached to a nonadhesive backing.

Accutane™ See ACNE.

acellular matrix A piece of skin from a cadaver, treated to clean away all living material, or cells, leaving an acellular (cell-free) framework to which new skin cells can cling as the body begins building a new layer of skin. Ordinarily, the body creates its own framework for new skin growth, a phenomenon that occurs every time the skin is injured. The exception is a burn severe enough to destroy several layers of skin. In this case, the surgeon uses the acellular matrix to provide the framework the patient's body cannot produce. Alloderm® is the brand name for one type of material processed from donated human tissue for use as an acellular dermal graft.

See also BURNS AND BURN RECONSTRUCTION; SKIN GRAFT.

acetic acid This clear liquid with a characteristic strong odor occurs naturally in many fruits such as apples and oranges, or in milk, or in wine exposed to oxygen. Concentrated acetic acid, known as glacial acetic acid, is highly corrosive, producing vapors that may damage the lungs, but mild solutions (5 percent acetic acid) are used in a variety of cosmetic products. For example, acetic acid is used as an acidifier in feminine hygiene products and as an exfoliant in skin toners, mildly irritating liquids that help flake off the top layer of dead skin cells, leaving behind a smoother surface. In fact, ancient Egyptian ruler Cleopatra's famous milk baths got their skin-smoothing power from acetic acid, and the Queen of the Nile is also rumored to have used vinegar, which is about 6 percent acetic acid.

acid See CHEMICAL SKIN PEEL; SKIN.

acne *Acne vulgaris;* skin condition most commonly triggered by increasing levels of androgens (male hormones), specifically testosterone, which rises at puberty for both boys and girls and fluctuates during pregnancy or when a woman starts or stops using birth control pills. Androgens stimulate sebaceous glands in the skin to produce large amounts of sebum, an oily, waxy material that keeps skin soft by preventing the loss of moisture from the surface. The excess sebum can block the opening (pore) to a pilosebaceous gland (a sebaceous gland attached to a hair follicle), allowing bacteria such as *Propionibacterium acnes* to multiply in the follicle. The bacteria release enzymes that inflame the follicle, which may swell and rupture, allowing bacteria to spread onto the skin, causing a pimple.

Acne cosmetica is acne caused by comedogenic (pore-blocking) ingredients in cosmetics; *acne medicamentosa* is acne aggravated by medical drugs; *acne rosacea* is a complication of the skin condition rosacea.

Symptoms and Diagnostic Path

The most common sign of acne is the comedo (plural, comedones), a plugged pilosebaceous gland. Whiteheads are "closed" comedones, meaning their plug is beneath the surface of the skin; blackheads are comedones whose plugs have reached skin level. Other signs of acne may include a papule (an inflammation that looks like small, light, red bump); a pustule (an infected papule); a module (a painful solid bump under the surface of the skin); a cyst (a small sac filled with solid or liquid matter); or an abscess (an infection under the skin in a close space).

Acne is characterized as *superficial* or *deep, mild, moderate,* or *severe* depending on the type of inflammation present. As a general rule, if the acne presents mostly as comedones, it is superficial or mild; a predominance of nodules and cysts is called deep or severe acne; moderate acne is somewhere in between.

Acneform eruption, a form of dermatitis that resembles acne, is triggered by exposure to certain drugs and/or environmental chemicals such as corticosteroids (cortisone, hydrocortisone, et al), iodides (medicines containing iodine), lithium (a sedative used to treat manic-depressive illness), or dioxin (a by-product in the manufacture of paper products). The most famous victim of this last reaction, a condition known as *chloracne,* was the former Ukrainian president Victor Yushchenko, who was believed to have been poisoned with dioxin in 2004 when he was an opposition candidate for president.

Treatment Options and Outlook

Simply keeping the face clean with plain toilet soap generally treats mild acne. Antibacterial soaps have no special benefit, and soaps containing abrasives may further irritate the skin. Over-the-counter (OTC) medications such as benzoyl peroxide, resorcinol, salicylic acid, and sulfur may be applied directly to the skin to kill bacteria and/or break down the sebum plug in pilosebaceous glands.

Various OTC and prescription products are used for moderate acne. For example, oral antibiotics (commonly tetracycline, minocylcine, and doxycycline) may be prescribed to combat infection, while topical retinoids or retinoidlike medicines such as tazarotene (Tazorac™) or ECoR adapalene (Differin™) may be used to break down the sebum plug and so that OTC topical medicines can reach into the follicles.

Severe acne may respond to topical or oral antibiotics. If the condition does not improve, an alternative is the retinoid drug isotretinoin (Accutane™), an altered version of vitamin A taken by mouth to shrink oil sebaceous glands and reduce the production of oily sebum, thus inhibiting the proliferation of bacteria.

Women with acne due to hormonal fluctuations are usually treated with low-dose estrogen birth control pills to reduce the amount of androgen produced naturally by the ovaries, or low-dose corticosteroids such as prednisone to reduce the amount of androgens produced by the adrenal glands, or an antiandrogen medicine such as spironolactone (Aldactone™) to lower sebum production.

Mild acne generally heals without scarring, but severe acne often leaves scars because the continuing inflammation and/or infection either destroy tissue or, paradoxically, increase production of collagen (supporting tissue under the skin). Excess collagen creates a raised scar called a KELOID. Tissue loss produces a recessed scar such as an ICE PICK SCAR (a small pit usually found on the cheek), or a depressed scar with sharp edges and steep sides, or a "soft scar" (so called because it feels soft to the touch and generally seems to blend into normal skin), or an atrophic macule, a soft mark colored by blood vessels just under the surface.

Once acne has cleared, several common plastic surgery techniques can help to smooth the scarred skin. FILLERS can be used to smooth superficial or soft scars, but the body eventually absorbs the filler, and the process must be repeated in about six months. The same is true of autologous fat transplants, injections of fat taken from the patient's own body to fill in deep scars from cystic acne. Like fillers, the body may absorb the fat and the process must be repeated in six to 18 months. DERMABRASION (a mechanical process that removes several layers of skin) and MICRODERMABASION (a mechanical process that removes only the top surface of the skin) can permanently eliminate superficial scars while reducing the depth of deeper scars. Laser treatments can also permanently smooth scars and reduce skin redness (although the laser itself will temporarily irritate and redden the skin). The type of laser and the number of treatments required depends on the size and depth of the scars. Individual ice-pick scars may be removed with "punch" surgery in which a small circle of skin and fat is excised, leaving a small wound to be closed with a single stitch or a small skin graft. Keloids require special care; people who form raised scars in response to acne may also develop scars after surgery. One alternative is to inject a steroid drug to smooth the skin around the keloid. A second alternative is to apply a topical retinoid. A third alternative is simply to leave the scar as it is.

Risk Factors and Preventive Measures

There is no sure way to prevent acne as hormones rise at puberty; avoiding the medication may prevent acne due to medication. The only way to reduce the risk of acne scarring is to treat the condition early so as to reduce inflammation and infection.

As for common folk remedies for acne, avoiding chocolate or spicy foods will not decrease the risk of acne. Moderate sun exposure might help dry up acne pustules, but more than moderate sun exposure makes them worse. Pregnancy, which increases the amount of estrogen circulating in a woman's body, may temporarily alleviate acne.

actinic keratosis   See KERATOSIS.

acupressure   See ACUPUNCTURE.

acupuncture   Asian healing technique to relieve discomfort and/or pain by inserting very thin metal (usually stainless steel) needles at one of a possible 2,000 specific points on the human body in order to stimulate the flow of *qi* (life force) through a *meridian,* one of 20 pathways through which *qi* moves.

In 2002, the World Health Organization (WHO) published "Acupuncture: Review and Analysis of Reports on Controlled Clinical Trials," a report concluding that acupuncture effectively relieves pain as well as a variety of medical conditions including adverse reactions to radiotherapy and/ or chemotherapy; allergies, such as hay fever; depression; intestinal disorders, such as acid reflux, constipation, diarrhea, duodenal ulcer, and esophageal spasms; and temporomandibular dysfunction (TMD).

Western physicians suggest that acupuncture works through the nervous system, enhancing the activity of the immune system and natural pain relievers such as endorphins, analgesics produced in the brain. This assumption rests on studies showing that acupuncture may alter brain chemistry by changing the release of neurotransmitters and hormones that affect the nerves and that these natural chemicals may alter the reaction of the central nervous system related to sensation and involuntary functions blood pressure, blood flow, and body temperature.

In plastic surgery, some suggest that acupuncture can be used as an alternative to a surgical face-lift and surgery for breast enlargement; there is no proof that these procedures are effective.

In most European countries, an acupuncturist must have a medical degree and be licensed to practice acupuncture. In the United States, most states have established training standards for acupuncture certification, but requirements for licensing of nonmedical personnel vary from state to state. The professional association for physicians trained in acupuncture in the United States is the American Academy of Medical Acupuncture.

Acupressure

Technique similar to acupuncture, except that it applies pressure on specific body points rather than inserting needles to relieve pain and/or discomfort.

See ACUPUNCTURE FACE-LIFT.

acupuncture face-lift   Insertion of slim metal (usually stainless steel) needles into the skin as a technique to reduce facial wrinkling.

Procedure

The skin is cleaned with alcohol and the needle, or needles, are inserted, sometimes at a site on the body far from the face. For example, if the acupuncturist believes that a specific wrinkle is caused by an imbalance of life force in the liver, the needles will be inserted in the skin covering the area over the liver.

Risks and Complications

Most people experience no pain with proper insertion of standard acupuncture needles; improperly placed needles may cause pain and/or injure internal organs. To reduce the risk of infection, the Food and Drug Administration requires that the needles be sterile, nontoxic, and labeled for use by qualified acupuncturists.

Outlook and Lifestyle Modifications

As of this writing, there are no rigorous scientific studies attesting to the success or failure of acupuncture to ameliorate facial wrinkles.

Adam's apple reduction   Also known as *Adam's apple shaving, tracheal shave, thyroid cartilage reduction (TCR),* or *chondrolaryngoplasty* (from the Greek *chondros,* meaning "cartilage," *larynx,* meaning "larynx, throat," and *plasso,* meaning "form."). Surgery to reduce the size of the Adam's apple (thyroid eminence), a V-shape cartilage structure in the neck (a secondary male sex characteristic) that juts out farther in men than in women, is most commonly performed as one in a series of alternations during male-to-female gender change.

Procedure

Once the patient is given local anesthesic, the surgeon cuts into a crease of skin on the neck, separates the muscles underneath to expose the cartilage, shaves cartilage from the front of the Adam's apple, the closes the incision and covers it with a dressing.

Risks and Complications

As with all surgery, bruising and swelling are common, and there is the possibility of blood clots and infection. Hoarseness and temporary changes in voice tone are common; permanent loss of voice is rare.

Outlook and Lifestyle Modifications

The scar eventually fades to a barely visible line in a crease of skin. The neck is smoother.

adhesion   From the Latin *adhaerere,* meaning to stick together. The process that enables two surfaces or edges such as two sides of a wound or surgical incision to grow together as the wound heals. In medical terms, the word *adhesion* is used to describe an unexpected, accidental joining of internal tissues either after surgery, for example after ABDOMINOPLASTY (tummy tuck), or as a result of a medical condition such as endometriosis, in which tissue from the uterus escapes and adheres to the lining of the abdomen. The surgical procedure used to repair or separate adhesions is called adhesiotomy (from the Greek *tome,* meaning "incision").

adipose tissue   From the Latin *adeps,* meaning fat. Tissue composed of fat cells, which are cells with a small nucleus (center), very little cytoplasm (the fluid inside cells), and one or more droplets of fat. Fat cells are created from stem cells in fatty tissue that develop into mature, long-lived fat cells that signal immature fat cells to divide and reproduce as needed throughout life to store excess calories as fat and to disappear when no longer needed. A lean adult has about 40 billion fat cells; an obese person, at least twice that amount; an obese person's fat cells are larger and more metabolically active than a lean person's.

White adipose tissue insulates the body against heat loss, cushions internal organs, and shapes the body. Brown adipose tissue serves as a source of stored energy. Brown adipose tissue, colored by plentiful blood vessels, releases stored energy as heat to warm a shivering body and provide energy when an individual is on a reducing diet. Note: Fetal adipose tissue develops in the third trimester of pregnancy; infants born premature may not yet have enough body fat to retain body heat and must be protected in warmed incubators.

The amount and distribution of adipose tissue is a genetically determined characteristic, based on family history and gender. Although males and females in the same family will have similar body shapes, overall, right from birth, males commonly have proportionately less adipose tissue than females do. Regardless of race or ethnicity, boys born full-term generally have less body fat than premature girls. At puberty, the difference becomes more pronounced; by adulthood, the average male body is 15 to 20 percent adipose tissue; the average female body, 20 to 25 percent. The extra female adipose tissue protects the more porous female bones and, after menopause, serves as a site for the synthesis of estrogen no longer provided by the ovaries.

A body site where adipose tissue accumulates is called a fat depot. A fat pad is a lump of adipose tissue under the skin that contributes to body contours. For example, there are fat pads on the eyelid, cheek, hip, buttock, thigh, and fingertip. Men commonly have fat depots on the upper body, in an "apple" figure, while women have fat depots at breast, hips, thighs, belly, and buttocks, a "pear" shape. After menopause, women may experience an increase in upper body fat. Excess upper body fat, specifically around the abdomen, is often linked to health problems such as heart disease, high blood pressure, and Type 2 (noninsulin dependent) diabetes. One way to measure this risk is to divide the circumference of the waist by the circumference of the hips. Women are considered to be at risk if the result, known as the waist-to-hip ratio, is 0.85 or higher; for men the risk ratio is 0.95.

The most common plastic surgery to reduce the size of fat depots is LIPOSUCTION; other more complicated procedures to reduce the accumulation of adipose tissue include ABDOMINOPLASTY, BREAST LIFT, and BUTTOCK LIFT.

advancement flap   Triangle-shaped piece of healthy skin adjacent to an injury. The broad base of the triangle is at the edge of the wound to be covered, the pointed tip at the far end. The skin is then advanced (pulled tip end forward, up, or down) to cover the injury, common in plastic surgery to repair a facial defect; for example, at the lip or the side of the nose.

The benefit of an advancement flap is that it creates a better cosmetic effect by eliminating the visible tension that might occur with a simple straight wound closure, hiding the closure in a natural skin fold, such as the creases at the nostril or beside the lips.

aesthetics   In cosmetic/PLASTIC SURGERY, the medical and nonmedical care of skin and hair. Medical procedures include laser therapy and pre- and post-operative care for plastic surgery. Nonmedical procedures include eyebrow shaping, eyelash application, facials, makeup, manicures and pedicures, hair and eyelash tinting, and hair removal.

An *aesthetician* (the modern term for cosmetologist) is a person with a high school diploma who has completed a certificate program in skin and hair care and is licensed to perform nonmedical preventative skin care and nonmedical and/or medical treatments to keep skin and hair healthy and attractive. Aestheticians offer an alternative for persons who wish to improve their appearance but do not wish to undergo invasive procedures. The certificate programs are accredited by the National Accrediting Commission of Cosmetology Arts and Sciences, an independent agency recognized by the U.S. Department of Education.

age factor   The effect of age on a medical condition or treatment. The age factor is an important tool for plastic surgeons when choosing a treatment and/or estimating a patient's successful recovery after cosmetic surgery.

The most basic part of the aging process is the slowing of the rate at which cells reproduce, a development with multiple consequences, including a less effective immune system and slower wound healing. At the same time, aging (and some illness, such as cancer, which are more common among older people) interferes with apoptosis, the process by which cells are programmed to die and exit from the body at an appropriate time so as to maintain healthy tissues. Perhaps the most visible signs of the age factor are the series of changes in the skin that become apparent later in life.

Aging skin is dryer and less elastic, with prominent lines, WRINKLES, and sagging not only on the face but also all over the body. The thin skin on the eyelids stretches and sags earlier than the thicker skin on the rest of the face. On the upper lid, the skin may fold downward, creating a hooded appearance. On the lower lid, the skin may droop to form swollen, puffy "bags." (As a rule, these changes are age-related, occurring most often in people older than 35; however, droopy or baggy eyelids may also be family trait that shows up at a younger age.) Skin color may change unevenly, and dark spots are common, particularly on parts of the body such as face and hands, which are exposed to sunlight. Loss of hair color is common, as is loss of hair on scalp, face, and body. Conversely, hair in ears and nostrils and on eyebrows may grow more profusely. Facial features such as the nose and brow may thicken; the fat pad under the cheek may shrink; the tip of the nose may dip; and the tip of the chin may protrude or recede.

For many people, cosmetic plastic surgery procedures such as a face-lift or a breast-lift or hair replacement are valuable tools in countering some of these visible signs of aging. The downside, of course, is that older patients have weaker, less elastic skin and therefore are likely to heal more slowly than younger patients after cosmetic surgery procedures, such as a CHEMICAL SKIN PEEL. In addition, the aging changes continue so long as life continues; to maintain the new appearance of the face or figure, the surgery must often be repeated.

See also BROW LIFT; CHEEK AUGMENTATION; CHIN RECONSTRUCTION; EYEBROW LIFT; FACE-LIFT; FILLER; HAIR LOSS.

age spot   See LENTIGO.

alarplasty   Plastic surgery to reduce the width of the nostrils (alar-wing nostrils) so as to create a shape more in line with the ideal of an isosceles triangle, a triangle whose base (bottom line) is shorter than the two equal length sides rising to the point at the top. Because the base of the nose (the nostrils) is often wider in men than in women, alarplasty is sometimes regarded as a procedure that makes the face look more classically feminine.

Procedure

Once the patient is sedated, the surgeon cuts an equal-size, wedge-shape piece of skin and underlying tissue from the base of each nostril. This is one of the few times that RHINOPLASTY (surgery on the nose) involves external surgery. Once the excess tissue is removed, the surgeon reforms the nostrils and sutures the remaining tissue in place to form a narrowed base.

Risks and Complications

Swelling and bruising are expected; as with all surgery, infection is a possible complication.

Outlook and Lifestyle Modifications

Once the swelling has subsided, a process that may take several months to be complete, the nose will look narrower; any scars left by removing the wedge-shape piece of tissue from each nostril will be hidden in the natural crease at the side of the nose.

alginate dressing   See ABSORBENT FOAM.

Alloderm™   See ACELLULAR MATRIX.

alloplast   From the Greek *allo,* meaning "other," and *plastos,* meaning "formed." Nonreactive material such as polyethylene, silicone, or stainless steel alloplastic implants used to build, rebuild, or add to a body tissue or part. Some alloplastic materials and implants such as the breast implants used in plastic surgery are easily shaped. Others, such as the molded implants used to create a firmed shape on the cheek, are not. All, however, are biocompatible, meaning that they will not provoke an immune system response. Polyethylene implants are porous; silicone and stainless steel implants, such as the artificial devices used to replace a hip or knee joint, are not.

alopecia   See HAIR LOSS.

ambiguous genitals   See INTERSEX.

ambulatory phlebectomy   See PHLEBECTOMY; VARICOSE VEINS.

analgesic   See ANESTHESIOLOGY.

anchor incision   This type of surgical incision is made in a shape often described as an anchor. A circle is cut around the areola (the dark tissue surrounding the nipple), followed by a straight line made down to the bottom of the breast, and then a curved line in the crease underneath the breast. This type of incision is used in BREAST REDUCTION surgery and BREAST LIFT procedures.

Andy Gump deformity   See CHIN RECONSTRUCTION.

anesthesiology   The medical specialty related to the practice of pain relief, including but not limited to

- evaluating and preparing a patient for anesthesia before surgery, including plastic surgery
- providing relief from pain during and after a medical procedure
- managing the patient in the period before, during and after surgery
- diagnosing and treating acute and/or chronic pain
- managing respiratory therapy
- supervising medical personnel involved in surgical procedures
- teaching and implementing anesthesiology techniques and practices

An anesthesiologist is a doctor specializing in anesthetics (anesthesiology); a person responsible for administering anesthesic and monitoring the patient's vital signs (respiration, heartbeat, blood pressure) during surgery, as well as keeping the patient comfortable and pain-free during recovery. A board-certified anesthesiologist is a person who has graduated from an accredited medical school, is licensed to practice medicine, has completed a residency in anesthesiology, and has passed the required tests administered by the American Board of Anesthesiology. Those who are already certified in anesthesiology may also apply to be certified in critical care medicine or pain medicine.

Anesthesiologists work with two broad classes of drugs, anesthetics and analgesics.

Anesthetics produce pain relief accompanied by a loss of consciousness, a state known as anesthesia, the interruption of one or more of the chemical reactions by which the body transmits pain messages from the site of an injury to the brain; anesthesia causes loss of consciousness.

Analgesics, on the other hand, reduce pain without causing a loss of consciousness, a situation known as analgesia, commonly used to reduce pain after surgery. Analgesics are classified as opioids or nonopiods. Opioids are natural derivatives of opium or synthetic imitators that inhibit the transmission of pain impulses from the brain. Opioids, which may be addictive, are available only by prescription. Nonopiods—acetaminophen and the nonsteroidal anti-inflammatories (NSAID) such as aspirin, ibuprofen, and naproxen—alleviate pain by reducing the body's production of prostaglandins, natural chemicals that enable the body to perceive pain.

History of Anesthetics

Early anesthetics such as alcohol and sedative plants such as cannibis, aka kif, hashish, hemp (active ingredient: tetrahydrocannabinols), coca (the source of cocaine), and poppies (the source of opium and morphine), were minimally effective but unreliable. The first modern anesthetics, inhaled gases such as ether or a mixture of nitrogen and oxygen (nitric oxide, "laughing gas") introduced in the later 19th century, rendered the patient temporarily unconscious, thus allowing painless surgery but they had unpleasant aftereffects such as nausea and vomiting. Modern anesthetics are designed to produce a quick loss of consciousness and an equally quick return to consciousness with minimal adverse effects when the anesthetic is withdrawn.

Types of Anesthetics

A local anesthetic is a substance applied to skin or mucous membrane or injected just under the surface to relieve pain in a small area of the body, such as a tooth. A regional anesthetic is a substance injected near or into a cluster of nerves to relieve pain in a larger area such as the pelvic region during childbirth. A general anesthetic, which may be inhaled or injected intravenously, is a substance that causes loss of consciousness, generally during major surgery. A short-acting anesthetic, which may be injected or inhaled, produces loss of consciousness that ends as soon as the administration of the anesthetic stops. Note: The smaller the area of the body affected by the anesthesia, the lower the risk of complications such as allergic reactions or respiratory failure.

An intercostal nerve block (from Latin *inter,* meaning "between," and *costa,* meaning "rib") is an injection of local anesthetic in the area between two ribs. It is used to relieve pain after chest surgery or discomfort due to a herpes zoster (shingles) infection. It may also be used as a diagnostic tool to locate the source of pain in the mid-body.

angel's kiss See HEMANGIOMA.

angioma See HEMANGIOMA.

antia-buch technique See EAR RECONSTRUCTION.

Apert's syndrome Genetic condition causing multiple physical defects, many of which may be repaired by plastic surgery. It is named for Eugene Apert (1868–1940), the French pediatrician who first described it in 1906.

Symptoms and Diagnostic Path
The visible features of Apert's syndrome include a cone-shape skull due to premature fusion of the skull bones, concave cheekbones, recessed nose, prominent eyes, misalignment of the jaws, and webbed fingers and/or toes. There may also be malformations of the heart and gastrointestinal tract; impaired vision due to weakness of the eye muscles; hearing loss due to frequent infections; and speech defects due to malformations of the palate.

Treatment Options and Outlook
Several surgeries may be required to repair these defects. The first is likely to be surgery to release the fused plates in the skull to allow the brain room to grow, a procedure usually done when the child is between three and 18 months old. Because the nose and cheeks may not grow as quickly as the skull, the facial bones may have to be repositioned during surgery that pulls back the bones surrounding the eyes and corrects any misalignment of the jaws. As the child's face grows, repeat surgery may be needed. Additional surgery is required to separate any webbed fingers and/or toes.

Risk Factors and Preventive Measures
Apert's syndrome is caused by a defect in Fibroblast Growth Factor Receptor 2 (*FGFR2*), a gene on chromosome number 10 that affects the development of fibroblasts, star- or spindle-shape cells in connective tissue. The condition may be inherited (the child of a person with Apert's has a 50–60 percent risk), or it may be the result of a spontaneous gene mutation. Apert's is a dominant trait; it appears only when an individual gets two damaged genes, one from each parent. Therefore, a child of a person with Apert's syndrome who does not inherit the condition has two healthy genes and is not at increased risk of passing the defect on to his or her own children. However, some studies show that the syndrome is more common among children of older fathers.

apocrine glands See HYPERHYDROSIS.

areolar reconstruction See BREAST RECONSTRUCTION.

arm lift Brachioplasty, from the Latin *brachium,* meaning arm, and the Greek *plastos,* meaning formed. Surgery to trim excess skin, at the back of the upper arm between the elbow and the shoulder, remaining after extreme weight loss or arising simply as a result of growing older.

Procedure
Once the patient is sedated, the surgeon makes an incision running along the spot on the back or underside of the arm where the excess tissue is to be removed. Depending on the length of the area to be treated, the incision may run from the bottom of the armpit to the top of the elbow. The surgeon cuts away the excess skin, tightens and sutures into place the supportive muscle and connective tissue underneath, and smooths and sutures the remaining skin into place using either absorbable sutures

or stitches that will be taken out once the wound has healed about one to two weeks after surgery.

Risks and Complications

The possible common complications of an arm lift include bleeding, bruising, infection, pain. Less common more serious complications may include poor wound healing, discolored skin, unusual scarring, and—if both arms are done—asymmetry (one arm larger than the other).

Outlook and Lifestyle Modifications

A successful arm lift gives the patient smoother, tighter upper arms almost immediately after surgery, but the final contours of the arm will not be visible until all swelling has receded, a process that may take up to several months.

arthritis Osteoarthritis, the most common form of arthritis, is a degenerative joint disease in which the cartilage that covers the ends of bones in the joint deteriorates. Rheumatoid arthritis is an autoimmune disease (a condition in which the body attacks its own tissues) characterized by inflammation of the lining of the joint that may destroy tendons and ligaments, the tissues that hold joints together. Plastic surgeons specializing in hand surgery may treat both forms of the disease.

Symptoms and Diagnostic Path

Both osteoarthritis and rheumatoid arthritis cause pain, stiffness, swelling, and difficulty in moving the hand, wrist, elbow, shoulder, foot, ankle, and knee. Rheumatoid arthritis may also cause bumps (rheumatoid nodules) over an affected joint; if the disease progresses, the loss of tendons and ligaments may result in deformities such as a hand turned inward at the wrist.

An X-ray showing destruction of a joint may be used to confirm a diagnosis of osteoarthritis. To confirm a diagnosis of rheumatoid arthritis, the physician may order a BIOPSY of fluid aspirated from a joint to rule out an infection, a biopsy of a rheumatoid nodule to rule out a malignant factor, and a blood test to confirm the presence of rheumatoid factor (antibodies characteristic of rheumatoid arthritis).

Treatment Options and Outlook

The least complex treatment for osteoarthritis and rheumatoid arthritis is either nonsteroidal anti-inflammatory drugs (NSAIDs such as aspirin and ibuprofen) and/or corticosteroids to relieve pain and reduce inflammation and swelling. Physical therapy can help increase muscle strength and keep the joint moving; splints may protect a joint during an episode of acute inflammation.

If these simple remedies do not succeed, plastic surgeons specializing in reconstruction may repair damaged joints via excision, fusion (arthrodesis), or arthroplasty (joint reconstruction) to relieve pain and restore mobility. The procedures are done with either general or local anesthesic, usually on an outpatient basis.

Excisions The surgeon cuts away inflamed or damaged soft tissue and closes the incision.

Fusion (arthrodesis) The surgeon joins two bones in the joint, fixing them in place with surgical screws and, if necessary, a bone graft. Because the joint will not bend once the bones grow together, the surgeon puts them into a position that is useful for the patient. For example, a straight finger that enables a patient to pick things up even without a bendable joint.

Arthroplasty (joint reconstruction) If the joint cannot be salvaged, the surgeon may replace or reposition tendons and ligaments that allow the joint to move. If the joint is damaged beyond repair, the surgeon removes the joint and replaces it with an artificial joint; occasionally an artificial joint may be used to restore movement to a previously fused joint. Artificial joints are commonly made of metal, plastic, or rubber. Note: In 2002, the Food and Drug Administration approved artificial finger joints made of pyrolytic carbon, the material found in most artificial heart valves.

Risk Factors and Preventive Measures

Osteoarthritis is most common after age 45, more common among women than among men. The known risk factors include a family history of osteoarthritis, a personal history of joint malformations or joint injuries, or obesity that stresses joints, or a health condition such as gout that affects the structure or formation of cartilage. Exercising to maintain or increase muscle strength lessens stress on joints, thus reducing the risk of osteoarthritis.

Rheumatoid arthritis most commonly appears in people age 25–45, more commonly among women than among men, and more common among Caucasians and Native Americans than among people of other races. The known risk factors include obesity that stresses joints, a family history of rheumatoid arthritis or another autoimmune disease, or a blood transfusion during which the patient receives incompatible cells that trigger an immune response.

See also HAND SURGERY; IMMUNE SYSTEM.

artificial skin See BURNS AND BURN RECONSTRUCTION.

Aufricht, Gustave (1894–1980) A native of Budapest, Hungary, who treated wounded soldiers during World War I and immigrated to the United States in 1923. There he practiced at Lenox Hill Hospital (New York), where he specialized in RHINOPLASTY and introduced the technique of geometric breast reduction, using lines drawn on the breast prior to surgery to create a surgical pattern that ensures a balanced breast with a viable nipple.

Aufricht, who trained under JACQUES JOSEPH, the German surgeon known as "the father of rhinoplasty," was a founding member of the American Society of Plastic and Reconstructive Surgeons (now the American Society of Plastic Surgeons) and a founder of the *Journal of Plastic and Reconstructive Surgery.*

See also BREAST REDUCTION.

autoimmune disease See IMMUNE SYSTEM.

autologous tissue breast reconstruction See BREAST RECONSTRUCTION.

autonomic nervous system See NERVOUS SYSTEM.

Aztec ear See EAR RECONSTRUCTION.

B cells   See LYMPHATIC SYSTEM.

bags (under eyes)   See EYE LIFT.

Baker-Gordon solution   Caustic solution created by American surgeons Thomas Baker and Hirsch Loeb Gordon in 1961. The liquid penetrates several layers of skin cells; as they heal, a thick new layer of collagen forms to fill in deep wrinkles. Adverse effects associated with phenol products such as the Baker-Gordon solution include an intense burning sensation that may last as long as six hours after application; permanent lightening of the treated skin, most noticeable in dark-skinned patients, with a clearly visible line separating treated from untreated skin; liver and kidney damage and/or irregular heartbeat due to absorption of phenol through the skin. As a result, the Baker-Gordon solution is used only by plastic surgeons performing a deep skin peel.

See also CHEMICAL SKIN PEEL.

baldness   See HAIR LOSS; HAIR REPLACEMENT SURGERY.

balloon expander   Expandable sac implanted under the skin prior to a variety of plastic and reconstructive surgeries. It is inflated to stretch the skin and encourage the growth of new skin to be used to cover a large wound, such as that left when a large tumor is removed or when CONJOINED TWINS are separated. Prior to surgery, the surgeons implant the balloon expanders so that living skin is available to cover the wound immediately when the tumor is removed or the twins are separated. The virtue of the balloon expander compared to transplanted skin taken from a donor is that the new skin created by the balloon comes from the patient's own body so that there is no risk of his rejecting the tissue.

See TISSUE EXPANSION.

barnacles of aging   See KERATOSIS.

bat ear   See EAR PINBACK.

BDD   See PLASTIC SURGERY.

beauty mark   See MOLE.

Becker breast prosthesis   See BREAST RECONSTRUCTION.

bell clapper deformity   Lack of a normal attachment between the testicle and other tissue inside the scrotum such as the epididymis (the storehouse for sperm) so that the testicle swings freely inside the scrotum, twisting the sperm ducts (tubes leading to the epididymis) and/or the vessels that carry lymph and blood to the testis. Prolonged twisting may result in loss of the testis.

Symptoms and Diagnostic Path
Bell clapper deformity is most commonly diagnosed at adolescence due to acute severe pain in the area of the scrotum and testes, which may be reddened, tender, and swollen so that the doctor

cannot feel normal scrotal structures when examining the patient. The condition may be diagnosed with an utlrasound examination, but tests must be done quickly to avoid serious damage to the testis.

Treatment Options and Outlook

This deformity is corrected with surgery to unwind the twist and suture the testis in place to prevent further turning.

Risk Factors and Preventive Measures

Bell clapper deformity is a congenital defect. There are no known risk factors or preventive measures.

belly button reshaping   See UMBILICOPLASTY.

bicoronal forehead lift   See FOREHEAD LIFT.

bifid nose   Cleft nose; a form of midline facial cleft; a birth defect resulting from the failure of the fetal facial bones to fuse properly; usually associated with CLEFT LIP AND/OR PALATE.

Symptoms and Diagnostic Path

The deformity, which may range from a small indentation in the tip of the nose to a complete separation of the nose, is diagnosed by physical examination.

Treatment Options and Outlook

Plastic surgery repairs or reconstructs the nose by repositioning existing cartilage and/or transplanting additional cartilage, bone, and skin. Successful surgery produces a normal-looking nose.

Risk Factors and Preventive Measures

As with cleft lip and/or palate, there is some evidence that parents born with a cleft nose have a higher risk of transmitting it to their children.

bikini wax   See WAXING.

Biobrane™   See BURNS AND BURN RECONSTRUCTION; CLOTTING FACTOR.

biofeedback   Behavioral modification techniques used to reduce tension and often to relieve pain, perhaps after a medical procedure such as PLASTIC SURGERY.

The technique is designed to increase the patient's ability to influence the normally automatic body functions such as blood flow, blood pressure, body temperature, brain wave activity, breathing, gastrointestinal functions, heart rate, and muscle tension; for example, by visualizing an iceberg in order to lower body temperature. As the patient practices biofeedback techniques, responses are transmitted via electrodes attached to the body onto a monitor that displays a visible record to both patient and therapist.

Biofeedback has been used successfully to lower blood pressure, alleviate chronic pain, relieve respiratory problems and sleep disorders, ease urinary incontinence and gastrointestinal disorders due to muscle spasms, and treat conditions such as migraine headaches or Raynaud's syndrome due to spasms of the blood vessels.

See NERVOUS SYSTEM.

biopsy   Diagnostic examination of body tissue, commonly, but not exclusively, to test for the presence of malignant cells. *Aspiration biopsy,* also known as a *needle biopsy* or a *fine needle biopsy,* obtains a specimen by inserting a hollow needle through the skin into the area to be examined. An *excision biopsy* surgically removes an entire LESION. A *punch biopsy* uses a sharp, round instrument to pierce the skin and remove a cylindrical-shaped piece of tissue. A *shave biopsy* uses a sharp blade to remove a lesion sitting above the surface of the skin. Most biopsies are done as out-patient procedures; all require at least a local anesthetic. Depending on the size of the sample to be removed, some excision, punch, or shave biopsies may require stitches to close the wound.

biosynthetic occlusive dressing   See BURNS AND BURN RECONSTRUCTION.

bird beak jaw   See CHIN RECONSTRUCTION.

bird face   See PARROT BEAK DEFORMITY.

birthmark   See MOLE.

Blair, Vilray Papin (1871–1955)   Pioneering American plastic surgeon who created techniques for repairing defects to the face and jaw. He was the author of *Surgery and Diseases of the Mouth and Jaw* (1912) and during World War I created the first specialized battlefield units for PLASTIC SURGERY. He developed techniques for split thickness skin grafting (i.e., the Blair-Brown graft). After the war, he served as chief of the first plastic surgery department at an American hospital, Barnes Hospital, the teaching hospital of Washington University in St. Louis, Missouri, and was a founder of the American Society of Plastic Surgeons.

blepharoplasty   See EYELID RECONSTRUCTION; EYE LIFT.

blood circulation   See CIRCULATORY SYSTEM.

blood count   See COMPLETE BLOOD COUNT (CBC).

blood gases   Also known as the *blood gas test,* a procedure to measure the levels of oxygen (O), carbon dioxide (CO_2), and bicarbonate (HCO_3) in the blood plasma, the clear liquid in blood. Blood gas measurements are used to monitor patients anesthetized for surgery, including PLASTIC SURGERY. It is also used to monitor patients with respiratory disease, kidney disease, and head or neck injuries that may interfere with respiration, or those on oxygen therapy.

CO_2 is a waste product eliminated through the lungs and kidneys. HCO_3, a compound that helps maintain a balance between acid and base, is regulated through the kidneys. Any imbalance between oxygen and carbon dioxide or any abnormal increase or decrease in bicarbonate upsets the body's pH (acid/base balance).

Respiratory acidosis (lower pH, too much CO_2) is an imbalance due to the inability of the lungs to eliminate CO_2 properly; *respiratory alkalosis* (higher pH, not enough CO_2) is a lack of CO_2 mainly caused by hyperventilation. Metabolic acidosis (low pH, too little HCO_3) is an imbalance in HCO_3 due to the kidneys' inability to regulate HCO_3. Metabolic alkalosis (elevated pH, too much HCO_3) is an imbalance in HCO_3 due to low blood levels of potassium, chronic vomiting, or an overdose of sodium bicarbonate (baking soda).

bloodless surgery   See BLOOD TRANSFUSION.

blood transfusion   The transfer of blood from one person to another. Originally a direct vein-to-vein transfer from donor to recipient, in modern times it is a transfer of donated blood either from an unknown donor via a blood bank or from a relative or other person known to the donor. Transfusions are often used to replace blood lost during surgery, including some extensive PLASTIC SURGERY procedures.

Procedure

A catheter (small tube) is inserted into the vein of the person to receive the blood and the blood flows through the tube into the vein.

Risks and Complications

Blood transfusion is a routine, safe procedure so long as the blood has been processed to screen out potentially hazardous contaminants, and the donor and recipient belong to the same blood group. Blood groups are identified by the genetically determined presence of one or more of the 200+ different immune system substances found on the surface of red blood cells.

Blood gathered from blood donations is preserved and stored after separating the red blood cells from the plasma, freezing the two separately, and reconstituting the blood when needed, a technique invented by Charles Drew (1904–1950), who established and led the American Red Cross blood bank. The U.S. Food and Drug Administration (FDA) is responsible for monitoring the safety of blood banks in the United States.

To that end, FDA requires that every unit of blood collected in the United States be tested for a number of infectious agents, including those linked to HIV-1 and HIV-2 (AIDS), hepatitis B, hepatitis C, TLV-1 (rare leukemia virus), and syphilis. All blood products, such as clotting factors, must also be treated to inactivate any virus that may be present. In addition, some potential donors are temporarily turned down because they have an infection or are taking medications that might cause a reaction in the recipient. Others are permanently excluded because they have a history of viral hepatitis or are HIV positive or have a history of male homosexual activity or intravenous drug use.

Once these tests are complete, the blood type of donor and recipient are matched so as to avoid the risk of a potentially fatal reaction due to incompatibility between blood types.

Note: Persons who prefer to avoid blood transfusions due to religious beliefs, health concerns, or other personal convictions may undergo bloodless surgery. This is usually done with the aid of several blood-conserving devices and techniques. Before undergoing bloodless surgery, the patient may spend some time in a hyperbaric chamber (an airtight enclosure filled with highly oxygenated air that increases the amount of oxygen in the patient's own blood cells) or take a drug that stimulates the production of red blood cells. During the bloodless operation, the surgeon may employ a cell saver to collect, clean, and return any blood the patient loses during surgery. A LASER, electrocautery, or a specialized vibrating scalpel may be used to seal blood vessels so as to minimize blood loss. Another option is use of a volume expander, nonblood intravenous fluid that increases the volume of the patient's blood so as to maintain adequate pressure in the blood vessels.

Outlook and Lifestyle Modifications

If the blood is free of contaminants and the blood type of donor and recipient match, the outlook is virtually always favorable.

See also BLOOD TYPE; IMMUNE SYSTEM.

blood type   Blood group; human blood is classified into types (groups) according to specific molecules called antigens (agglutinogens) on the surface of red blood cells that trigger the production of

specific substance called antibodies (agglutinins) that cause blood to aggluntinate (clot).

The most important classification of blood types is the ABO system created by Austrian scientist Karl Landsteiner (1868–1943), who won the Nobel Prize in physiology/medicine (1930) for identifying the human blood types A, B, and O. A fourth human blood type, AB was identified in 1902. The red blood cells in Type A blood carry antigens called Type A agglutinogens that stimulate the production of produce antibodies called Type B agglutinins. Type B blood is exactly opposite, with antigens called Type B agglutinogens that stimulate the production of Type A agglutinins. Type AB has both Type A and Type B agglutinogens and agglutinins. Type O has neither. (Note: Because a person receives two genes for blood type, one from each parent, technically Type A = AA or AO; Type B = BB or BO; Type AB = AB; and Type O = OO. In the United States, approximately 42–45 percent of the population is Type O; 38–42 percent is Type A; 9–10 percent is Type B; and 4 percent is Type AB.)

Including the ABO system, there are more than 20 known human blood groups, each with its own agglutinogens and agglutinins. To date, the list includes Auberger, Bg, Bombay (H), Cartwright, Chido/Rogers, Colton, Cost-Sterling, Diego (positive found only among East Indians and Native Americans), Dombrock, Duffy (negative provides some immunity to malaria), Gerbich, H, Ii, JMH, Kell, Kidd, Knops, Landsteiner-Wiener, Lewis, Lutheran, MNSs (used in maternity and paternity tests), Rapf, Rh (rhesus factor), Scianna, Stoltzfus, Vel, Wright, Xg.

Determining a person's blood type is essential to safe blood transfusion. If a person with Type A blood gets a transfusion of Type B or Type AB blood, the Type B agglutinins in the recipient's blood will attack the donor's blood cells, causing them to agglutinate (form blood clots). Similar reactions occur if a person with Type B blood gets a transfusion of Type A or Type AB blood or if a person with Type O blood gets a transfusion of Type A, Type B or Type AB blood. The red blood cells in Type O blood has neither A nor B agglutinogens or agglutinins, so it attacks them both as invaders in the body.

As a result, a person with Type A blood can donate blood to a person with Type A or Type AB and receive blood from a person with Type A or Type O. A person with Type B blood can donate blood to a person with Type B or Type AB and receive blood from a person with Type B or Type O. A person with Type AB blood can donate blood only to a person with Type AB, but is a universal receiver who can take blood from a person with Type A, Type B, or Type AB because both A and B antigens are a natural part of his/her body. A person with Type O blood is a universal donor who can donate to anyone but can receive blood only from a person with Type O.

Blood groups other than ABO are less problematic. Unlike A, B, and O agglutinogens, which trigger the immediate production of agglutinins, none of the antigens in the other blood type system react unless the recipient has been sensitized by previous exposure to the blood. This may occur via an earlier transfusion or, in the case of the Rh factor, by the fetus's exposure to the mother's Rh+ or Rh- blood during pregnancy.

See also BLOOD TRANSFUSION.

body contouring See ABDOMINOPLASTY; LIPO-SUCTION.

body dysmorphic disorder (BDD) See PLASTIC SURGERY.

body fat See ADIPOSE TISSUE.

body piercing Cosmetic procedure; puncturing the skin with a hollow needle to make a hole into which the patient may insert a piece of jewelry, most commonly at the earlobe, lip, tongue, nipple, navel, or genitals.

Procedure

The site to be pierced is cleaned with an antiseptic, pierced, and cleaned again with an antiseptic and a temporary post (small metal rod) is inserted to keep the hole open as it heals.

Note: Although body piercing is considered a cosmetic procedure, it is an invasive procedure.

The person who does the piercing must wash his/her hands with a germicidal soap, wear disposable gloves, and use disposable or sterilized instruments.

Risks and Complications

People who get piercings may experience pain, swelling, or scarring around the pierced area. There is a risk of allergic reaction to jewelry made of nickel or brass rather than nonreactive titanium, 14-carat gold, or surgical-grade steel. The pierced area may also become infected, leading to poor healing, and there is a possibility of transmission of blood-borne disease such as hepatitis and HIV/AIDS via nonsterile instruments or procedures. Some complications are specific to the site of the piercing.

Complications specific to *ear piercing* may include a higher risk of infection from piercing the rim of the ear than from piercing the lobe. Reusable ear piercing "guns" often exert excessive pressure when piercing tissue and are more likely than hollow needles to cause injury and infection. In addition, "studs" inserted with these guns may be made of materials not approved by the Food and Drug Administration (FDA) or a stud covered with nontoxic gold plating may release material from the underlying metals if the studs corrode, are scratched, or have imperfections on the surface.

Complications specific to *tongue piercing* may include chipped teeth, receding gums, irritation under the tongue, and excess scar tissue. Nerve pain (trigeminal neuralgia) may be triggered by the stud in the tongue irritating a nerve under the tongue connected to the trigeminal nerve. Finally, the tongue is supplied with multiple blood vessels through which an infection may spread to major organs including (but not limited to) the heart and brain.

Complications specific to *genital piercing* may include contamination of the pierced area during unprotected sex.

Regardless of the piercing site, complications from body piercing are least likely to occur when a surgeon or a trained professional does the procedure. Currently, 43 states have legislated regulations for training nonmedical persons who do piercing and the facilities in which they work, and/or requirements for parental consent for body piercing for minors.

Outlook and Lifestyle Modifications

Pierced skin commonly heals within two months or less; to speed healthy healing, patients are advised to avoid handling and moving the jewelry.

body temperature   See FEVER.

bolt foot   See CLAW FOOT.

bone   Hard, multilayer connective tissue and the major component of the skeleton. PLASTIC SURGERY plays an important role in the management of bone malformation due to birth defects or bone loss due to injury or illness, many of which are commonly repaired with reconstructive surgeries such as bone grafts and bone lengthening.

Building and Losing Bone

Bone is active, living tissue. Cells called osteoclasts continually destroy old bone, and cells called osteoblasts continually build new ones via bone morphogenetic protein, a natural or engineered growth factor identified and named in 1965 by orthopedic surgeon and researcher Marshall Urist (1914–2001). With age, the destruction continues, but the rebuilding slows, leading to an inevitable weakening of the bones. This is more prominent in older women, because the female hormone estrogen (whose production declines at menopause) is vital to the preservation of existing bone.

Through natural processes, the body absorbs and discards old bone cells, which are then replaced with new cells. This is called bone resorption. As the body ages, it continues to resorb old cells at the normal rate, but the production of new cells declines, thus leading to weaker, less dense bones in older bodies.

Examining a Bone

The top layer of bone, a thin outer covering called the periosteum, contains nerves and blood vessels. The second layer is dense hard cortical bone (also known as compact bone), which accounts for

nearly 80 percent of the bone in the human body. Cortical bone is made of osteons, long cylinder-shape weight-bearing units with a central canal for nerves and blood vessels. Under the cortical bone, some bones—the pelvis, the ribs, the spine, the skull, and the knobby ends (epiphyses) of the long arm and leg bones—have a layer of more elastic cancellous bone (also known as trabecular bone because it is built like a mesh with units called trabeculae, from the Latin *trabs*, meaning beam). Cancellous bone accounts for about 20 percent of the bone in the human body. The center of many bones, such as the long bones and the pelvic bones, is filled with soft tissue called bone marrow. The yellow marrow in the center of the hard long bones of the arms and legs contains hematopoietic stem cells that become blood cells and stromal stem cells that grow into bone, cartilage, fat, and nerve cells. The red marrow in the center of the spongy bone in the rounded knobs at the ends of the long bones does contain hematopoietic stem cells.

Counting and Classifying Human Bones

At birth, human beings have as many as 300 different bones; as the body matures, some bones, such as those in the skull, wrist, and ankle, fuse, leaving the adult human body with 206 bones, accounting for about 15 percent of the body's weight. The longest bone is the thighbone, which is about one-quarter of the adult body's height; the smallest, the stirrup bone in the middle ear, is about one-tenth of an inch long.

The long bones of the arms and legs are tubes filled with bone marrow. The shorter bones of the fingers and toes are similar to long bones but have no central cavity with bone marrow. The flat bones of the skull and ribs are two layers of compact bone with some cancellous bone in between. Some oddly shaped bones such as the vertebrae (the sections of the spine) are called irregular bones.

See also BONE BIOPSY; BONE REPLACEMENT; LIMB-LENGTH DISCREPANCY.

bone biopsy   Examination of a sample of bone tissue, most commonly to diagnose a bone tumor or to identify the cause of bone pain or the condition of bone. In some cases, a plastic surgeon may order a bone biopsy to ascertain the health of the bone before performing a reconstructive procedure.

Procedure

For a BIOPSY requiring only a small sample, the surgeon numbs the area with a local anesthetic, cuts a small incision in the skin, and inserts a biopsy needle into the bone. A biopsy requiring a larger sample or one where a malignant tumor is suspected is performed under general anesthesia so that the tumor can be removed immediately if necessary.

Risks and Complications

Common complications include soreness and/or swelling at the site. Less frequent complications may include a bone fracture, infection of the skin or bone, or excessive bleeding (an occasional consequence of bone disorders).

bone lengthening   See LIMB-LENGTH DISCREPANCY.

bone morphogenetic protein   See BONE.

bone replacement   PLASTIC SURGERY to replace or rebuild bone lost to injury or to disease or missing from birth due to a congenital defect.

Procedure

The common procedures to replace bone are a bone graft, a bone flap, or an implant of a synthetic network to support new bone cells.

Bone graft   The preferred replacement is a graft from the patient's own body; the tissue is easily accepted by the patient's body and provides factors essential to the growth of new bone. A graft of bone harvested from another person, usually a cadaver, is not quite as good because it carries the risk of an immune reaction. Bone paste is a filler material prepared from powdered bone taken either from the patient or a donor. Bone preserved by chilling and dehydration for use as a graft is called a freeze dried graft.

Bone flap   In some cases, the replacement of choice may be an osteocutaneous flap, a piece of tissue composed of skin and bone, often with an

artery. The bones most often taken for skin-bone-artery flaps, commonly used to repair or reconstruct damaged or defective jaw, arm, or leg, are the radius (the bone in the forearm that runs from the elbow to the thumb); the fibula (the smaller of the two calf bones); the scapula (the flat bone that connects the humerus [upper arm bone] with the clavicle [collar bone]); and the iliac crest, the top of the hip bone.

Synthetic scaffold   Alternatively, the surgeon may implant a network frame made of synthetic material to provide a scaffold on which the patient's own bone can grow; once the new bone grows in, the synthetic material is absorbed by the body. The benefit of this technique is that the synthetic material is easily available; it does not provoke an immune reaction; and it has a low risk of infection. To replace a missing bone close to a joint, the surgeon may chose a metallic implant.

Risks and Complications

Postsurgical pain and/or discomfort is common. As with any surgery, the most common serious complication is infection that may destroy tissue, causing the replacement to fail.

Outlook and Lifestyle Modifications

Successful surgery restores the bone structure and normal functioning.

See also IMMUNE SYSTEM; SKIN FLAP; SKIN GRAFT.

bone resorption   See BONE.

bone scan   Diagnostic test for abnormalities in the bone, including the spread of cancer from an organ to the bones. Like a BONE BIOPSY, a bone scan may be performed prior to reconstructive plastic surgery to confirm the health of the bone on which the surgeon will be working.

Procedure

First, the doctor or medical technician injects a radioactive substance (radionuclide) injected into the bloodstream.

After the injection, the patient is free to move about for about four hours, to allow the radioactive material to circulate through the body, collecting in "hot spots" in bone, places where the bone is breaking down or repairing itself. To aid the circulation of the radioactive arterial, the patient will drink plentiful amounts of liquid.

After four hours, the patient returns for the scan, first urinating to get rid of any radioactive material in the bladder that might otherwise show up on the film. The scan is performed with a gamma camera, a device sensitive to radioactivity. The gamma camera takes pictures of the entire skeleton, a procedure that takes about an hour.

Risks and Complications

The test material injected prior to a bone scan is considered safe for adult men and women who are not pregnant. Women who are pregnant rarely get this test because the radioactive material might cross the placenta.

Once the scan is finished, it takes about a day for all the radioactive material to be cleared from the body via the urine, so the patient is usually advised to drink a lot of fluids. Women who are nursing are usually advised to express sufficient milk before the test so that the baby can be fed away from the mother's body (the milk itself is considered safe within six hours after the test).

bone shortening   See LIMB-LENGTH DISCREPANCY.

bone substitute   See BONE REPLACEMENT.

bone transplant   See BONE REPLACEMENT.

bone wax   A sterilized mixture of wax (beeswax), antiseptics, and softeners such as oil, applied to the bone during surgery, including reconstructive PLASTIC SURGERY, to control bleeding from bone surfaces. Also known as Horsley's bone wax after its inventor, British surgeon Victor Alexander Haden Horsley (1857–1916). Bone wax works by physically blocking the flow of blood. Because it is a foreign substance, it can have adverse effects if left in place, including worsening an infection and inhibiting bone regeneration.

Botox®   Brand name, injectible form of processed botulinum toxin A, a protein secreted by *Clostridium botulinum* bacteria that binds to nerve endings at the site where nerves join to muscles, preventing the nerves from signaling muscles to contract.

In 1989, the U.S. Food and Drug Administration (FDA) approved the use of Botox injections to relieve severe muscle spasm or uncontrollable blinking. In 2000, the FDA approved Botox injections to treat spasmodic torticollis (spasms that twist the head and neck to one side). In 2002, the FDA approved the use of injections of very small doses of Botox—about 10 percent of the amount used to treat muscle spasms—as a cosmetic procedure to relieve deep vertical grooves between the eyes, and it is now used to relax deep vertical grooves between nose and mouth.

Botulinum toxin injections also reduce hyperhydrosis (unusually profuse underarm sweating), sometimes for as long as 10 months per treatment, but are not yet FDA-approved for this purpose. In 2006, researchers at the Mayo Clinic in Rochester, Minnesota, reported that injecting botulinum toxin A at the site of a facial wound early in the healing process might reduce the severity of scarring.

Note: Dysport, a less potent form of botulinum toxin A, has been approved in Europe for the treatment of muscle disorders including cervical dystonia (twisting of the neck), limb spasm in cerebral palsy, involuntary spasm of the eyelid and other facial muscle spasm and is currently in clinical trials in Europe and the United States for use in smoothing facial WRINKLES and lines.

Procedure

The surgeon marks lines on the face where the skin wrinkles when the patient smiles or frowns or forms other expressions. He then cleans the patient's face with an antiseptic (commonly alcohol) and may numb the sites with ice. He then injects the Botox with a very fine needle.

Risks and Complications

Common complications include spreading of the Botox to other areas on the face and/or a temporary asymmetry in the face and/or a drooping muscle, such as an eyelid. A rare but serious complication is difficulty in swallowing due to injections in the neck. *Caution: Botox should be administered only by a person trained in its use either by the drug's maker or by an accredited medical institution.* The introduction of "Botox parties" at which untrained and sometimes unlicensed personnel perform Botox injections strongly increases the risk of complications.

Outlook and Lifestyle Modifications

Botox is most effective for younger patients whose skin is still elastic; older patients are likely to find the results of a surgical FACE-LIFT more satisfying and longer lasting.

botulinum toxin type a complex   See BOTOX.

boutonniere deformity   See FINGERS AND TOES, CONGENITAL STRUCTURAL DEFECTS.

bovine collagen   See FILLERS.

brachioplasty   See ARM LIFT.

brachydactyly   See FINGERS AND TOES, CONGENITAL STRUCTURAL DEFECTS.

brandy nose   See ROSACEA.

Brazilian waxing   See HAIR REMOVAL.

breast augmentation   Surgery to insert an implant to enlarge the female breast or to make the breasts equal in size.

Procedure

The surgery, which generally takes one to two hours, is performed either with general anesthesic or local anesthesic and sedatives. The surgeon makes an incision either in the inframammary fold, the crease under the breast; or at the edge of the areola, the brown tissue surrounding the nipple; or under the armpit (a transaxillary incision); or at the navel. Reaching through the incision, the surgeon separates the skin from the underlying muscle or the muscle from the underlying tissue and inserts the implant either in between the muscle and the skin or underneath the muscle. With the implant in place, the surgeon may insert tubes to drain excess fluids. The incision is closed, and the process is repeated on the other breast. When both incisions are closed, the surgeon wraps the breasts in a gauze bandage. The tubes, stitches, and bandages are usually removed within a week. Strenuous physical activity is usually prohibited for up to six weeks.

Risks and Complications

Patients may experience bruising, soreness, swelling, and increased sensitivity, particularly around the nipple. There is also a risk of infection and/or scarring.

Complications related specifically to the implant may include seroma, a pooling of fluid around the implant that delays healing and may allow the implant to emerge through the skin. The breast tissue may thin or shrink due to pressure from the implant. Scalloping, ripples in the surface of the implant, may appear due to overfilling with saline solution. Implants may slip toward the center of the chest, or become deflated, or rupture. Formation of scar tissue around the implant, a phenomenon known as capsular contracture, occurs in as many as 33 percent of all women with implants.

Shifting, rupture, or capsular contracture may require corrective surgery. Capsular contracture occurs when a layer of scar tissue forms around the implant and hardens, which is painful and can change the shape of the breast. According to clinical studies submitted to the U.S. Food and Drug Administration (FDA) by implant manufacturers, the incidence of additional surgery is one in eight for women who have undergone breast augmentation.

Outlook and Lifestyle Modifications

To protect the incisions and reduce scarring, the patient is usually advised to avoid strenuous activity (lifting, sports, or sex) for up to six weeks after surgery.

The presence of breast implant may affect the accuracy of future mammography. For example, the implant may block some views of the breast, requiring additional films, or calcium deposits in the tissue around the implant may be mistaken for tumors, requiring a diagnostic BIOPSY. Only a radiologist experienced in the techniques required to obtain and read the picture should perform a mammogram of a breast with an implant.

Breast implants may reduce a woman's ability to breast-feed; some studies suggest that as many as two-thirds of women with breast implants are unable to breast-feed versus only 7 percent of women without implants. Breast implants do not prevent the breasts from sagging after pregnancy.

breast implant   There are two basic modern breast implants, the silicone gel implant created in 1961 by Houston plastic surgeons Thomas Cronin and Frank Gerow and the saline implant, a silicone envelope filled with a sterile saline (saltwater) solution, first manufactured in France in 1964. Both devices were virtually unregulated until 1976, when the U.S. Food and Drug Administration (FDA) was given the right to regulate medical devices. The agency immediately labeled implants as such. In 1988, the FDA tightened the rules, suggesting that as with medical drugs, the agency could require manufacturers of breast implants to submit studies on safety and effectiveness.

Silicone gel breast implants   In 1992, reacting to series of reports linking leakage from silicone gel breast implants to medical problems such as autoimmune and connective tissue disorders, the FDA banned the use of the devices for cosmetic surgery, restricting them to use in clinical studies on BREAST RECONSTRUCTION after MASTECTOMY. However, over the years, various scientific reviews, including a 1999 report from the Institute of Medicine, an independent research organization, have shown that breast cancer, autoimmune diseases such as lupus, and connective tissue disorders such as scleroderma are no more common among women with implants than among those who have not had implants. As a result, in 2006, the FDA approved the use of silicone gel-filled breast implants, one manufactured by Allergan (formerly Inamed) and

the other by Mentor, for breast reconstruction in women of all ages and BREAST AUGMENTATION in women ages 22 and older. (The metal platinum is used as a catalyst [a substance that hastens a chemical reaction but is not itself involved in the reaction] to convert silicone oil into silicone gel for breast implants. In rare cases, platinum may leak from the implant, collecting in the bone marrow, from which it is carried by blood cells to other parts of the body where it binds easily to nerve endings. It may cause nervous system disorders, including involuntary tics and loss of vision or hearing.)

Saline breast implants   The saline breast implant may be either smooth or textured, round or contoured silicone sac/shell filled with a sterile saline (saltwater) solution, produced in varying sizes to match the healthy breast after mastectomy or to enlarge both breasts during breast augmentation. The empty shell is surgically implanted under the chest skin and filled either through a self-sealing valve on the front of the implant or through a valve on the back that allows the surgeon to add saline solution after surgery so as to change the size and/or shape of the implant after it is in place. Because saline breast implants are relatively new medical devices, there are no conclusive studies of long-term safety and effectiveness; the implants are not considered a lifetime device. They wear out over time, and problems such as deflation or rupture of the implant may require additional surgery to remove or replace the device.

breast lift   Mastopexy; surgery to lift and reshape sagging breasts and/or to reduce the size of the areola.

Procedure

Before surgery, the surgeon may recommend a mammogram to rule out the possibility of a tumor and donation of a unit of the patient's own blood in the (unlikely) event that a transfusion may be required.

The breast lift is most commonly performed via an incision shaped like an anchor with a circle around the areola (the dark tissue surrounding the nipple), a straight line down to the bottom of the breast, and a curved line in the crease underneath the breast. The surgeon separates the skin from the underlying tissue and removes as much glandular and fatty tissue as required. Next the nipple and areola (with blood vessels and nerves intact) are moved up into their new position on the breast. Excess skin is cut away and incision closed to create a smooth, firm surface.

For patients with less distinct drooping, the surgeon may use a doughnut incision, cutting two concentric circles around the areola, lifting out a doughnut-shape piece of skin, removing some underlying tissue, and closing the circular incision to form a smooth, firm surface.

In either case, if the patient is having an implant inserted, during surgery the surgeon places the implant into a pocket between the skin and the muscle underneath or underneath the muscle itself (see BREAST AUGMENTATION). After closing the incision, the surgeon covers the wound with gauze and fits the patient with an elastic bandage or a specially designed surgical bra.

Breast lift via an anchor incision is commonly done under general anesthesia and may require a one-to-two day stay in the hospital; breast lift via a doughnut incision may be done with local anesthesia plus a sedative and is generally an outpatient procedure. Within a week after surgery, the bandages and surgical bra will be replaced with a layer of gauze and a support bra to be worn 24 hours a day for up to four weeks. The stitches are removed within two weeks, but to avoid stress on the incision, the patient usually should avoid strenuous activity or heavy lifting for up to four weeks.

Risks and Complications

Common side effects of the surgery include bruising, swelling, discomfort, and/or temporary or loss of sensation in the breast, particularly around the nipple. For most patients, sensation returns as the swelling subsides; for some women, however, the loss may be permanent.

Breast lift surgery leaves extensive scarring, red and thick in the months immediately after surgery, then slowly fading to thinner, lighter lines, depending on the patient's skin type. As healing progresses, the nipples may be unevenly positioned, requiring corrective surgery.

Outlook and Lifestyle Modifications

This surgery may be done on any size breast, but the most successful and long-lasting results are achieved on smaller breasts. Because the nipples and milk ducts remain intact, the surgery will not interfere with nursing in the future, but a future pregnancy, like any significant change in weight, will stretch the breast tissue.

breast reconstruction Surgery to reconstruct a breast after MASTECTOMY, most often done to treat or prevent breast cancer. Most women who have had a mastectomy are candidates for breast reconstruction, but the timing of the surgery may vary with the patient. The benefits of immediate reconstruction, which is done at the time of the mastectomy, include less surgery and skin that has not been damaged by scarring or follow-up radiation treatment for cancer. Delaying reconstructive surgery gives the patient time to consider all options, including whether to have reconstruction; if the patient requires radiation therapy after mastectomy, delaying reconstructive surgery allows the skin additional time to heal.

Procedure

Breast reconstruction, which is most commonly performed under general anesthesic, may be done in one of three ways:

1. by inserting an implant immediately after mastectomy,
2. by expanding the skin after mastectomy and then inserting a breast implant during a second surgery, or
3. by building a new breast with a graft of skin and supporting tissue from another part of the patient's own body, either immediately after mastectomy or during a second surgery.

Reconstructing the breast with an immediate implant After mastectomy, the surgeon inserts an implant between skin and muscle just before closing the incision or grafts a piece of skin from another part of the patient's body to cover the implant or takes a graft of skin and underlying fatty tissue to build a new breast (see below). The candidate for

this procedure is a woman whose cancer has presumably been removed completely, who does not require follow-up radiation, and who has enough healthy breast skin to cover the implant.

Reconstructing the breast by expanding skin tissue After mastectomy, the surgeon inserts a temporary or permanent expandable sac such as a tissue expander under the skin and the chest muscle, leaving a small opening to a valve through which the surgeon can periodically inject a saltwater solution to fill the balloon and stretch the skin. The first permanent tissue expander for this purpose, created in 1984, is called the Becker breast prosthesis. After several weeks/months, when the skin has stretched sufficiently to cover a reconstructed breast, the opening is closed and the expander is left in place as an implant or the expander is removed, replaced with a permanent implant, and the incision closed. Finally, the nipple and the areola (the pigmented area surrounding the nipple) are reconstructed with a graft taken from another part of the body or tattooed on. This is called areolar reconstruction.

Reconstructing the breast with a tissue graft The surgeon lifts a tissue flap from the patient's abdomen, back, buttocks, or thighs to cover an implant or to build an entire breast. The tissue may be fixed in place on the chest while still attached to its original site so that it retains its original blood supply until it has grown firmly into place and establishes a new blood supply at the breast. Or the skin may be lifted entirely free from the original site and immediately attached to blood vessels and nerves at the site of the new breast. One flap used in reconstructing the breast is the latissimus dorsi flap, an oval piece of skin, underlying fat, and muscle lifted from the back, behind the armpit just under the shoulder, and moved around to the front of the body, where it is shaped into a breast, and sutured into place. Because there is little body fat in the back, this flap works best for women with small- to medium-size breasts. In most cases, an implant is also inserted during the surgery. Generally, this procedure produces excellent results with few complications; however, the skin on the back is often a different color and texture from the skin on the breast.

Note: Reconstructing the breast after breast surgery using only tissue from the patient's own body is called total autogenous latissimus (tal) breast reconstruction.

Before closing the incisions required for any of these three procedures, the surgeon is likely to insert a surgical drain to allow fluid to flow out rather than collect under the skin. The drain and the stitches are removed within a week to 10 days after surgery.

Risks and Complications

Patients may experience bruising, soreness, swelling, increased sensitivity, and/or scarring.

Complications related specifically to the implant may include seroma, a pooling of fluid around the implant that delays healing and may allow the implant to emerge through the skin. Thinning and shrinkage of the breast tissue may occur, caused by pressure from the implant. An implant may slip toward the center of the chest, or become deflated, or ruptured. Formation of scar tissue around the implant, known as capsular contracture, occurs in as many as 33 percent of all women with implants. Shifting, rupture, or capsular contracture usually requires corrective surgery. According to clinical studies submitted to the Food and Drug Administration by implant manufacturers, the incidence of additional surgery is 1 in 2.5 for reconstruction patients.

Outlook and Lifestyle Modifications

To protect the incisions and reduce scarring, the patient is usually advised to avoid strenuous activity (lifting, sports, or sex) for up to six weeks after surgery.

The rebuilt breast may feel firmer than a natural breast and may not match the remaining breast; occasionally, a surgeon will recommend surgery to reshape the natural breast to match the new one. Reconstruction of the breast lost to cancer does not affect the risk of a recurrence or the choice of treatment if the cancer recurs. However, the presence of a breast implant may affect the accuracy of future mammography. For example, the implant may block some views of the underlying tissue, requiring additional films, or calcium deposits in the tissue around the implant may be mistaken for tumors, requiring a diagnostic biopsy. Only a radiologist experienced in the techniques required to obtain and read the picture should perform a mammogram of a breast with an implant.

See also BREAST AUGMENTATION; BREAST IMPLANT.

breast reduction   Surgery to reduce the size of the breasts, or one breast, when the two are of unequal size, a condition called macromastia. It is done by removing glandular tissue, fatty tissue, and excess skin; for women who experience back pain, neck pain, skin irritation, or respiratory problems due to large, pendulous breast. Prior to surgery, the surgeon may recommend a weight-loss diet to reduce the size of the breasts, a mammogram to rule out the possibility of a tumor, and donation of a unit of the patient's own blood in the (unlikely) event that a transfusion may be required.

Procedure

The two-to-four hour surgery may be done in a hospital or in an outpatient center, usually under general anesthesic. Once the patient is sedated, the surgeon makes an incision in one of three shapes: an anchor, a doughnut, or a lollipop.

Anchor incision   The surgeon cuts a circle around the areola (the dark tissue surrounding the nipple), a straight line down to the bottom of the breast, and a curved line in the crease underneath the breast, and removes glandular tissue, fat, and skin. In most cases, the nipple and areola are moved up into position on the reshaped breast still attached to their own blood vessels and nerves. If the breasts are extremely large, the nipple and areola are lifted entirely off the breast and put into place as a skin graft. As with all successful skin grafts, new attachments to blood vessels will form to nourish the tissue, but there will be a loss of sensation due to the loss of nerve tissue.

Doughnut incision   The surgeon makes an incision around the areola, lifts a circular-shape piece of skin with a hole in the center (the areola/nipple) off the breast, removes excess tissue to make the areola smaller, and moves the nipple higher on the breast.

Lejour breast reduction   To perform this procedure, created by Madeline Lejour of the department of plastic surgery at the University of Brussels (Belgium), the surgeon marks the breast with guide-lines before surgery. She then uses liposuction to remove fatty tissue and creates a short vertical scar that does not extend below the inframammary fold (IMF), the fold under the breast.

Short scar incision ("lollipop")   The surgeon makes an incision in a circle around the areola, with a short straight line partway down the breast, and removes tissue from the sides and under part of the breast, leaving the upper part intact.

Once the correct amount of tissue has been removed and the nipple and areola are in place, the surgeon closes the incision, covers the wound with gauze, and wraps the area in an elastic bandage to reduce the risk of swelling. A small tube may be inserted in each breast and left there for a day or two to drain off blood and fluids, again to reduce the risk of swelling. Bandages and drains are usually removed within two days after surgery; stitches are removed within three weeks; a surgical or athletic bra is worn 24 hours a day for several weeks or until swelling and bruising are gone.

Z mammoplasty   In this technique for surgical breast reduction, the surgeon makes an incision around the nipple and areola (the pigmented area around the nipple). The surgeon then peels back the skin, relocates the nipple and areola, and removes tissue at the base of the cone formed by the breast. She next uses a Z-shape incision to pull the skin together and reduce tension on the nipple/areola area. The procedure works best in young women who do not have striae gravidarum (stretching due to the pull of gravity), a natural consequence of aging.

One tool available to surgeons planning breast reduction surgery is geometric breast reduction, a system created by American plastic surgeon GUSTAVE AUFRICHT; a diagram of lines drawn on the breast prior to surgery to create a surgical pattern that ensures a balanced breast with a viable nipple.

Risks and Complications

Swelling, bruising, mild discomfort (especially during the first menstrual period after surgery), pain, minor bleeding and drainage of liquid from the wound, infection, small sores around the nipple, and temporary loss of sensation in nipple and/or breast due to swelling of the tissues are relatively common. A moisturizer may be useful to relieve dry skin after surgery so long as it is not used near the sutures. The patient may be told to avoid sexual activity for a week or longer because sexual arousal may cause the incisions to swell.

More serious complications may include heavy bleeding or drainage that require medical treatment, slightly mismatched breasts and/or unevenly positioned nipples and/or permanent loss of sensation in nipple and/or breast, or persistent pain. In rare cases, the blood supply to the transplanted nipple and areola may fail. If the tissue dies, it must be removed and the nipple and areola reconstructed with tissue grafts from another part of the body.

Outlook and Lifestyle Modifications

Most swelling, bruising, and discomfort fade within a few weeks, but it may take as long as a year for the breasts to assume their final shape, which, like their original shape, may change with weight gain/loss and/or hormonal shifts during the menstrual cycle or pregnancy.

Breast reduction may leave extensive scarring; as its name suggests, the short scar incision leaves the least. In the months immediately after surgery, scars may be red and thick, and then slowly fade to thinner, lighter lines, depending on the patient's skin type.

Because the surgery removes many of the milk ducts leading to the nipples, it may not be possible for women who expect to become pregnant to then breast-feed their infants.

bromelain See CHEMICAL SKIN PEEL.

brow lift See FOREHEAD LIFT.

Brown, James Barrett (1899–1971) American plastic surgeon. In 1925, he joined Vilray Papin Blair to develop one of the first plastic surgery centers in the United States, at the University of Missouri. He served as chief of plastic and reconstructive surgery to the U.S. Army during World War II and authored more than 300 scientific articles, 30 book chapters, and eight books on plastic and reconstructive surgery.

browplasty See FOREHEAD LIFT.

buccal fat pad extraction Facial contouring; a PLASTIC SURGERY procedure to slim the shape of the cheeks by removing part of the fat pad, the fatty deposit that creates the curve of the cheek. This procedure is done most commonly for persons older than 23 to 27, an age at which the fat pad begins to shrink naturally; rarely performed in people older than 50.

Procedure

The fat is removed through two incisions inside the mouth, between the upper molars and the mucous membrane of the cheek, and then the incisions are closed.

Risks and Complications

After surgery, soreness, swelling, and numbness are common; the stitches are removed within a week, but it may take up to four months for the swelling to subside completely. Other possible complications include infection, a starved appearance if too much tissue is removed, unequally sized cheeks, scarring, or nerve damage.

Outlook and Lifestyle Modifications

The surgery produces a more finely sculpted face.

buffalo hump See KYPHOSIS.

Bunnell, Sterling (1882–1957) American hand surgeon, author of *Surgery of the Hand* (1944), organizer of nine U.S. Army Hand Centers during World War II, and a founder of the American Society for Surgery of the Hand. He also created the Bunnell sutures, surgical stitches used to tie tendons together in a manner that preserves their ability to move and turn.

See also HAND SURGERY.

burns and burn reconstruction A burn is any injury caused by contact with chemicals, electrical current, heat, or radiation. Burn damage may be characterized by the severity of the burn or the burn's effect on the surrounding tissue. A first-degree (superficial) burn reddens the epidermis (top layers of skin cells) and causes some swelling. A second-degree (partial thickness) burn damages both the epidermis and the dermis (the second layers of skin cells), causing blisters and perhaps some tissue death with minimal scarring but not enough to prevent the regrowth of skin. A third-degree (full thickness) burn destroys all layers of the epidermis and the dermis and extends into the fat and muscle or bone below, causing deep scarring.

Burn reconstruction is a multistage medical and surgical treatment to prevent or reduce scarring and tissue contraction immediately after a burn and/or to increase function and decrease disfigurement once the burn has healed.

Procedure

Burn reconstruction occurs in three stages: evaluation of the wounds, prevention of further damage or deterioration, and reconstruction.

Evaluation In evaluating damage to the tissue surrounding a burn, the zone of hyperemia is an area where the burned tissue is injured but can still be saved. The zone of status is an area where the tissue can be saved with immediate treatment such as cooling and fluids to preserve the blood vessels. The zone of coagulation is an area where the blood vessels have been destroyed, leaving the tissue irreversibly damaged.

To estimate the size of the area damaged by a burn and plan appropriate treatment, burn specialists and plastic surgeons use one of two diagrams, the Wallace Rule of Nines and/or the Lund and Browder Chart.

The Wallace Rule of Nines, created by A. B. Wallace and published in the British medical journal *The Lancet* in March 1951, divides the body into units assigned numerical values related to the number nine that enable the physician to calculate the extent of a burn as a percentage of the surface of the body. For adults, the head and neck (front and back) account for 9 percent of the body surface; each arm (front and back), 9 percent; chest and abdomen (front), 18 percent; abdomen (back), 18 percent; genital area, 1 percent; leg (front and back), 18 percent.

The Lund and Browder chart, created by C. C. Lund and N. C. Browder and published in the medical journal *Surgical Gynecology and Obstetrics* in 1944, assigns to body areas a percentage of the total body surface that varies according to the age of the patient and divides the leg into three distinct areas: thigh, leg, and foot. This chart is more accurate, especially for children, whose head and abdomen are proportionately larger and whose legs are proportionately smaller than an adult's. For example, on the Lund and Browder chart, a five-year-old child's face or the back of the head is estimated to be 6.5 percent of the total body area; for an adult, 3.5 percent. Similarly, the front or back of the five-year-old child's thigh is estimated to be 4 percent of the total body surface; for an adult, 4.75 percent.

Prevention To reduce the risk of thick, disfiguring scars, the burned area is immediately covered with a skin substitute. These synthetic dressings, which remain in place 24 hours a day (except for bathing), prevent fluid loss, thus helping to keep the tissue moist and supple. They also reduce the risk of infection by protecting the burned skin against contaminants.

Two skin substitutes used to cover burns that damage only the epidermal (top) layers of skin cells are TranCyte™ Human Fibroblast Derived Temporary Skin Substitute and Biobrane®. Transcyte is a two-part dressing with a clear top layer that allows air and fluids to flow in and out and an inner layer of NYLON mesh impregnated human fibroblats (cells that produce other skin cells) coated with bovine or porcine collagen and human growth factor. When the dressing produces enough human cells to create a layer of skin, the synthetic material is removed and, if neccessary, a skin graft is put in place. Biobrane® is nylon with a gel that interacts with human clotting factors in the wound to create a protective covering that keeps fluids in and microorganisms out. Like Transcyte, Biobrane is removed when the wound heals.

A dressing used to cover areas damaged by third-degree burns is Integra™ Dermal Regeneration Template, a two-layer product with a silicone sheet on top and a mesh template underneath that encourages the growth of cells in the dermis, the layer under the epidermis. When the body has produced enough cells to create a stable layer of skin, the silicone sheet is removed and a graft of epidermal skin is put in its place (the mesh is eventually absorbed by the body).

As the skin heals, new connective tissue forms and may tighten the adjacent tissue (extrinsic contracture) or the internal tissue at the site of the wound itself (intrinsic contracture). To reduce the risk of contracture, the patient is wrapped in elastic bandages or custom-made COMPRESSION GARMENT that may be worn for up to 23 hours a day for as long as 18 months after the burn. Splinting may be used to keep limbs straight. Some cases may require serial casting, a series of casts that move joints/limbs into increasingly normal positions, or ranging (moving the joints), which prevents tendons and ligaments around the joint from contracting, thus preserving the ability to move.

Reconstruction About a year after the burn, when the scars have stabilized, PLASTIC SURGERY to repair burn damage can begin. The simplest procedure is one or more Z-shape or Y-shape incisions to relieve the tension on the scar. Or the surgeon may remove the scar tissue and cover the wound with a graft of skin from the patient's own body, preferably a full thickness graft, especially for sites such as the fingers where the skin is often bent. If the patient does not have enough healthy tissue for grafting, a thin split-thickness graft can be placed over a cell-free, or acellular, frame to strengthen the thinner graft.

Alternatively, the surgeon may lift a SKIN FLAP from the chest or groin and move it to cover an adjacent area, leaving the flap connected to the original site so as to keep the flap alive in its new site.

Risks and Complications

As with all surgery, grafts and flaps carry the risk of infection and additional scarring, including the formation of heavy scar tissue that may impede the patient's movement.

Outlook and Lifestyle Modifications

The cosmetic and success of burn reconstruction and the restoration of mobility (and in fingers and hands) depends in large part on the severity of the burn.

See also KELOID.

Burow, Karl August (1809–1874) German surgeon; creator of Burow's operation, a technique for increasing the flexibility of an advancement flap by cutting small triangular incisions at the wide base of the flap to make it easier to lift the skin up and move it forward. He also created Burow's solution, an astringent antiseptic solution of an aluminum compound in water that is used to relieve inflammations and itching of minor skin irritation due an allergic reaction to insect bites, cosmetics, household chemicals (most commonly, detergents), or to metals in jewelry (most commonly, nickel), and plants (most commonly poison ivy and poison oak).

butt lift   See BUTTOCK LIFT.

buttock augmentation   Glutealplasty; cosmetic surgery to firm and shape the buttocks, the rounded surfaces of the lower back created by the bulk of the three-layer muscle that controls the movement of the thighs: the gluteus maximus (top layer), gluteus medius (middle layer), and gluteus minimus (inner layer).

Procedure

The procedure may be performed either by inserting soft implants through an incision at the base of the spine or by injecting into the buttocks fatty tissue removed by liposuction from other parts of the patent's body. It is most commonly performed as outpatient surgery with either regional (epidural) or general anesthesic.

Once the patient is sedated and lying on the stomach, the surgeon makes an incision either in the crease where the buttock meets the top of the back of the thigh or in the gluteal crease or fold, the horizontal groove where the lower edge of the buttock meets the top of the thigh. Reaching in through the incision, the surgeon makes a pocket either beneath or on top of the gluteus maximus muscle (the largest of the three muscles that make the curve of the buttock), slightly above the area on which the patient will sit so as to reduce the risk of the implant's shifting after surgery. When one side is done, the surgeon repeats the procedure on the other side, examines the buttocks to be sure they are the same in size and shape, and sutures the incisions. The patient is usually awake and ready to leave within two hours.

Alternatively, the surgeon may use liposuction to remove excess fat from another area of the patient's body, usually the thigh or "love handles" (lower part of the back). The fat is cleaned, purified, and injected into the buttocks, checking to be certain that the result is symmetrical. This procedure, which is usually done with regional anesthetic, is not practical for patients with little extra body fat.

Risks and Complications

Common risks are bleeding, bruising, discomfort, infection, and reaction to the anesthetic.

After buttock implants, the risk of infection is higher if the implants are inserted through an incision at the center crease in the buttocks. Discomfort when sitting, standing, walking, or lying on the back is common for several weeks, and patients may require an elastic COMPRESSION GARMENT for support. The implants may shift or break, requiring additional surgery.

Outlook and Lifestyle Modifications

As swelling recedes over several months, the true shape of the new buttocks becomes clear. After fat grafts into the buttocks, the body may eventually absorb the fatty tissue; the buttocks may look unbalanced, necessitating another round of liposuction and another series of fat injections.

buttock lift   Surgery to remove excess skin and fat just under the buttock and/or on upper thigh; usually performed as an outpatient procedure under general anesthesia or local anesthesia plus sedatives.

Procedure

Once the patient is sedated and is lying facedown on the operating table, the surgeon makes an incision either at the top of the buttock or in the crease where the buttock meets the top of the back of the thigh or (less frequently) in the gluteal crease or fold, the horizontal groove where the lower edge of the buttock meets the top of the thigh. He then lifts the skin, removes excess fat (if necessary), and removes excess skin to tighten and firm the buttock. When one side is done, the surgeon repeats the procedure on the other side and examines the buttocks to be sure they are the same in size and shape. A COMPRESSION GARMENT may be used to reduce swelling and help speed the natural tightening of the skin.

Risks and Complications

Bleeding and bruising are common, but bruises usually fade within three to four weeks. Discomfort when sitting, standing, walking, or lying on the back are likely to last for several weeks. To relieve discomfort and speed healing, patients are often told to lie on the stomach, not the back, for the first week after surgery.

The risk of infection is higher if the incisions are made in the gluteal crease.

Outlook and Lifestyle Modifications

The final shape of the buttocks becomes evident within six months. The improvement may last as long as 10 years, subject to the continuing natural age-related loss of skin elasticity and/or gaining or losing significant amounts of weight.

buttock reduction   See BUTTOCK LIFT.

buttonhole flap   See LASIK.

butyl-2-cyanoacrylate   See WOUND ADHESIVE.

cable graft   See NEUROPLASTY.

cadaver skin graft   See SKIN GRAFT.

café au lait macule (CALM)   Light-to-dark-brown coffee-colored mark of varying size, from a small freckle to more than three inches across. In the United States, about 0.3 percent of whites, 3 percent of Hispanics, and 18 percent of blacks are born with at least one CALM, which may not be clearly visible until the child is two-to-three years old. After that, the size and number of CALMs tend to increase with age. The marks are easily removed with a yellow or red light LASER.

Individual CALMs are rarely a health problem, but multiple CALMs may signal an underlying illness such as neurofibromatosis ("Elephant Man Disease"), a genetic condition characterized by numerous nerve tumors. They may also indicate McCune-Albright syndrome, an endocrine disorder; Fanconi anemia, a congenital blood disorder associated with mental retardation; or tuberous sclerosis, an inherited disorder linked to nerve and skin tumors, seizures, and mental retardation.

See also MOLE.

Cagot ear   See EAR RECONSTRUCTION.

calf augmentation   Surgery to improve the shape of the calf, the curve of flesh at the back of the lower leg, below the knee. The calf is created by the layering of two muscles: the gastrocnemius muscle, which comes down from the rounded end of the femur (the long bone of the thigh), and the soleus muscle, which is attached to both the tibia (the large, long

bone in the front of the lower leg) and the fibula (the smaller, nonweight-bearing bone behind the tibia). Note: The fibular is usually called the calf bone, a term also used in PLASTIC SURGERY to describe bone taken from the leg of a young cow and processed for use as bone implants for human beings.

Procedure

Once the patient is given general anesthesic, the surgeon makes an incision at the bottom of the back of the knee and separates the muscle tissue from the overlying skin and fatty tissue. He next slides a calf implant, a rounded packet of silicone, through the incision into the space between muscle and the overlying tissues, and then pushes and massages the implant into place. The procedure is repeated on the other leg. When both inserts are in place and the legs appear symmetrical, the incisions are closed.

Risks and Complications

Patients are usually advised to avoid strenuous exercise for two months prior to surgery to reduce the risk of an injury that might delay the operation. After surgery, they may be told to stay in bed for up to 48 hours to keep the implants from shifting.

Swelling and bruising may last for up to three weeks. Walking in shoes with heels may be more comfortable than flat shoes because the heels put weight on the front of the foot, taking pressure off the calf. When sitting, the calves should be below the knees to avoid pooling blood in the calf.

Outlook and Lifestyle Modifications

Most patients wind up with the cosmetic improvement of a well-rounded calf and require no follow-up treatment.

See BONE REPLACEMENT.

camouflage cosmetics Makeup formulated specifically to conceal imperfections, correct skin color, or shade the face so as to disguise swelling or emphasize facial contours.

Cosmetic concealers are thick, opaque liquids or creams used to cover a birthmark, scar, bruise, or post surgical discoloration.

Color correctors are liquids or creams used under a regular foundation/base to neutralize natural skin color or to cover bruising or redness after a cosmetic procedure such as a CHEMICAL SKIN PEEL; lavender hides yellow skin tones, green hides red.

Shading cosmetics, also known as *contouring cosmetics,* are powders used to create the illusion of light and shadow so as to accent or deemphasize facial bone structure. Light shades (highlighters) make an area more prominent; dark shades (shadows) make a naturally prominent area seem to recede.

Cannon, Bradford (1906–2005) A graduate of Harvard Medical School (1933), Dr. Cannon joined Massachusetts General (1940), where he created the hospital's first residency in PLASTIC SURGERY and became its first chief of plastic and reconstructive surgery. He served as president of the Boston Surgical Society, New England Society of Plastic and Reconstructive Surgery, and the American Association of Plastic Surgeons (1957). Following the 1942 fire that killed more than 500 people at the Cocoanut Grove nightclub in Boston, Cannon developed a new treatment method for burns. By wrapping burned areas with petroleum-coated gauze containing boric acid, he was able to preserve burned skin, and he used grafts of cadaver skin to cover large damaged areas. During World War II, Cannon served as a military surgeon, treating soldiers disfigured by burns or shell fire while chief of plastic surgery at Valley Forge General Hospital in Pennsylvania. After the war, he helped create a pediatric plastic surgery clinic at Mount Auburn Hospital in Cambridge, Massachusetts, and became a consultant to the Atomic Energy Commission, investigating the health effects of radioactive weapons tests in the South Pacific Marshall Islands.

canthus The angled point on either side of the eye just above where the upper and lower lids meet. The medial canthus is the area just above the medial commissure, the corner of the eye nearest the nose that houses the tear drainage system and the medial canthal tendon. The lateral canthus is the area just above the lateral commissure, the corner of the eye nearest the ear that contains the lateral canthal tendon, along with other supporting muscles and ligaments.

Canthal reconstruction (*canthoplasty*) is surgery to repair damage due to an injury or a defect in the canthus. *Canthopexy* is surgery to tighten the canthus with one suture so as to reposition/lift the lower eyelid. Canthopexy is less invasive than canthoplasty, but its results do not last as long.

See also EYE LIFT.

cantilever bone graft See RHINOPLASTY.

cap technique See FINGERTIP REPAIR.

carpal tunnel syndrome The carpal tunnel is the passage through the wrist for tendons and a major nerve for the hand; pressure within the passage causes the discomfort called carpal tunnel syndrome.

Symptoms and Diagnostic Path
Carpal tunnel syndrome is diagnosed by its most common symptoms: tingling, numbness, or aching in the hands plus loss of free movement of the hand and fingers.

Treatment Options and Outlook
In moderate cases, NSAIDS (nonsteroidal anti-inflammatory drugs such as aspirin or ibuprofen) and/or splinting the hand may provide relief. More severe disability may require PLASTIC SURGERY. The surgeon makes an incision across the center of the palm from the edge of the fingers up to the wrist and releases or cuts back the tissue underneath that is pressing on the nerve; when the wound is closed, the surgeon applies a splint dressing to keep the hand still as it heals. The surgery leaves a scar that is barely visible. The results of the surgery—relief from pain, freedom of motion—depend on the extent of the damage; the earlier carpal syndrome is treated, the better the outcome.

Risk Factors and Preventive Measures

Carpal tunnel syndrome most commonly occurs after an injury. It is also associated with rheumatoid arthritis and with fluid retention during pregnancy. The role of repetitive motion, such as typing on a computer keyboard, once considered a serious risk factor, has been called into question by new studies.

Carpue's operation   Indian rhinoplasty; surgery to reconstruct a damaged or defective nose with a SKIN FLAP lifted from the forehead. Carpue's operation originated in India. It is so named because it was brought to Great Britain (1814) by Joseph Constantine Carpue (1764–1846), the first British military plastic surgeon.

See also RHINOPLASTY.

cartilage (connective tissue)   A highly resilient material found between the bones in the joints and spine, at the ends of the long bones in the arms and legs, and in tubelike body structures such as the bronchi (the windpipes leading into the lungs). Cartilage cushions bones and prevents their rubbing against each other. It also provides a firm but flexible framework to hold open internal tubes such as the larynx (throat) and bronchi and a firm but bendable frame for the outer ear.

In PLASTIC SURGERY, grafts of cartilage, most commonly from the patient's own body, are used to build a supporting framework on which to reconstruct and/or repair a cartilaginous organ such as an ear or nose missing from birth or damaged by an injury.

See also EAR RECONSTRUCTION; RHINOPLASTY.

catgut   See SUTURE.

cat's ear   See EAR RECONSTRUCTION.

cauliflower ear   See EAR RECONSTRUCTION.

central nervous system   See NERVOUS SYSTEM.

cervicoplasty   See NECK LIFT.

cheek augmentation   The cheek is the part of the mid-face area from the side of the nose to the ear, between the eye and the upper lip. It is shaped by a four-part cheekbone (two bones on each side of the face) and rounded by a natural fat pad under the skin. Cheek augmentation is a term used to describe either a reconstructive procedure to repair or reshape this area when the bone is missing or a procedure to replace the contour lost when the fat pad under the cheek has been reduced as the patient ages.

Procedure

The surgeon makes an incision either in the lower eyelid or inside the mouth on one side of the face, then inserts either a permanent silicone or Gore-Tex™ implant or a graft of fatty tissue that will eventually be absorbed by the body. To ensure proper fit, an implant may be inserted, evaluated, then removed and reshaped to fit the patient's face before being fixed in place; the fat graft is massaged into place. Depending on the extent of the defect, the procedure may be repeated on the other cheek.

Risks and Complications

After surgery, swelling and bruising may last up to two weeks. Discomfort while eating is more common when the incision is inside the mouth.

Other possible complications include infection, a reaction to an implant, rejection of the implant, or slippage of the implant. If the infection does not respond to antibiotics, the implant may have to be removed and replaced after a suitable waiting period. If the implant shifts significantly, a second surgery may be required to reposition it. If the patient's body reacts to or rejects the implant, it must be removed and cannot be reinserted.

Outlook and Lifestyle Modifications

The patient will experience soreness and swelling for several days after the surgery; the final contours of the face are not visible until all swelling has resolved, a period which may take up to several months. The fat graft may eventually be absorbed by the body, requiring another surgery to maintain the contour of the cheek.

cheek implant   See CHEEK AUGMENTATION.

cheiloplasty   See LIP REDUCTION.

chemical skin peel   Use of a chemical agent to produce a controlled injury to the skin so that the skin heals and grows new skin cells, new blood cells, and new collagen (connective tissue), eventually creating a tighter, smoother skin surface with fewer discolorations.

Skin peels are described as *superficial, medium,* or *deep,* depending on how far the chemical peeling agent penetrates into the layers of skin cells. A superficial chemical skin peel penetrates only the first layer of the epidermis, the outermost layer of skin cells.

The peeling agents used for a superficial skin peel are alpha hydroxy acids, solid carbon dioxide (CO_2), Jessner's peel, salicylic acid, or a low (10–35 percent) concentration of TCA (trichloroacetic acid). Bromelain is a proteolytic (protein-destroying) enzyme in pineapples, often used as an ingredient in cosmetic exfoliants. Over-the-counter products for a mild skin peel may include alpha hydroxy acids (AHA), a group of naturally occurring acidic compounds in food such as citric acid found in fruits; glycolic acid, found in sugarcane and fruits; lactic acid, found in milk; and malic acid, found in apples. Alpha hydroxy acids are natural exfoliants that flake away the top layer of dry skin cells. Processed or synthetic alpha hydroxyl acids are commonly added to over-the-counter cosmetics designed to make the skin feel smoother; they are used in PLASTIC SURGERY to produce a superficial chemical skin peel, a procedure that removes only the top layers of skin cells.

A medium depth chemical skin peel penetrates through the epidermis to the first layer of the dermis, the two-level layer of cells just under the epidermis. The peeling agents used for a medium depth skin peel are a combination of CO_2 plus TCA or Jessner's peel plus TCA or TCA plus glycolic acid.

A deep chemical skin peel penetrates into the middle of the stratum reticulare, the second layer of the dermis. The chemical peeling agent used for a deep skin peel is the Baker-Gordon solution, a phenol-based liquid. Note: Laser skin resurfacing produces results similar to the deep chemical skin peel with fewer adverse effects such as long-term redness.

Conditions that respond well to a chemical skin peel are light WRINKLES such as "crow's feet" (fine lines radiating outward from the corners of the eyes caused by exposure to sunlight or smoking or repeated smiling and squinting), light scarring, discolored spots due to exposure to sunlight, eruptions and related discoloration, and some forms of ACNE. Defects on the skin surface such as fine wrinkles are treated with a superficial peel. Defects such as damage from long-term exposure to sunlight that extend into the top layer of the dermis are treated with a medium depth peel. Deep wrinkles such as those between the eyebrows or between nose and mouth may require a deep peel.

Other factors that influence the type of peel recommended for a specific patient are: skin color, as determined by the FITZPATRICK SKIN TYPE CLASSIFICATION scale; the degree of sun damage (as measured by the Glogau Photoaging Classification); and the patient's medical history. For example, people who scar easily or form KELOIDS (thick, raised scars) or whose skin has been severely damaged, as by a deep burn, are generally not considered good candidates for medium or deep skin peels. Any recent procedure such as facial surgery or dermabrasion that irritates or injures that skin may rule out any peel, at least temporarily. People who have recently had radiation treatment usually should have a skin biopsy performed to make sure the hair follicles (small pits from which individual hairs grow) are intact because the regrowth of skin cells begins in these follicles.

Finally, some medical drugs may adversely affect the success of a skin peel. Anticoagulants ("blood thinners") may increase bleeding after a deep peel; for the same reason, doctors may advise patients taking aspirin, which is a mild anticoagulant, to stop for one week prior to a deep peel. Isotretinoin (Accutane™) increases the risk of scarring; it is usually avoided for up to six months before a chemical peel. Using oral contraceptive pills may cause chloasma (brownish pigmentation on the face); taking oral contraceptives after a peel may darken the skin, reversing the effects of the peel. On the other hand, a patient with a history of herpes simplex (cold sores) may be advised to begin taking the antiviral drug acyclovir (Zovirax) two days before the peel and to continue for five days afterward.

Procedure

The surgeon cleans the skin and wipes the skin surface with a solution of acetone or rubbing alcohol or a combination of the two in order to remove fatty material to allow the peeling agent to penetrate. Areas of delicate skin such as the lips, inside the nose, and the corners of the eye are protected with petroleum jelly.

Next, the paste or foam chemoexfoliant/peeling agent is applied with a special brush or sponge or cotton pads/swabs, starting at the forehead and moving down the face to the chin, being careful to ensure that the peeling agent does not drip onto other areas or pool in the folds of the face.

As the peeling agent begins to work, it causes a sharp tingling sensation, and keratins (proteins in the skin) clump together, forming a whitish-to-gray tint called frost. A superficial peel that destroys only the top layer of skin produces a bright white frost; a deeper peel produces a gray-white frost. If the frost is uneven—heavier or lighter in some places than in others—the doctor may reapply the peeling agent. How long the peeling agent stays on the skin affects the depth of the peel. Once enough time has elapsed or the color of the frost shows that the peel has reached the proper depth, the doctor will stop the peeling action by neutralizing the peeling agent with cold water, a cold wet compress, a bicarbonate spray, or a soap-free cleanser. (Some peeling agents, such as salicylic acid and trichloroacetic acid, are neutralized by the skin itself.) Note: A deep peel with a phenol-based product such as Baker-Gordon solution requires the surgeon to monitor the patient's heart during the procedure because absorption of phenol through the skin may cause an irregular heartbeat.

When the peel is complete and the peeling agent has been neutralized, the doctor will cover the skin with a dressing to protect the skin from air. Follow-up visits will be scheduled to check for any sign of infection; a person who has had a superficial peel will come back a week after the procedure; a person who has had a deep peel may be scheduled to return two or three times in the first week.

Risks and Complications

After a peel, as the chemical injury heals, the skin will exfoliate (flake and peel). The deeper the peel, the longer the period of exfoliation is likely to last.

Redness may last for up to three months after a peel. Severe redness or redness that lasts longer than three months can be treated with an anti-inflammatory medication such as a cortisone cream. The healing skin is very sensitive to sunlight, so the patient should stay out of the sun or wear a protective hat and apply a strong sunscreen when exposure to sunlight is unavoidable.

As healing continues, the skin may turn darker or lighter than it was before the peel. Medium and deep peels, which penetrate to the dermis, may stimulate the formation of keloids (thick, white scar tissue). Picking at the healing skin may also cause scars.

Topical antibiotic creams and disinfectant wash reduce the risk of a bacterial infection. Fungal (Candida) infections are treated with an antifungal drug, commonly ketoconazole (Nizoral). Cold sores may be prevented or treated with the antiviral medication acyclovir (Zovirax).

Ointments that protect the skin can clog the sebaceous glands (glands that secrete sebum, a natural skin lubricant) and cause small cysts (milia) two to three weeks after the peel. Acne may also occur.

Pigmentation mismatch is a potentially permanent complication of skin treatments such as a skin peel, in which the treated skin heals lighter or darker than the normal skin color.

Outlook and Lifestyle Modifications

The chemical skin peel provides a noticeable but temporary change in the texture and sometimes the color of the skin. However, to maintain the effect, the procedure must be repeated at intervals that vary depending on the patient's natural skin type and lifestyle. For example, repeated exposure to sunlight after the peel has healed will restart the process of skin damage.

chemoexfoliation See CHEMICAL SKIN PEEL.

cherry hemangioma See HEMANGIOMA.

chin augmentation See CHIN RECONSTRUCTION.

chin lift Surgery, most commonly performed on an outpatient basis, to remove excess sagging skin and fat around and beneath the chin, so as to tighten the chin line for a more youthful appearance. The fat pad under the chin is called a *buccula* and may create a double chin when it becomes too large.

Procedure
The patient is given general anesthetic. The surgeon makes two incisions, one under or behind each ear, trims away excess skin, and lifts the skin into place and closes the incision with stitches or surgical glue. Afterward, the surgeon may wrap a dressing around the head and under the skin to exert pressure on and protect the incision.

Risks and Complications
Bruising, swelling, and mild discomfort are common following this surgery.

Outlook and Lifestyle Modifications
Successful surgery eliminates excess sagging skin to produce a smooth chin line.

chin reconstruction Surgery to reconstruct, enlarge, or reduce the rounded lower edge of the face, the skin-and-fat-covered lower jaw. This is done to balance the features of the face, for example, to bring the chin forward into line with the nose when the face is seen in profile. When done for cosmetic purposes, this is usually called chin augmentation or chin reduction. Chin reconstruction is similar, but its aim is medical rather than cosmetic, to replace chin bone and/or tissue destroyed by an injury or the removal of a tumor or to repair a deficit or deformity due to a birth defect. An example of the former is Andy Gump deformity, a receding chin and lower face resembling those of a 1930s cartoon character, caused by the surgical removal of part of the back of the lower jaw to excise a tumor or infected tissue or to repair serious injuries. Examples of the latter are bird beak jaw, a birth defect characterized by an abnormally underdeveloped lower jaw with overhanging upper jaw, and Pierre Robin anomaly, an abnormally small jaw (micrognathia), cleft palate, and large tongue, first identified by French dental surgeon Pierre Robin (1867–1950).

Procedure
The patient is given general anesthetic. The surgeon makes an incision either inside the mouth between the lower lip and the lower jaw or underneath the chin, then inserts either tissue from the patient's own body (usually a piece of calf bone plus surrounding muscle, skin, and blood vessels) or a silicone or polyethylene implant, custom made for the individual patient. The tissue or implant is manipulated into place over the existing chin bone, and the incision is closed, usually with absorbable sutures.

Surgery to reduce the size of the chin so as to bring it into alignment with the nose when seen in profile or to reduce a very large lower jaw is the same as for chin augmentation except that the surgeon removes part of the bone rather than inserting implants.

Risks and Complications
For several days after surgery, the patient may be uncomfortable when moving the mouth to smile or talk. Bruising and swelling subside as the incisions heal, but it may require several months for the swelling to disappear completely so that the final shape of the new jawline is visible.

The most common complication after chin augmentation or reduction is a loss of feeling in the lower lip due to nerve damage during surgery. Other possible complications include infection, a reaction to an implant, rejection of the implant, or slippage of the implant. If the infection does not respond to antibiotics, the implant may have to be removed and replaced after a suitable waiting period. If the implant shifts significantly, a second surgery may be required to reposition it. If the patient's body reacts to or rejects the implant, it must be removed and cannot be reinserted.

Outlook and Lifestyle Modifications

An incision inside the mouth leaves no visible scar; an incision under the chin leaves a minimal scar.

chin reduction   See CHIN RECONSTRUCTION.

chin tuck   See CHIN LIFT.

chloasma   Mask of pregnancy, melasma (from the Greek *mela,* meaning "dark"). This is a temporary brown pigmentation, usually over a woman's forehead, cheeks, and upper lip.

Symptoms and Diagnostic Path

Chloasma, diagnosed simply by its distinctive appearance, occurs most frequently during pregnancy, especially among with women with darker (olive) skin. The pigmentation fades a few months after delivery, but may intensify with subsequent pregnancies. Chloasma occurs most frequently due to a mild natural increase in estrogen levels, as occurs during pregnancy. It may also occur due to the use of hormonal contraceptives such as oral contraceptives or contraceptive patches or injections, or it may be linked to an interaction between ultraviolet light (sunlight) and some medicines and/or cosmetics. It is most likely to occur among women with naturally darker (olive) skin.

Treatment Options and Outlook

Camouflage cosmetics will hide the pigmentation. Bleaching creams containing hydroquinone may slightly lighten the color, as may cosmetic creams containing an alpha hydroxy acid. Medical remedies include prescription cream containing tretinoin (Retin-A™) or a superficial CHEMICAL SKIN PEEL. Laser treatment is sometimes considered, but it may reduce the pigmentation or make it worse.

Risk Factors and Preventive Measures

Using a sunblock with a high protection number or makeup with sunscreen and a mild cleanser that does not irritate the skin reduces the risk of chloasma.

chondrolarnygoplasty   See ADAM'S APPLE REDUCTION.

circulatory system   The heart, lungs, and blood vessels (arteries, veins, and capillaries) make up the circulatory system. Plastic surgeons are often in attendance at procedures to repair structural damage to the heart. Most commonly, they repair or replace blood vessels, for example, in surgery to ameliorate varicose veins.

The circulatory system governs the circulation of blood around the body. It was first accurately described by British physician William Harvey (1578–1657) in a 1628 treatise entitled *Exercitatio Anatomica de Motu Cordis et Sanguinis in Animalibus* (*Anatomical Exercise on the Motion of the Heart and Blood in Animals*).

Blood flows from the right ventricle (lower right chamber of the heart) through the pulmonary artery into the lungs, where red blood cells pick up oxygen. The oxygenated blood flows back through the pulmonary veins to the left ventricle (lower left chamber of the heart) and up into the left atrium (upper left chamber of the heart). From there it is pumped out through the coronary artery to veins and capillaries through which it travels to every body organ, tissue, and cell, delivering nutrients and oxygen and picking up waste products. Ultimately, oxygen-depleted blood flows through large veins (inferior vena cava and superior vena cava) into the right atrium (upper right chamber of the heart) and then back down into the right ventricle as the circle begins anew.

circumcision reversal   See FORESKIN REPLACEMENT.

claw foot   Deformity which may be present at birth or acquired due to a muscle disorder in the foot or damage to the nerves of the leg or spinal cord. It is sometimes associated with cerebral palsy or rheumatoid arthritis.

Symptoms and Diagnostic Path

Claw foot is diagnosed by physical examination. The arch of the foot is abnormally high, the toe joints nearest the foot bend up, and the furthest joints of the toe bend down, giving the entire foot a clawlike appearance.

Treatment Options and Outlook

The first level of treatment for claw foot is a change in footwear, including cushioning to relieve pain and/or calluses where the toes push up against the shoe. Surgery to reduce the arch of the foot so that more of the bottom of the foot touches the ground may be appropriate if severe pain is present in the toes or a badly deformed foot interferes with daily activities. The results, however, vary with the type of surgery and/or the severity of the deformity. Surgery is not recommended for athletes, children, and people with circulatory problems (including people with diabetes), those with neuromuscular disorders, or those with rheumatoid arthritis.

Risk Factors and Preventive Measures

Claw foot is a birth defect, for which there is no known risk factor or preventive measure.

claw hand Deformity in which the fingers are bent so as to resemble an animal's claw. Claw hand condition may be congenital (present at birth) or occur later in life due to nerve damage, damage to the underlying muscles and tendons, or to contraction of the skin following burns of the hand.

Symptoms and Diagnostic Path

Claw hand is diagnosed by physical examination.

Treatment Options and Outlook

Claw hand due to a birth defect may be treated with surgery to straighten the finger.

The primary treatment for claw hand due to nerve or muscle injury is nonsteroidal anti-inflammatory drugs and splinting to straighten the hand. The treatment for claw hand due to contracture of the skin following a burn is burn reconstruction.

Risk Factors and Preventive Measures

There is no known risk factor or preventive measure for a claw hand birth defect.

See also BURNS AND BURN RECONSTRUCTION; CLAW FOOT.

cleft earlobe   See EAR RECONSTRUCTION.

cleft lip and/or palate   A birth defect resulting in separation in the upper lip and/or palate (roof and back of the mouth) due to the failure of embryonic tissues to fuse properly to form the face and jaw.

Symptoms and Diagnostic Path

A cleft in the lip may be minimal, simply an indentation in the upper lip, or it may be a complete separation of the lip that extends all the way up to the bottom of the nose. The cleft may be unilateral (on one side) or bilateral (on both sides). A median cleft lip is an opening in the center of the upper lip, often accompanied by a cleft in the nose (bifid nose).

More than seven of every 10 infants born with a cleft lip also have a cleft palate, a failure of the two halves of the top of the mouth to fuse. The cleft may involve only the soft palate (the back of the mouth), or it may come forward into the hard palate (the roof of the mouth). It may be complete, going all the way through the tissues of the palate, or it may penetrate only part way. It may also be a submucosal cleft (occult cleft palate), a separation in the muscles under the surface of the palate without a visible separation on the surface of the palate. Like a cleft in the lip, a cleft in the palate may be either unilateral or bilateral.

Cleft lip and/or palate make it difficult for an infant to swallow food and to learn to speak clearly. In addition, infants with cleft lip and/or palate are at higher risk for middle ear infections and dental problems.

A coloboma (from the Greek *koloboma,* for "a part taken away" is a small notch in the lower eyelid due to an extension of a cleft lip and/or cleft palate. It can be repaired during surgery for lip and/or palate.

A mid-face (nose and mouth) framed by a protruding forehead and chin, called a dish face deformity, is also associated with cleft lip or palate, although it may sometimes be due to facial injury.

Treatment Options and Outlook

Cleft lip The treatment for cleft lip is surgery to close the separation, usually within the first three months of life. The surgical technique used to repair a cleft lip depends on whether the cleft is unilateral or bilateral. In general, repairing a unilateral cleft produces an asymmetrical lip; a repaired bilateral cleft produces a symmetrical lip.

To repair a lip with a unilateral cleft, the surgeon may lift a triangular piece of skin and mucous membrane from the other side of the lip (Mirault-Blair-Brown method); or lift a rectangular flap from the cleft side to create a cupid's bow in the center of the lip (Hagadorn–Le Mesurier method); or a Z-shape incision in the edge of the cleft lip to reposition the center of the lip (Tennison-Randall method); or simply an incision that loosens the lip tissue and enables the cupid's bow to move down into a natural position.

In repairing a lip with a bilateral cleft, if the patient has some columella tissue (the vertical ridges between mouth and nose), the simplest method is with a V-Y flap, an incision in the shape of a V with the bottom sewn together in a straight line to form a Y. If there is no columella tissue, the surgeon will use a forked flap (a piece of lip tissue with two points on top) to create a more normal shaped lip.

Cleft palate In very rare cases, as when the patient has other medical conditions that preclude surgery or when no qualified surgeon is available, a cleft palate may be covered with a dental appliance, but the standard treatment for cleft palate is surgery to close the gap and lengthen the palate (a short palate may interfere with the ability to speak distinctly). Surgery to repair a cleft soft palate is usually performed at age three to four months; for the hard palate, usually between nine and 18 months.

There are four common techniques used to repair a cleft palate: the von Langenbeck technique, the Furlow technique, the three-flap/V-Y technique, and the Vomer flap.

The von Langenbeck technique closes the cleft with two flaps lifted from the palate itself. The disadvantage of this surgery is that it can only be used to close one cleft and that it does not lengthen the palate. The Furlow technique, also known as the double reversing z-plasty technique, closes narrow clefts and/or clefts underneath the surface of the palate with a Z-shape incision that produces two flaps, one in the mucous membrane of the back of the mouth, the other on the side of the nasal mucous membrane. Half of each flap includes the underlying muscle. When the flaps are joined along the Z ("reversing"), the palate is lengthened, with muscle tissue along its entire length. The three-flap/V-Y technique (also known as the Wardill-Kilner-Veau technique) is most commonly used to repair an incomplete cleft by taking triangular flaps from the top of the mouth to close the cleft and lengthen the palate. The Vomer technique lifts tissue from the thin bone that forms the lower part of the membrane dividing the passage inside the nose, rotates the tissue downward and attaches it to the palate. This technique is used most frequently with wide clefts or bilateral clefts.

In addition to the tissue used to close the cleft, bone grafts taken from the hip, ribs, or other parts of the body may be used to close clefts involving the back of the upper jawbone. The bone grafts create a supporting structure to prevent tissue flaps from collapsing after surgery. Note: In November 2004, surgeons at Cardinal Glennon Children's Hospital in St. Louis, Missouri, performed the first repair of a cleft lip and palate without a bone graft, inserting a collagen sponge impregnated with genetically engineered bone morphogenic protein into the gap between the nose and gum. The protein is a growth factor that encourages the formation of new bone cells to anchor the sponge and fill it with new bone to close the space between the nose and mouth. This procedure will require fewer surgeries and heal more quickly than current techniques.

After surgery to repair cleft lip or palate, swelling, bleeding, and pain are common; infants and young children may need restraints to keep them from putting their fingers in their mouths.

In the days right after surgery, a child is usually fed liquids or very soft foods from a cup or Breck feeder (a red rubber tube attached to a syringe) rather than from a bottle or a spoon, because the child's sucking on the bottle's nipple or gumming/chewing the spoon might interfere with healing. Depending on the extent of the surgery and how quickly the incisions heal, a normal diet may be resumed in two to three weeks. Rinsing with clean water will keep the mouth clean; gentle brushing may be resumed after a week.

As the child grows, additional surgeries may be required, as well as consultations with an otolaryngologist (ear, nose, throat doctor), a dentist or dental surgeon, a speech therapist, an audiologist (a person specializing in hearing problems), and a psychologist and/or social worker.

Risk Factors and Preventive Measures

Together, cleft lip and/or cleft palate are the fourth most common birth defects in the United States, occurring in one of every 500 Asian, Latino, and Native American babies; one in every 700 American white babies of European ancestry; and one in every 1,000 African-American babies; more frequently among boys than in girls. Cleft palate alone is less common among white and African-American babies; the incidence, respectively, is 1.4 and 0.4 in every 1,000 live births. Among Asians, however, the incidence may be as high as 3.2 in every 1,000 live births. In all cases, the defect is more common among girls than among boys.

As many as one in every seven infants with cleft lip and/or palate has other birth defects. Recent multinational studies of cleft lip and/or palate among babies in Brazil, Denmark, Japan, and the United States suggest that half of all babies born with cleft palate alone may have other defects, and that half of those may be due to a mutation in a gene governing the production and use of the immune system chemical interferon regulatory factor 6 (IRF6).

The risk of a parent with cleft lip and/or palate having a child with a similar defect is between 3 to 9 percent; the risk if higher if both parents have a cleft. If parents who do not have a cleft have one baby with cleft lip and/or palate, the risk that a second child will have the same defect is 2 to 8 percent.

Other risk factors for cleft lip and/or palate include a viral infection during pregnancy; a nutritional deficiency, specifically a deficiency of the B vitamin folic acid (also associated with an increased risk of spina bifida, incomplete closure of the spinal tube); and a pregnant woman's use of certain medicines, including, but not necessarily limited to, antiseizure drugs, steroids, insulin, salicylates (aspirin), sedatives (phenobarbitol), and tretinoin (Accutane). Note: Although some medicines are risky for the fetus, no pregnant woman should stop taking any medicine for a chronic illness except as directed by her physician.

There are currently no hard-and-fast rules for preventing cleft lip and/or palate; some studies suggests that taking a multivitamin containing folic acid before conception and during the first two months of pregnancy may reduce the risk.

clitoroplasty Cosmetic plastic surgery to reduce and reconstruct an abnormally large clitoris.

Procedure

Once the patient is anesthetized, the surgeon makes an incision above the clitoris, frees the clitoris, shortens the shaft of the clitoris, and recovers the tip with the original tissue so as to preserve sensation.

Risks and Complications

As with any surgery, the patient may experience swelling bleeding, bruising, and discomfort. The risks associated with clitoroplasty also include nerve damage.

Outlook and Lifestyle Modifications

Successful surgery produces what the patient considers a more natural and/or attractive result.

See also PHALLOPLASTY; VAGINOPLASTY.

clotting factor Naturally occurring substances in blood required for blood coagulation; essential to healthy healing of tissue after any injury, including the incisions made during PLASTIC SURGERY.

The clotting factors in human blood include

- factor I: fibrinogen, a protein that converts to fibrin in blood clots
- factor II: prothrombin, precursor of thrombin

- factor III: thrombokinase/thromboplastin, an enzyme that converts prothrombin to thrombin
- factor IV: calcium ION
- factor V: proaccelerin, a compound that hastens the action of prothrombin
- factor VII: cothromboplastin/proconvertin, coagulant
- factor VIII: antihemophillic factor/Hemofil™ coagulation factor missing in hemophilia A
- factor IX: coagulation factor missing in hemophilia B
- factor X: prothrombinase, coagulation factor associated with thrombin
- factor XI: thromboplastin antecedent, coagulation factor that prevents hemorrhage
- factor XII: Hageman coagulation factor, reduces clotting time for bleeding from veins
- factor XIII: fibrinase, enables fibrin to form a stable clot

The absence of any of these clotting factors may be considered a bar to elective surgery such as cosmetic plastic surgery procedures. (No factor VI is included above because it is considered a subset of factor V.)

See HEALING PROCESS.

club finger/toes See FINGERS AND TOES, CONGENTIAL STRUCTURAL DEFECTS.

club foot Talipes; foot (or feet) that turns in and down rather than projecting straight out from the leg, due to abnormally short or tight tendons in the foot and ankle.

Symptoms and Diagnostic Path

Club foot is diagnosed by physical examination; the physical characteristics of a patient's specific deformity is confirmed with X-ray pictures.

Treatment Options and Outlook

If the foot is flexible, it may be moved into the correct position and set in a splint, preferably right after the baby is born and tendons, ligaments, and bones are still relaxed. The cast, which stretches the foot into a normal position, is removed periodically over a period of several months so that the foot can be stretched farther and a new cast applied to hold it in the new position.

If the foot is rigid at birth, surgery may be required to lengthen or shorten tendons so the foot bones and joints may be aligned normally. After surgery, a cast is used to keep the foot in the correct position as it heals. Follow-up physical therapy helps to strengthen the foot, make it more flexible, and keep it in a normal position. Occasionally, a club foot and the calf above it may remain smaller than the other leg.

Risk Factors and Preventive Measures

Club foot is the most common congenital defect of the legs, occurring in about one in every 1,000 live births in the United States. There are no clear preventive measures.

club hand Also known as radial club hand; a hand bent inward and up due to a congenital defect of the radius, a bone in the lower part of the arm that extends from the elbow to the base of the thumb. The defect, which may be inherited, is associated with other genetic problems such as defects of the heart, kidney, and gastrointestinal tract and genetic disorders such as extra chromosomes.

Symptoms and Diagnostic Path

There are four types of radial club hand.

- In Type 1 radial club hand, there is only a minor bend in the wrist, with very little loss of motion.
- In Type 2 radial club hand, the radius may not grow long enough, causing the ulna (the second bone in the forearm) to bend outward; some of the wrist bones may be shorter than normal, and the thumb may not develop fully.
- In Type 3 radial club hand, as much as two-thirds of the radius may not develop; the bent ulna and wrist do not fully support the hand, and some or all of the fingers may be deformed.
- In Type 4 radial club hand, the radius is completely absent, the ulna is severely bent, the thumb is

missing, the fingers are deformed or missing, and there is limited movement in the elbow.

Club hand is visible on physical examination. The physical characteristics of a patient's specific deformity are confirmed with X-ray pictures.

Treatment Options and Outlook

The hand may be repositioned through manipulation soon after birth, or the bone may be surgically repositioned or reconstructed to move the hand into normal position. Successful surgery gives the patient use of the hands.

Risk Factors and Preventive Measures

There are no known preventive measures for club hand.

cold pack Any one of several types of cold applications used to relieve pain, swelling, and inflammation. The cold pack numbs the area to which it is applied, constricts local blood vessels, and slows the leakage of fluid from body cells, thus reducing inflammation and swelling due to an injury or to a chronic condition such as ARTHRITIS.

The simplest cold pack is an old-fashioned ice bag filled with ice cubes or a plastic freezer bag filled with ice cubes with a bit of water to cover the cubes. A wet towel folded into a plastic food bag and chilled in the freezer or a plastic bag of frozen peas or corn kernels may also be used. Commercial, plastic, or fabric-covered cold packs filled with silicone gel are flexible even when solidly chilled in the freezer and remain cold for up to 30 minutes.

For the first day or two after an injury, the ice pack may be applied for 10 minutes, once an hour. As pain, swelling, and inflammation diminish, the pack can be used three times a day or after any strenuous activity involving the affected site. Regardless of type, the ice pack should be applied over a cloth such as a towel, never directly to the skin, and never for longer than 15 to 20 minutes.

See also CRYOSURGERY.

collagen dressing See ABSORBENT FOAM; COLLAGEN REPLACEMENT THERAPY.

collagen replacement therapy Collagen is the network of large protein molecules found in skin, cartilage, bone, and other connective tissue; the primary constituent of the dermis (the second layer of skin, just under the epidermis). It accounts for more than one-third of the protein in the body and about three-quarters of the protein in skin tissue, providing a frame that ties cells together so that new cells can grow to heal wounds and broken bones.

With aging, the body begins to produce collagen more slowly, leading to loose or sagging skin, especially on the face. Collagen replacement therapy is designed to remedy this with injections of purified bovine (cow) collagen that firm the skin and eliminate fine facial WRINKLES. Some fillers, such as Dermalogen, are made from cadaver skin, which is less likely than filler made from bovine collagen to cause allergic reactions.

Procedure

The collagen is mixed with lidocaine, a local anesthetic, but the surgeon may also use an anesthetic cream or spray to numb the injection site. Depending on the extent of the wrinkling, more than one series of injections may be required.

Risks and Complications

An allergic reaction to the collagen is possible. Bovine collagen is compatible with human tissue, but it may be allergenic or irritating for some individuals. Before starting the treatment, the doctor will test the collagen on the patient's skin, usually on a small spot on the underside of the arm between the elbow and wrist, and then check the area over a period of several weeks to see if any adverse reaction occurs.

Outlook and Lifestyle Modifications

The collagen is slowly absorbed into the body; on average, injections may be required twice a year to maintain the effect.

See also FILLER.

coloboma See CLEFT LIP AND/OR PALATE.

complete blood count (CBC) Group of tests to quantify and classify the blood cells in a cubic milliliter (ml) of blood. It is used to screen for various diseases and medical conditions, to monitor the effectiveness of certain drugs. Plastic surgeons, like surgeons, usually order a presurgical CBC as a guide to the patient's health and fitness for the surgical procedure.

For example, a higher-than-normal number of white blood cells may suggest an infection; a lower-than-normal number of red blood cells may suggest anemia; a higher- or lower-than-normal number of platelets may explain excessive bleeding or unusual clotting; a lower-than-normal number of white blood cells may be the result of cancer chemotherapy that suppresses the production of new cells in the body.

The tests included in a CBC are

- *white blood cell count,* the number of white blood cells in the sample
- *white blood cell differential,* the number of the different types of white blood cells present
- *red blood cell count,* the number of red blood cells in the sample
- *hemoglobin levels,* the amount of the oxygen-carrying protein in the sample
- *hematocrit,* the percentage of space in the sample occupied by red blood cells
- *platelet count,* the number of platelets in the sample
- *mean corpuscular volume/MCV,* the size of the red blood cells in the sample
- *mean corpuscular hemoglobin/MCH,* the amount of hemoglobin inside the red blood cells
- *red cell distribution width/RCDW,* the number of red cells of different sizes

compression garment   Elasticized wrap, bandage, facial mask, shirt, vest, legging, stocking, abdominal binder, lower body garment, or full body garment worn 24 hours a day for a period ranging up to several months. The garments are used to protect the skin and prevent fluid loss after a severe burn or to speed healing after surgery, including PLASTIC SURGERY.

The garments provide support, decrease discomfort, and speed healing after procedures such as ABDOMINOPLASTY, BREAST AUGMENTATION, BREAST LIFT, BREAST REDUCTION, FACE-LIFT, facial implants, LIPOSUCTION, and NECK LIFT. They reduce edema (swelling caused by the collection of fluid at the site of the incision), improve the flow of blood and lymph, keep the skin cool and dry, hold injured tissues together, and relieve tension on the sutures, thus reducing scarring.

conjoined twins   Two individuals who develop from a single fertilized egg that has failed to separate completely; the babies are born joined at one part of the body such as the chest or the top of the head and may share one or more organs such as the liver or heart.

Whether conjoined twins can be successfully separated into two independent bodies depends on the extent of the shared tissue. Infants joined simply by a band of tissue are usually easily parted. Those who share a single nonvital body part such as one leg may be separated and the deformity repaired with prostheses. Those joined at the head, like Carl and Clarence Aguirre, Filipino conjoined twins separated at Montefiore Medical Center in New York in 2004, are extremely difficult to treat due to possible brain damage, which the Aguirre children have since experienced. Those who share a vital organ, such as a heart, cannot be separated into two living persons.

The primary surgery to separate conjoined twins is performed by physicians specializing in various fields such as orthopedics or neurosurgery, but PLASTIC SURGERY is often used to improve the appearance of the separated twins.

connective tissue   Material that shapes or supports the body and its various parts, stores fat cells, and manufactures blood cells. Fat, CARTILAGE, and BONE are forms of connective tissue. The term is usually reserved, though, for collagen or elastin fiber networks such as the loose connective tissue found under the skin and in the covering around the heart, lungs, and muscles; the denser connective tissue around organs such as the kidneys; in ligaments, the tissues holding bones and joints in place; and in tendons (tissues connecting muscles to bone).

The healthy growth and maintenance of connective tissue is vital to healing, including healing after PLASTIC SURGERY, because the growth of new connective tissue anchors the repair or reconstruction in place.

constriction band syndrome   Growth of fibrous bands around a developing fetal hand or limb that may interfere with normal fetal development, leading to visible congenital defects such as fused fingers, scoliosis (abnormally curved spine), or a missing limb. Some of these defects may be corrected through PLASTIC SURGERY.

Symptoms and Diagnostic Path
Bands are diagnosed via prenatal ultrasound.

Treatment Options and Outlook
Treatment may include surgical removal of the bands and corrective plastic surgery such as separation of fused fingers soon after birth.

Risk Factors and Preventive Measures
Constriction band syndrome occurs spontaneously in approximately one in every 10,000 to 15,000 births. There are no known risk factors or preventive measures.

consultation   Meeting between doctors to discuss diagnosis and treatment options for a particular patient or a meeting between doctor and patient to discuss all aspects of treatment.

For patients considering PLASTIC SURGERY, the American Society of Plastic Surgeons (ASPS) recommends asking two distinct sets of questions, the first related to the surgeon and the facility in which the procedure will be done, and the second, about the procedure.

Questions about the doctor and facility include:

1. Is the doctor board-certified by the American Board of Plastic Surgery?
2. How many procedures of the type the patient is planning has the doctor performed?

3. Does the doctor have hospital privileges to perform this procedure? If so, at which hospitals?
4. Is the surgical facility accredited by the Joint Commission, an independent agency that accredits more than 15,000 hospitals and health care facilities in the United States?

Questions about the procedure include:

1. Is the patient a good candidate for the proposed procedure?
2. What are the risks involved with this procedure?
3. What must the patient do to improve the success of this procedure?
4. What is the expected recovery time after this procedure? What care will the patient need? Will the patient be required to stay home from work?

In addition, at the consultation, the patient should ask the doctor to spell out all financial costs and arrangements, including whether or not the procedure is covered by the patient's insurance.

Finally, before proceeding with cosmetic surgery to alter the patient's appearance, many plastic surgeons require a psychological evaluation to ascertain the patient's readiness for the proposed procedure.

contouring   See LIPOSUCTION.

copper nose   See ROSACEA.

coronal lift   See FOREHEAD LIFT.

corset platysmaplasty   See NECK LIFT.

Cosmoderm®   See FILLER.

CosmoPlast™   See FILLER.

Crazy Glue   See SUTURELESS CLOSURE.

Crikelair, George (1920–2005)   One of the group of surgeons who established the practice of PLASTIC SURGERY in the United States and a leading advocate for reforms in the production of fabrics so as to reduce flammability, a major cause of disfiguring skin injuries among children. Crikelair was director of the plastic surgery service at Columbia-Presbyterian Medical Center from 1959 to 1977; chair, American Board of Plastic Surgery; president, the American Society of Plastic and Reconstructive Surgeons; and a prominent member of the national advisory committee that helped draft and promote the 1972 Flammable Fabrics Act ratified in 1972.

Crouzon syndrome (Crouzon disease)   Group of congenital facial defects including broad forehead, beaked nose, and large jaw due to premature fusion of the bones of the skull caused by a mutation (change) in a gene on chromosome 10 that enables the body to make and use a growth factor. Identified by French physician Octave Crouzon (1874–1938).

Symptons and Diagnostic Path
Crouzon syndrome is diagnosed by its appearance.

Treatment Options and Outlook
Plastic surgery to reconstruct the features can offer cosmetic improvement.

Risk Factors and Preventive Measures
Crouzon syndrome is a genetic disorder, a dominant trait that occurs is one parent passes along the mutated gene or if one of the responsible genes on the child's two copies of chromosome 10 mutates spontaneously. There is no known risk factor for the condition, other than its appearance earlier in a family group, and no known preventive measure.

crow's feet   See CHEMICAL SKIN PEEL.

cryosurgery   Use of liquid nitrogen or carbon dioxide to freeze and destroy body tissue; widely used to remove premalignant or malignant tissue such as basal cell skin cancers or to freeze and destroy tumors in organs such as the liver and kidney. Cryosurgery is used in PLASTIC SURGERY for cosmetic procedures such as removal of a wart or darkened age spots.

Procedure
The surgeon applies liquid nitrogen to the skin with either a cotton-tip swab or as a spray for a very short period of time, about five seconds.

Risks and Complications
Immediate redness and slight swelling, followed in a day or two by the formation of a scab that drops off, leaving a pink spot that usually fades to vary light pink barely visible on light skin. After short cryosurgery, the spot on dark skin may be darker than the surrounding area; prolonged exposure to the liquid nitrogen kills melanocytes (pigmented skin cells), leaving a pale spot on dark skin.

Outlook and Lifestyle Modifications
Successful cryosurgery removes small spots without producing noticeably visible change in skin color.

CT-scan (obsolete: CAT-scan)   Picture produced by computerized axial tomography, a noninvasive, painless, quick-imaging technique that creates images of soft tissue, organs, and other internal structures via an X-ray camera that rotates around the axis (center line) of the body. CT-scans are useful in instances of complicated PLASTIC SURGERY such as separating CONJOINED TWINS and repairing the area where the individuals were once connected.

The CT-scanner, an X-ray camera invented in 1972 by the British engineer Godfrey N. Hounsfield and South African physicist Alan Cormack, joint recipients of the Nobel Prize in medicine or physiology (1979), is a large, rotating, square machine with a hole in the middle. Inside the scanner are an X-ray tube on one side and a fan-shape detector on the other. The patient lies on a table that slides into the hole in the scanner. Each time the scanner rotates a full circle around the body, the X-ray camera sends beams through the body, transmitting an image to the detector. The X-ray camera continues to circle the body, recording images at 5 to 10 millimeter (0.2 to 0.4 inch) intervals. The detector sends the images to a computer that puts them together to create a picture showing a cross section of the part of the body being scanned.

The images created by a CT-scanner are about 100 times clearer than those of a conventional X-ray machine, enabling a surgeon to plan reconstructive procedure in advance of actual surgery, or to evaluate a tumor or an injury to internal organs, such as kidney or spleen without performing invasive surgery. Doctors may also use a CT-scanner to plan and administer targeted radiation treatment or biopsies.

Procedure

The patient may (or may not) remove his/her clothes but must remove all metal objects such as clothes with metal closures and—depending on the area of the body that will be imaged—hairpins, jewelry, eyeglasses, hearing aids, and removable dentures.

Depending on the area to be imaged, the patient may be told not to eat or drink for several hours before the CT-scan or may be required to use a contrast material to make structures such as blood vessels or kidneys more visible or show the difference between adjacent tissues. The contrast material may be injected through an intravenous needle or swallowed or given by enema. The patient lies on a table that can move up or down and in and out of the center of the CT-scanner. Once the patient is settled in place, the technologist leaves the room but can speak to the patient over an intercom.

During the scan, the X-ray camera inside the machine takes pictures as the table moves. A *regular CT-scan* usually takes less than an hour. *Spiral computerized axial tomography,* an advanced form of imaging also known as the spiral CT-scan or the fast CT-scan, can scan an entire chest of abdomen in less than 10 seconds. Spiral CT-scans are most often used to detect blockages in blood vessels such as the coronary arteries without the need for an invasive procedure such as angiography (the insertion of a minuscule camera into an artery).

When the scan is finished, the patient may be asked to wait until the images are examined to determine if more pictures are needed.

Risks and Complications

A CT-scan exposes a patient to radiation equal to about three years' worth of normal background radiation, the radiation occurring naturally on Earth. Women who are pregnant (or think they may be) should inform their doctor before having the scan. The contrast material used in some CT-scans can cause flushing due to dilated small blood vessels or mild itching or a metallic taste in the mouth. Ordinarily, these symptoms disappear quickly.

In rare cases, the contrast material (which contains iodine) may trigger serious allergic reactions in persons allergic to fish and/or shellfish. It may also be hazardous for patients with a history of asthma, diabetes, heart disease, kidney problems, or thyroid conditions. Women who are nursing should wait 24 hours after contrast injection before resuming breast-feeding.

See also MAGNETIC RESONANCE IMAGING (MRI); RADIATION; ULTRASOUND SCAN; X-RAY EXAMINATION.

cultured skin   See SKIN GRAFT.

Cutler-Beard bridge flap   See SKIN FLAP.

cyclosporine   See IMMUNE SYSTEM.

Cyrano nose   See HEMANGIOMA.

cytokines   See IMMUNE SYSTEM; IMMUNOTHERAPY.

Dacron™ Synthetic filament (thread), woven into a material that resists stretching, bleaching, and tearing. British chemist J. R. Whitfield invented the filament and then sold it in 1941 to ICI/Imperial Chemical Industries, which named the material made from Whitfield's filament Terylene®. In 1945, DuPont was given the right to market it in the United States and changed the name to Dacron™. Modern plastic surgeons use Dacron to build artificial blood vessels; in surgery it also serves as a material for blood transfusion filters designed to catch particles that might otherwise clump together to form a posttransfusion blood clot.

Dardour flap See HAIR REPLACEMENT SURGERY.

Davis, John Staige (1872–1946) First surgeon with a practice entirely devoted to PLASTIC SURGERY and author of the first American plastic surgery textbook, Davis was responsible for the first formal training program for surgeons specializing in plastic surgery. He was also the first chairman of the American Board of Plastic Surgery. Davis's innovations include the Davis graft used to close the wound after surgery to clean out or remove an infection, inflammation, or tumor in the ear and the Davis-Crowe mouth gag, a device (invented with Samuel J. Crowe [1883–1955]) that rests against the inside of the upper jaw and depresses the tongue to hold the mouth open during surgery.

degloving A term used to describe either a specifc injury or a technique used to harvest tissue for a transplant.

A degloving injury, most commonly of a hand or foot, is one in which much or most of the skin and underlying fat layers are peeled away in a manner similar to removing a glove or sock, to expose the bone structure underneath.

The degloving surgical procedure is used as part of the evolving technique for a partial or total face transplant. The plastic surgeon deliberately peels off the skin and underlying fat tissue of the face from the donor, taking care to remove the important blood vessels as well. The surgeon performs the same degloving procedure on the recipient and then covers the patient's exposed bone structure with the donor tissue.

See also FACE TRANSPLANT.

dental bonding Cosmetic dental procedure employing composite resins, a material commonly used to fill dental cavities, to repair chipped or cracked teeth; to replace the surface on discolored teeth; to fill in gaps between teeth; to reshape or lengthen teeth; or to protect a tooth root that has been exposed due to gum recession.

Procedure
First, the tooth is etched with a mild acid solution to roughen the surface, which is then painted with a conditioning liquid that helps the bonding material stick to the surface. Next, the dentist applies one or more layers of a durable, puttylike resin (plastic material) colored to match the natural teeth. The tooth is exposed to a high-intensity light that cures (hardens) the plastic. Finally, the surface is shaped to match the other teeth and polished.

Caring for Bonded Teeth
While bonding typically lasts from three to 10 years, exactly how long it remains intact depends both on

how it is applied, how it relates to the bite, and how it is protected. The resin is durable, but breakable, liable to damage from biting on hard food or ice or chewing on hard objects such as a pen or pencil and habits such as bruxism. Regular checkups can catch small chips or cracks, enabling the dentist to repair the defect before the entire veneer is dislodged.

Comparing Risks and Benefits

Bonding with resins is a relatively simple and inexpensive procedure that removes less dental enamel than porcelain veneers or dental crowns (caps). Porcelain veneers or caps must be made in a dental laboratory and require additional visits. Bonding can be done in one session in the dentist's office. Resin veneers may stain or crack/chip more easily than porcelain veneers or crowns.

dental crown (dental cap)   Ceramic, metal, or ceramic-and-metal restoration cemented over a tooth that has been significantly reduced in size. It covers the tooth above the gum line. Dental crowns are used to repair worn, broken, or decayed teeth, or to improve the appearance of the teeth. Dental crowns are more durable but more expensive than resin or porcelain dental veneers.

dental implant   Dental endosteel implants are used to anchor replacement teeth. Endosteel implants are surgically placed in alveolar bone and allowed to integrate with bone as a secure retainer for various prosthetic (replacement) needs, such as crowns, fixed bridges, and retainers for removable dentures.

See also PERIODONTAL DISEASE.

dental veneer   Porcelain veneers, dental porcelain laminates; thin pieces of dental porcelain or composite resins custom made to cover the front surface of the tooth so as to improve the appearance of chipped, discolored, misaligned, misshapen, or unevenly spaced teeth.

Procedure

On the first visit, the dentist prepares the tooth for the veneer by reducing a small amount of dental enamel from the front of the tooth. He then makes an impression of the tooth to create a model from which the dental technician works. Depending on the condition of the teeth, this may or may not require local anesthetic. The model is sent to a dental technical laboratory, which manufactures the veneer and returns it to the dentist, who approves the fit and color, both of which can be adjusted before the veneer is fixed on the tooth. (If the prepared teeth are unsightly, the dentist may apply a temporary layer of plastic resin.)

On the second visit, the dentist cleans and polishes the tooth surface, then etches it with a weak acid solution to provide an appropriate surface for attaching the veneer. The dentist applies a resin to the back of the veneer, sets the veneer in place, and exposes the tooth to a high-intensity light or a laser that "cures" (hardens) the resin. Finally, the dentist removes excess cement, makes adjustments as necessary so as to ensure that the teeth meet properly, and schedules a third visit to check the placement and reaction to the veneer.

Risks and Complications

Veneers are not a good choice for people who do not have sufficient tooth structure or whose teeth are weakened by decay or large dental fillings. They are also not indicated in cases where the opposing teeth are in an interfering location or if the patient has excessive tooth grinding habits.

Outlook and Lifestyle Modifications

The advantages of porcelain veneers are that they are more stain resistant than resin veneers (see DENTAL BONDING). The color is easier to match to natural teeth, and porcelain reflects light more like natural teeth. The disadvantages are that porcelain veneers are more expensive than resin veneers, that applying them requires the dentist to remove dental enamel, and that it is difficult to repair them if they chip. Typically, porcelain veneers may last five to 10 years or more. Porcelain is durable (resistant to wear) but breakable, liable to damage from biting on hard food or ice or chewing on hard objects such as a pen or pencil or clenching and grinding the teeth.

dentistry   Dentistry is the practice of prevention, diagnosis, and treatment of disease, injuries, and oral functions of the mouth, jaws, and teeth. A *dentist* is a person licensed to practice dentistry. An *endodontist* (from the Greek *endo,* meaning "in") treats conditions affecting the interior tissues of the tooth. An *orthodontist* (from the Greek *ortho,* meaning "correct") treats irregularities in the position of the teeth. A *periodontist* (from the Latin *peri,* meaning "around") treats conditions and diseases of the gums and surrounding bone. Each of these specialists may have a role to play in *cosmetic dentistry,* the use of dental procedures to enhance appearance, often in conjunction with plastic surgery.

denture A dental prosthesis. A device that replaces missing teeth. A *partial denture* replaces several teeth; a *full denture* replaces all the teeth in the upper or lower jaw, or both jaws. A partial denture is attached to existing teeth or endosteel implants. A full denture may be held in place by suction, with the help of a pastelike adhesive substance, or it may clip onto implant devices in the patient's jaw. Dentures may be used in PLASTIC SURGERY to alter facial features. In cosmetic or restorative dentistry, a two-part clip, called an extracoronal attachment, is sometimes used to attach a permanent or removable partial denture to the top (crown) of a tooth next to the denture or to another restoration. One part of the clip goes on the denture; the other on the tooth or restoration next to it.

depression Treatable mental illness that may affect people of any age, any race or ethnic group, and in any walk of life. Because depression may be a factor in a person's decision to seek PLASTIC SURGERY, modern plastic surgeons usually perform a PSYCHOLOGICAL EVALUATION of prospective patients to identify those whose expectations of the surgical outcome are unrealistic.

If depression is present prior to surgery, the surgeon may suggest that the patient seek psychiatric counseling or treatment so as to approach the operation with a realistic view of the outcome. POSTSURGICAL DEPRESSION, a common phenomenon sometimes called "third day blues," generally fades as the incisions heal and the patient sees the outline of the changes in his/her appearance. If the

postsurgical depression lasts longer than the surgeon deems reasonable, once again he may suggest psychological counselling and/or treatment.

Symptoms and Diagnostic Path

According to the National Institute of Mental Health, in any one year about one in 10 American adults older than 18 will experience an episode of depression. About 10 million will suffer a major depression; another 11 million will have dysthymic disorder (mild, chronic depression); and another 2.3 million will have bipolar disorder, a condition in which episodes of depression alternate with episodes of elation (mania). Major depression and dysthymic disorder affect twice as many women as men; bipolar disorder is equally common among men and women.

The symptoms of depression are feelings of sadness and anxiety, worthlessness, or inappropriate guilt; difficulty in thinking clearly or making decisions; preoccupation with death or thoughts of suicide; changes in appetite leading to spontaneous weight gain or loss; alterations in sleep patterns (either sleeping too much or sleeping too little); restlessness; and irritability. Many people experience one or more of these symptoms in reaction to a life crisis such as a major illness or the loss of a job or the death of a loved one, but for people with depression the symptoms are not linked to another condition such as an illness, nor do they lessen with time.

Treatment Options and Outlook

Depression may be treated with psychotherapy ("talk therapy") or with antidepressants (medical drugs that correct the imbalance in brain chemicals) or with a combination of the two.

Antidepressants are medical drugs that alleviate emotional depression by balancing the supply of neurotransmitters, naturally occurring chemicals in the brain, such as serotonin and dopamine that facilitate the transmission of impulses among brain cells. Antidepressant drugs act only on these brain chemicals; they are not sedatives, tranquilizers, or stimulants; they are not habit-forming; and they have no effect on people who are not depressed.

The most commonly prescribed antidepressant drugs are tricyclics such as amytriptyline (Elavil ™)

that restore normal levels of norepinephrine and serotonin and SSRIs (selective serotonin re-uptake inhibitors) such as fluoxetine (Prozac™), paroxetine (Paxil ™), and sertraline (Zoloft™), which prevent the body from absorbing and inactivating large amounts of the calming neurotransmitter serotonin.

Antidepressants may take up to six weeks to reach full effectiveness, although many patients begin to feel better within three weeks. The American Psychiatric Association recommends taking the medicine for some time after symptoms have improved so as to prevent a relapse. Antidepressants may also be useful in relieving the temporary depression that often follows surgery, including plastic surgery.

Risk Factors and Preventive Measures

The causes of depression may be both physical and psychological. For example, low levels of serotonin and norepinephrine, two chemicals that facilitate the transmission of signals in the brain, are believed responsible for symptoms such as anxiety, irritability, and fatigue. People easily overwhelmed by stress or generally pessimistic seem to be at risk for depression; continuous stress, such as exposure to violence or abuse, may trigger depression in susceptible individuals. Finally, genetics plays a role; depression appears to run in families.

Dermabond™   See WOUND ADHESIVE.

dermabrasion   Use of a high-speed, rotating surgical brush or a sandpaper-covered device to remove the top layers of the skin so as to smooth out fine WRINKLES and scars, or remove tattoos. A dermabrader is any device used in dermabrasion.

Procedure

Dermabrasion is commonly done on an outpatient basis in a surgeon's office or hospital outpatient center with local anesthesic plus a sedative. The surgeon numbs the skin and scrapes away the top layer of roughened skin to the proper depth. For deep scars or very rough skin, the procedure may be performed in stages, several weeks apart. When the surgery is finished, depending on the depth of the dermabasion, the skin is may be covered with a protective ointment, a wet dressing, a wax dressing, or a dry dressing.

Risks and Complications

Redness and swelling, as well as pain, burning, and aching are possible but likely to subside within a few days. Increasing redness and discomfort may signal the formation of unusual scar tissue.

Outlook and Lifestyle Modifications

As the skin heals, a crust/scab forms over the treated area, allowing new skin to form underneath. When the crust/scab falls away, the skin appears tight and pink. The color and tightness gradually diminishes over a period of up to three months, during which the patient is advised to avoid all irritating substances such as various cosmetics, shaving, and/or strenuous activities. Until the normal skin color returns, a process that may take as long as a year, the skin should be protected from sunlight.

See also TATTOO REMOVAL.

dermal electrosurgical shave excision   Electrosurgical shave excision; the use of an instrument emitting a low voltage electrical current to slice ("shave") away a very thin layer of skin.

Procedure

The surgeon uses this technique to remove a raised lesion such as a mole or to smooth ("feather") the edges of a wound or scar so as to make it level with the surrounding tissue.

Risks and Complications

None other than a possible lightening of skin color when the wound heals.

Outlook and Lifestyle Modifications

Successful surgery removes the lesion or reduces the scar, leaving behind a level surface.

dermaplaning   Use of an instrument called a dermatome to smooth away the top layers of roughened skin, remove thin pieces of skin for grafts, remove small skin lesions, or remove damaged layers of burned skin. A drum dermatome is a hand-operated cutting instrument used for harvesting split thickness skin grafts or to debride small burn wounds. An air-driven or electricity-driven dermatome is a powered instrument used to harvest split thickness skin grafts or debride large burn wounds.

Procedure

Cosmetic dermaplaning is customarily done in a doctor's office or in a hospital outpatient center. Therapeutic dermaplaning, such as the removal of burned skin, is an inpatient hospital procedure. The surgeon numbs the skin and removes the top layers of skin to the proper depth.

Risks and Complications

Redness and swelling, as well as pain, burning, and aching, are possible but are likely to subside within a few days. Increasing redness and discomfort may signal the formation of unusual scar tissue.

Outlook and Lifestyle Modifications

As the skin heals, a crust/scab forms over the treated area, allowing new skin to form underneath. When the crust/scab falls away, the skin appears tight and pink. The color and tightness gradually diminishes over a period of up to three months, during which the patient is advised to avoid all irritating substances such as various cosmetics, shaving, and/or strenuous activities. Until the normal skin color returns, a process that may take as long as a year, the skin should be protected from sunlight.

dermis See SKIN.

dermolipectomy See ABDOMINOPLASTY.

Dermologen® See COLLAGEN REPLACEMENT THERAPY.

Dieffenbach, Johann Friedrich (1792–1847) German plastic and reconstructive surgeon, he was the director of the surgical clinic at the Berlin Charite and the author of the comprehensive two-volume *Die operative Chirurgie*. He was the first surgeon to use ether as anesthesia for PLASTIC SURGERY (RHINOPLASTY) and the creator of the Dieffenbach flap (also called the Dieffenbach method) and the Dieffenbach operation. The former is a surgical technique for repairing a defect in the lip by moving the lip tissue to the side without completely detaching it from the lip. A Dieffenbach flap may also be used in repairing defects to the nose. The Dieffenbach operation is a surgical technique to replace missing skin with a pedicle flap (a piece of skin that retains a stalk through which blood circulates).

dietary fat An essential nutrient in food; rich in energy, with more than twice as many calories per gram as protein or carbohydrates, (nine calories per gram for fat v. four calories per gram for the other two).

Food provides three kinds of fat: triglycerides, phospholipids, and sterols. Triglycerides, the primary fat in ADIPOSE (fatty) TISSUE, are made of one unit of glycerol (a water-soluble carbohydrate that carries fats through blood) and three (tri=three) units of fatty acids. Phospholipids are fat molecules that contain phosphorus, a mineral that enables fats to dissolve in water; phospholipids such as lecithin can carry fat-soluble compounds such as hormones through the blood and the watery fluids that flow through cell membranes. Sterols are ring-shape fat and alcohol compounds used to manufacture bio-chemicals such as bile, hormones, and vitamin D.

In addition, the fats derived from food become part of every body cell membrane (the outer "skin" that holds the cell together); a component of myelin, the material covering nerves and nerve cells; and the principal material from which brain tissue is built.

All dietary fats (fats in foods) are combinations of fatty acids, but the fats are classified according to the predominant number of fatty acids. For example, a saturated fat, such as butter, has mostly saturated fatty acids; a monounsaturated fat, such as olive oil, has mostly monounsaturated fatty acids; and a polyunsaturated fat, such as corn oil, has mostly polyunsaturated fatty acids.

Fatty acids are chainlike molecules of carbon atoms with hydrogen atoms attached to each carbon plus a carbon-oxygen-hydrogen group at one end of the chain. An essential fatty acid is one the human body cannot put together from other fats but must obtain from food; linoleic acid, found in vegetable oils, is an essential fatty acid.

Fatty acids are classified as saturated, monounsaturated, or polyunsaturated, depending on the number of hydrogen atoms attached to each carbon. All fatty acids have an even number of carbon atoms. Each carbon atom has four sites available to form attachments (bonds) to other atoms. The first carbon in the chain has three bonds to hydrogen atoms and one to the next carbon. The last carbon in the chain has two bonds (a double bond) to an oxygen atom and one to a hydrogen atom.

In a saturated fatty acid, every carbon atom other than the first and the last has one bond to each of two hydrogen atoms and one bond to the carbon atom before it and the one after it in the chain. A monounsaturated fatty acid (*mono*, meaning "one") has two fewer hydrogen atoms than a saturated fatty acid because two carbon atoms in the chain share a double bond, leaving them with one bond each to the next carbon and one bond to a hydrogen atom. A polyunsaturated fatty acid (*poly*, meaning "many") has two or more double bonds between carbon atoms in the chain and four or more fewer hydrogen atoms than a saturated fatty acid.

dish face deformity   See CLEFT LIP AND/OR PALATE.

dominant gene   See GENETICS.

Doppler effect   See ULTRASOUND SCAN.

double chin   See CHIN LIFT.

doughnut lift   See BREAST RECONSTRUCTION; BREAST REDUCTION.

dowager hump   See KYPHOSIS.

Down syndrome   Genetic disorder identified by British physician John Langdon H. Down (1828–1896). Group of physical and mental characteristics arising from the presence of additional material on chromosome 21 that alters fetal development, leading to mental retardation as well as such physical signs as

- slanted eyes
- an eyelid fold normally found only in persons of Asian descent
- small flattened nose
- abnormally shaped ears
- large protruding tongue
- deep crease across the palm
- lax muscles
- extremely flexible joints
- missing joint on fifth finger
- extra space between first and second toes

Some physical signs of Down syndrome may be ameliorated with plastic surgeries such as procedures to alter the shape of the eyelid or the size and thrust of the tongue or to correct the positioning of the fingers.

See also MACROGLOSSIA.

dumbo ear   See EAR PINBACK.

Duoderm™   Brand-name latex-free porous adhesive dressing that absorbs excess moisture from a deep skin wound and protects the wound from contamination while allowing air to circulate to the wound to speed healing; commonly used by plastic surgeons to bandage skin ulcers and bed sores (pressure sores) as a preventive measure to reduce the risk of the sore's growing steadily larger and destroying more tissue.

Dupuytren's contracture   Involuntary flexing of the fourth (ring) and fifth (little) fingers due to thickening and/or shrinkage of the fibrous connective tissue (fascia) on the palms along with similar contraction of the tendons. The condition was identified by French anatomist, surgeon, and pathologist Baron Guillaume Dupuytren (1777–1835), assistant surgeon to the Hôtel-Dieu (Paris), professor of operative surgery, professor of clinical surgery at the École de Médecin, and head surgeon to the Hôtel-Dieu, who endowed the chair of anatomy at the École de Médecine and established a home for physicians in distress.

Symptoms and Diagnostic Path
The flexed fingers and tightened skin are clearly visible on physical examination.

Treatment Options and Outlook
Heat, massage, and stretching exercises may provide some relief, but there is no effective permanent treatment other than fasciectomy, PLASTIC SURGERY performed with local anesthesia to lift the skin and cut apart the thickened tissue underneath. Occasionally skin grafts are required to replace the previously shrunken and tightened skin.

While the success of the surgery may be relative to the original condition, the hand will look better. Follow-up physical therapy and splinting the hand at night should return full motion to the fingers.

Risk Factors and Preventive Measures
Dupuytren's contracture occurs most commonly in middle age, most often in women, and may run in families. It has been associated with diabetes or liver disease (cirrhosis of the liver) or antiseizure drugs for epilepsy, but no direct cause has been identified.

dynamic wrinkles   See WRINKLES.

Dysport™   See BOTOX.

Eagle Barrett syndrome Also called prune belly syndrome and triad syndrome, this birth defect is characterized by missing or weak abdominal muscles; abnormal development of the urinary tract, particularly the ureters (the tubes through which urine flows from kidneys to bladder); and cryptorchidism (failure of the testicles to descend into the scrotum). Plastic surgeons can repair or ameliorate these defects with the specific surgeries, described below.

Symptoms and Diagnostic Path

The defect may be diagnosed via prenatal ultrasound showing abnormal development of the urinary tract and an extended, wrinkled fetal belly due to weak abdominal muscles and pooling of fluid in the abdomen.

Treatment Options and Outlook

Reconstructive surgery early in life can repair the ureters and correct the position of the testes; recently surgeons have been developing procedures to do this surgery while the fetus is still in the uterus.

Frequent urinary tract infections are treated with preventive antibiotics; kidney failure, if it develops, requires dialysis or a kidney transplant.

Risk Factors and Preventive Measures

Eagle Barrett syndrome occurs once in every 40,000 live births in the United States, most commonly among boys (95 percent). One in five fetuses with Eagle Barrett syndrome die before birth. One in three children born with the syndrome die from kidney problems before age two, and half of those who live go on to develop urinary problems. There is no known cause and no cure other than corrective surgery.

ear See EAR PINBACK; EAR RECONSTRUCTION.

ear pinback Otoplasty; surgery to flatten abnormally protruding ears, a feature known colloquially as "Dumbo ear," after the hero of the 1941 Disney movie based on Helen Aberson and Harold Pearl's 1939 children's book, or bat ear. The story is about a baby circus elephant ostracized because his very large ears make him different from the other elephants, but who becomes the star of the show when he learns to spread his ears and fly.

Ear pinback was first performed by Edward Talbott Ely at Manhattan Eye, Ear and Throat Hospital in New York City (1881). A related, nonsurgical approach to flattening protruding ears, called ear splinting, wraps a bandage around a newborn's head to bend the still-flexible cartilage frame of the outer ear closer to the side of the head. The bandage is left in place for days or weeks; if it fails to alter the protrusion, the most likely remedy is ear pinback.

Procedure

Ear pinback may be done under local or general anesthetic, most commonly on an outpatient basis, with the patient going home the same day. The surgeon makes an incision in the natural crease behind the ear, removes excess skin and cartilage from the rim of the ear, and stitches the ear in place closer to the head. The head is then wrapped in a turbanlike dressing to protect the ear.

Risks and Complications

The most likely complication specific to this operation is that the ear will fall back into its original protruding position. The general risks of surgery, such as infection, also apply.

Outlook and Lifestyle Modifications

Bruising and obvious swelling usually disappear within two weeks. As with any PLASTIC SURGERY, the final results are not apparent until all swelling has disappeared, a process that may take several weeks or even months. At that point the thin scars from the incision are barely visible in the folds of skin behind the ear.

See also EAR RECONSTRUCTION.

ear reconstruction   Surgery to replace, rebuild, or repair a missing, deformed, or injured ear. Among the deformities addressed with reconstructive plastic surgery are

- *Cagot ear*   Ear with a missing earlobe; inherited birth defect named for the Cagot area of the Pyrenees Mountains between France and Spain where the defect is most common. A new lobe can be built with PLASTIC SURGERY.

- *cat's ear*   Birth defect in which the outer edge of the ear folded over toward the face rather than lying flat against the head; corrected by plastic surgery to flatten and anchor the ear against the head.

- *cauliflower ear*   Ear whose shape has been distorted by repeated injury to the tissues; named for its resemblance to the lumpy vegetable. May be repaired by plastic surgery.

- *cleft earlobe*   Congenital indentation or notch in the fleshy part of the earlobe; repaired by building a new earlobe with transplanted tissue.

- *cup ear*   Also known as *lop ear*; an ear with a small helix (CARTILAGE-stiffened outer rim of the ear) that stands away from the head rather than lying flat and a large central depression around the opening into the ear; together, these make the ear look like a small cup. May be repaired with plastic surgery to enlarge the helix and anchor the ear more closely to the head.

- *Darwinian ear*   Congenital defect in which the cartilage rim around the shell-shape external ear is flat rather than folded over. It is considered an evolutionary remnant of a time when the human ear was upright, pointed, and controlled by muscles that made it possible to move the ear in different directions. It is named for British biologist and evolutionist Charles Darwin (1809–82).

- *microtia*   Birth defect in which one or both ears are partially or wholly missing.

- *question mark ear*   A rare birth defect that may be an inherited trait, characterized by an ear that stands out from the head and has a cleft between the lobe and the ear's cartilage outer rim. The defect is also known as Cosman's ear for New York plastic surgeon Bard Cosman (1931–83), who first identified it.

- *scroll ear*   A birth defect in which the outer edge of the ear bends forward and in, folding the ear toward the head.

- *Stahl's ear*   Also called Vulcan ear after the *Star Trek* character Mr. Spock; a congenital deformity; an abnormal fold in the skin and cartilage of the ear so that the upper edge of the rim of the ear is pointed rather than round.

- *Wildermuth ear*   A congenital defect in which the helix (the curved outer cartilage border of the ear) turns backward, pushing the ante-helix (inner ridge of the ear) forward. It is named for German neurologist Hermann A. Wildermuth (1852–1907).

Procedure

The procedure varies with the problem. A torn earlobe may simply be stitched together. A small injury or deformity in the rim of the auricle (the outer ear) may be repaired with a piece of skin drawn down from the scalp. Multiple surgeries may be required to reconstruct an entire ear. Surgery for children with microtia usually occurs around age six when the normal ear is near its adult size and can serve as a pattern for the new ear. An ear lost to injury may be repaired or reconstructed when the tissue in the area of the injury is sufficiently healed. Surgery may not be feasible for patients whose skin is badly damaged after a burn or previous surgeries.

In general, to rebuild an entire ear or part of the cartilage rim of the ear, the surgeon begins by removing cartilage from around the patient's ribs. He then bends the cartilage to form a frame for the outer ear and implants the cartilage frame under the skin at the side of the head so that the skin folds around the frame. Using multiple sutures to hold the frame firmly in place, the surgeon creates an ear that looks as natural as possible. Subsequent surgeries over a period of several months are required to form an earlobe, separate the reconstructed ear from the head, and build a tragus, the small rounded projection in front of the external canal leading to the inner ear.

Reconstruction with rib cartilage may not be possible for people born with multiple birth defects or who do not have enough cartilage for grafts due to previous use of the same tissue. One alternative for a lesser deformity is the *Antia-Buch technique,* a reconstructive procedure for the ear that moves tissue from the back/underside of the rim of the ear around and forward to repair a defect on the front rim of the ear.

For more severe deformity, a practical alternative is to use a prosthetic, a plastic frame covered with a flap of skin from the forehead and then sutured to the side of the head. A second alternative is to anchor a completely artificial ear to the bone at the side of the patient's head. In the future, a third alternative may be available; in experimental studies, natural cartilage ear frames have been grown under the skin of laboratory mice, but to date no ear strong enough to be implanted in a human being has been produced.

The surgeon may also choose to reconstruct a damaged or missing ear with polyethylene, a porous synthetic material also used to reconstruct the bones around the eye. Once the polyethylene is in place, natural body tissue can grow into it, anchoring the polyethylene securely to the face/head.

Risks and Complications

The most common side effects are discomfort, pain, infection, and damage to the skin, the transplanted cartilage, or the ear frame itself.

If the skin covering the ear frame does not remain healthy after surgery, the surgeon may pull a flap of skin down from the side of the forehead to cover exposed cartilage on the frame and then attach the skin to the side of the head. Differences of skin color, texture, and thickness between the skin in the flap and the side of the head are less obvious as the wound heals.

After surgery, part of the rib cartilage may be absorbed into the surrounding area on the side of the head or the cartilage in the frame may shift so that the ear looks unbalanced. Removing rib cartilage leaves a painful wound and sometimes a caved-in appearance.

Outlook and Lifestyle Modifications

Thick scars may form at ear and chest; the most common remedy is scar revision (surgery to release or remove the scar) or an injection of long-acting anti-inflammatory drugs. A prosthetic ear may feel unnatural because it does not transmit sensation.

ear splinting   See EAR PINBACK.

eccrine glands   See HYPERHYDROSIS.

ectropion   See EYE LIFT.

elasticity   The ability of a substance to resume its original shape after being stretched. Many PLASTIC SURGERY procedures, such as ABDOMINOPLASTY, CHEMICAL SKIN PEELS, and FACE-LIFTS are necessitated by the age-related loss of skin elasticity leading to wrinkles and sagging.

Skin and some body structures, such as the walls of the blood vessels, are able to expand due to the presence of elastic fibers. These slender filaments, or threads, in the tissue are woven into a network that forms stretchable membranes of elastin, the major protein in the connective tissue in expandable body structures such as skin, muscles, and the walls of blood vessels. The age-related loss of elastin is a major component is the appearance of aging skin.

"Elastic skin" is a nonmedical term for skin that stretches farther than normal without injury due to the presence of abnormal connective tissue. This condition is usually accompanied by joints that are also highly elastic and is associated with Ehlers-Danalos syndrome, a group of inherited connective tissue disorders.

elastic skin See ELASTICITY.

electrodessication The use of electric current to remove skin lesions or to seal off blood vessels; in PLASTIC SURGERY, a procedure to remove small, usually benign growths such as warts or skin cancers on the surface of the body. The name comes from the Latin *desicco*, meaning "dry."

Procedure

The surgeon injects a local anesthetic and then scrapes off the growth with a tool that delivers the electric current. She then cauterizes the area to stop bleeding and covers the wound with a dressing to protect it from contamination.

Risks and Complications

The wound forms a scab that drops off relatively quickly as the wound heals. If the growth recurs, the process may be repeated.

Outlook and Lifestyle Modifications

The patient will have a small mark at the site of the surgery that is lighter than the surrounding skin.

electrolysis Hair removal technique employing a machine called an epilator to remove hairs by inserting a thin probe into a hair follicle, the small indentation in the skin from which a hair grows. The probe destroys both the hair and the follicle so that the hair cannot grow back. There are three types of epilators: thermolysis (from the Greek *therm*, meaning "heat" and *lysis*, meaning "break") epilators, galvanic epilators, and blend epilators.

Procedures

Before starting electrolysis, the doctor or electrolysis technician may apply a local anesthetic to the skin. During the procedure, he inserts the very thin epilator probe into a hair follicle to destroy the hair and the cells from which it grows.

Thermolysis epilators emit high-frequency radio waves that heat and kill hair-growing cells, a process known as electrocoagulation. Thermolysis, which takes from one to 15 seconds to destroy one hair, is most commonly used on fine facial hair.

Galvanic epilators deliver an electrical current to the follicle, producing a chemical reaction that converts salt and water in the skin around a hair to sodium hydroxide (lye) that destroys the hair and the hair follicle. Galvanic epilators, which may require up to two minutes to destroy one large follicle, are most commonly used on body hair rather than facial hair.

Blend epilators deliver both heat and electrical current through a single probe. The combination technique, which takes up to 12 seconds for a large follicle, is considered more effective than either treatment alone.

The patient usually requires multiple visits to remove a sufficient number of hairs.

Risks and Complications

Electrolysis may cause scarring, irregular pigmentation, and infection, including a flare-up of herpes ("cold sores") in susceptible individuals.

Outlook and Lifestyle Modifications

For most people, electrolysis provides permanent hair removal; a minority may see the hair grow back.

Ellenbogen criteria Five general standards for ideal eyebrow shape and position on the face developed by American plastic surgeon Richard Ellenbogen in 1983 as an aid to surgeons repositioning the eyebrows during a FOREHEAD LIFT.

First, the thicker end of the left (or right) eyebrow should start at a point on the top of a line drawn straight up from the left (or right) nostril to the inner edge of the left (or right) eye, i.e., the edge of the eye closest to the nose.

Second, the thinner end of the left (or right) eyebrow should end at a point on the top of a line extending from the outer edge of the left (or right) nostril to the outer edge of the left (or right) eye, i.e., the edge nearest the ear.

Third, the ends of the eyebrow should be at about the same height above the eye.

Fourth, the highest point of the eyebrow should be directly above the outer edge of the pupil (the edge nearest the ear).

Fifth, a woman's eyebrow should arch above the bone over the top of the eye; a man's brow should run along the bone.

endoforehead lift   See FOREHEAD LIFT.

endomidface lift   See ENDOSCOPY; FACE-LIFT.

endonasal rhinoplasty   See RHINOPLASTY.

endoscopy   Minimally invasive diagnostic or surgical procedure performed via a slim rigid or flexible tube that accommodates a TV camera that transmits images to a television screen. The endoscopist, a physician trained in the use of endoscopic instruments, can examine the body's internal structures by inserting the tube either through a very small incision or into a natural opening such as the mouth (to examine the esophagus) or the anus (to examine the colon). The endoscope also accommodates various surgical tools such as tweezers or scalpels, enabling a surgeon to perform various procedures without cutting a large incision.

Procedure

Plastic surgeons perform various endoscopically assisted cosmetic procedures, including (but not limited to) endoscopically assisted ABDOMINOPLASTY, BREAST AUGMENTATION, FACE-LIFT, and FOREHEAD LIFT. Endoscopy is also used for reconstructive surgeries, including (but not limited to) the placement of SKIN FLAPS and the insertion of tissue expanders.

Endoscopic breast augmentation   The surgeon inserts an endoscope through a small incision made under the arm or at the navel to visualize the correct placement of a breast implant. The technique is also used to evaluate existing implants or to examine scar tissue that has compressed an implant, making it uncomfortably hard.

Endoscopic face-lift, endoscopic forehead lift   The surgeon makes multiple small incisions rather than the traditional long incision along the hairline. For example, the surgeon may use one small incision behind the hairline above the ear and a second small incision inside the mouth to free the facial fat pad (cheek), which is then lifted and stitched into its new, higher position. Incisions in the lower eyelid and upper gum line may be used to tighten muscles and skin at midface; incisions under the chin and behind the ears may be used to tighten the neck.

Endoscopic flap surgery   The surgeon uses an endoscope to lift a piece of skin from a donor site via two or three short incisions rather than one or more longer ones. When the surgery is finished, the surgeon applies a pressure dressing that remains in place for several days. Ordinarily, the patient goes home the day of the surgery; the incisions heal, and the stitches come out within seven to 10 days.

Risks and Complications

The known risks of endoscopy and/or endoscopically assisted plastic surgery are similar to those of traditional surgery: infection, fluid accumulation beneath the skin (which must be drained), damage to blood vessels or other internal tissues, and nerve damage leading to loss of sensation.

However, regardless of the site of the diagnostic procedure or surgery, the smaller endoscopic incisions leave smaller scars and are less likely than long scars to cause accidental nerve damage. The anesthesia is usually a local anesthetic rather than general anesthesia. As a result, healing is quicker, and there is less bleeding, bruising, and swelling than with a standard incision; any bruising, numbness, and swelling usually disappear within two weeks.

See also LAPAROSCOPY; MINIMALLY INVASIVE SURGERY.

end-to-end anastomosis   From the Greek *anastomosis*, meaning "opening." Surgical joining of the ends of two open body tubes, such as two blood vessels or two open ends of the digestive tube after removal of an intervening section.

This procedure is used by plastic surgeons to establish a succesful connection between existing blood vessels and those found in tissue transplanted as skin grafts so as to ensure normal blood ciculation to the new tissue. This is vital to the success of the graft; without a continuous plentiful blood supply, the graft/transplant will fail.

See also SKIN GRAFT.

entropion See EYE LIFT.

enzyme A protein that causes chemical changes in a specific substance without being changed itself. Enzymes are often named by adding -ase to the name of the substance the enzyme affects. For example, collagenase is the enzyme that breaks down collagen; protease is an enzyme that breaks down protein; lipase is an enzyme that breaks down fats (from the Greek *lipo*, meaning "fat"). In cosmetic surgery, naturally occurring proteases such as bromelain, a proteolytic enzyme extracted from pineapples, are used as mild exfoliants, substances that flake away dead cells from the surface of the skin.

epaulet flap See SKIN FLAP.

epicanthal fold This fold of skin runs from the top of the nose over the upper eyelid to the farther end of the eyebrow, giving the eyelid a smooth rather than a naturally creased appearance. The epicanthal fold is a normal feature of the eye in people of Asian descent. In other racial groups, it may be present right after birth and then disappear, or it may be present as a characteristic of Down syndrome, a form of mental retardation. The term *epicanthal* comes from the Greek *epi*, meaning "on" and *canthus*, meaning "corner of the eye."

epidermis See SKIN.

epilation See ELECTROLYSIS.

epilator See ELECTROLYSIS.

erbium yag laser See LASER.

excessive wound healing See KELOID; SCAR FORMATION.

excisional back lipectomy See BUTTOCK LIFT.

exfoliation Natural shedding of the top layer of cells from skin or mucous membranes. In PLASTIC SURGERY, a mechanical or chemical process designed to remove dead cells so as to smooth and soften the skin.

Mechanical exfoliants such as bath brushes, loofah pads and sponges, washcloths and towels, and facial scrubs with tiny hard particles such as ground nut pits rub off the top cells. Razors scrape them away. Astringent cosmetic liquids (exfoliants, toners) dry the skin so that dead cells flake away easily when skin is washed and dried with a towel.

See also CHEMICAL SKIN PEEL.

external radiation therapy Radiation such as cobalt-60 gamma rays, an electron beam, neutron beams, proton beam, or X-rays aimed at the body to treat cancer or some kinds of skin diseases. The opposite would be the implantation of radioactive particles into the patient's tumor, as is often done to treat localized prostate cancer, a tumor contained wholly within the prostate gland. External radiation therapy may occasionally damage healthy tissue. If the damage is severe, PLASTIC SURGERY may be used to repair the injured tissue.

Procedure

The first step in external radiation therapy is simulation, the use of imaging studies such as CT-SCANS to pinpoint the tumor and define a treatment port or field, the site at which the radiation will be aimed. The port may be tattooed or marked with permanent ink to ensure the radiation's being delivered to the same spot each treatment. If treatment requires total stillness, immobilization devices such as molds may be used to keep the patient in the correct position during the radiation treatment.

The treatment itself delivers a series of small doses of radiation separated by a rest period to protect healthy cells and tissues; the typical schedule for external radiation treatment is five days a week for five to seven weeks. The exact dose and timing depend on the size, site, and type of the tumor, as well as the patient's general health.

During the treatment, the patient sits or lies on a special chair or treatment table positioned so as to enable the radiation to reach to treatment port. Depending on the site, the therapist may put shields on the patient's body to make sure that the radiation hits only the treatment port. The therapist then leaves the room to deliver the radiation from a nearby site that allows him/her to monitor the patient via television or through a window in the wall of the treatment room. The session may last as long as 30 minutes, but the actually delivery of radiation takes up only one to five minutes at most.

A specialized, computer-controlled miniature radiation machine with a robotic arm that circles the patient's head to deliver multiple small doses of radiation to a brain tumor is called a Cyberknife.

Risks and Complications
Skin irritation, burns, or increased sensitivity to sunlight; lower-than-normal levels of red blood cells, white blood cells, or blood platelets (small particles that enable blood to clot); and fatigue. Note: External radiation therapy does not make the body radioactive.

Outlook and Lifestyle Modifications
Effective destruction of the tumor.

extreme makeover ("X-treme" makeover) *Makeover* is a lay term for multiple cosmetic and/or plastic surgery procedures to improve appearance. An extreme makeover is a radical change in appearance requiring multiple cosmetic procedures, including PLASTIC SURGERY on the face and body, plus cosmetic and/or reconstructive DENTISTRY; changes in diet and exercise, makeup and hair styling; and wardrobe consultation. On television shows such as *Extreme Makeover,* the surgeries appear to be performed either simultaneously or within a few days of each other. In reality, these operations are best performed over a period of several months so

as to allow sufficient time for healthful healing and recovery.

See also BREAST IMPLANT; FACE-LIFT; LIPOSUCTION.

eye See EYE LIFT.

eyebrow lift See FOREHEAD LIFT; TATTOO (MEDICAL).

eyebrow replacement PLASTIC SURGERY to replace an eyebrow lost to alopecia or to an injury, most commonly a burn.

Procedure
To replace a lost eyebrow, the surgeon may use a SKIN FLAP lifted from the scalp with hair intact or 100 to 150 micrografts, very small pieces of skin containing one to two hairs each. To mask the loss of scalp hair and reduce the visibility of scars, the grafts are usually taken from the area behind the ear. The surgery, done with LOCAL ANESTHETIC, usually lasts less than two hours, and the patient goes home the same day. Once the brows heal, a second procedure is occasionally required to fill out or balance the eyebrows.

Cosmetic tattooing to simulate a complete eyebrow or fill in gaps in an existing one is a nonsurgical alternative.

Risks and Complications
Mild bruising or swelling of the eyelids, as well as tiny scabs at the implant sites may occur. The scabs fall off, and the bruising and swelling recede within a week. A more serious complication is the failure of the grafted skin to grow into place at the new site.

Outlook and Lifestyle Modifications
As in hair replacement on the scalp, most of the hairs in grafts fall out soon after transplant but will resume a regular schedule of growth and replacement within several months. After that, the hair must be trimmed periodically to keep it short enough to resemble a natural eyebrow.

See also HAIR REPLACEMENT SURGERY; TATTOO (MEDICAL).

eye-ear plane The orbitomeatal (*orbit*, meaning "eye socket," and *meatal*, meaning "inside of the ear") plane; an imaginary reference line on the skull, drawn from the upper edge of the external opening of the right ear, through the ear canal, across the top of the edge of the bone under the right eye, through the nasal bone, across the top of the edge of the bone under the left eye, through the canal of the left ear to the external opening of the left ear. A measurement used in planning facial and/or head and neck plastic surgery.

eyelash transplant PLASTIC SURGERY to make the lashes on the upper lid look fuller or to replace lashes lost to alopecia or to an injury, most commonly a burn.

Procedure

The surgeon numbs a small area on the scalp, either behind the ear or in the back at the hairline, where neck meets scalp. He then lifts a piece of hair-bearing skin from the scalp, removes excess skin and underlying fatty tissue from the hair-bearing skin, and divides the skin into pieces holding one hair. He numbs the upper eyelid with LOCAL ANESTHETIC; fits the patient with an eyeshield to protect the eye; and uses a fine needle to implant single hairs, one at a time, into the edge of the lid. The surgeon may implant up to 50 single hairs in a procedure lasting about an hour.

Risks and Complications

Swelling and bleeding, though rarely, may occur. Ordinarily, there are no visible scars.

Outlook and Lifestyle Modifications

Because the transplanted hairs come from the scalp, they continue to grow and must be trimmed periodically so that they resemble natural lashes. Perhaps more important is not to brush into and irritate the eye. Note: An alternative to eyelash implants is a cosmetic tattoo of tiny dots on the edge of the eyelid.

See also TATTOO (MEDICAL).

eyelid lift See EYE LIFT.

eyelid reconstruction Surgery to repair or replace a defect due to an injury or the removal or a malignant tumor from the eyelid or to create an upper eyelid crease on an Asian eyelid.

Certain medical problems such as hypothyroidism (abnormally low secretion of thyroid hormones), Graves' disease (thyroid disorder associated with bulging eyes), dry eye, high blood pressure or heart disease, diabetes, a detached retina or glaucoma may complicate this surgery.

Procedure

The first step is to evaluate the defect. An injury that does not extend through all layers of the skin cells and that covers less than half the eyelid is usually repaired with a SKIN FLAP, commonly a semicircular piece of skin from the adjacent area of the lid (Tenzel flap). A defect that stretches over more than half the eyelid and/or an injury that goes through all layers of the skin may be repaired with a graft of skin lifted from the lower eyelid (Cutler-Beard flap) or skin from the opposite eyelid.

Regardless of the type of flap or graft required, the surgery is performed more easily on older patients, because they are more likely to have excess loose skin on the eyelid. Whichever graft is chosen is stitched into place; a pressure dressing is applied to reduce swelling and bleeding while holding the flap or graft in position.

Risks and Complications

Common problems include bruising, discomfort, swelling and tightness, dryness or excessive tearing, gumminess, itching, or burning. Temporary sensitivity to light or double vision or blurred vision may occur, and patients may be unable to wear contact lenses for at least two weeks. Sensitivity to sunlight, wind, and irritants such as perfume and difficulty closing eyes completely are also possible. Keeping the head elevated for several days and applying cold compresses may help reduce the swelling and bruising that commonly lasts from a week to a month. Eyedrops may relieve dryness and/or gumminess; dark glasses will protect against bright light and/or irritants in the air.

Rare complications include severe pain or the permanent inability to close the eyes completely, requiring additional surgery.

Outlook and Lifestyle Modifications

The scars on the constructed or repaired eyelid may be visibly pink for six months or more after surgery, eventually fading to a thin white line. After reconstructing an eyelid, the surgeon may implant single hairs or draw an "eyeliner tattoo," small tattooed dots, to replace or simulate eyelashes.

See also TATTOO (MEDICAL).

eyelid surgery See EYEBROW REPLACEMENT; EYELASH TRANSPLANT; EYELID RECONSTRUCTION; EYE LIFT; TATTOO (MEDICAL).

eye lift Blepheroplasty; surgery on the eyelid to remove fat, excess skin, and muscle from the upper and lower eyelids so as to tighten a drooping upper lid ("hounddog eyes") or remove "bags under the eyes," the permanent sagging under the lower lid due to age-related loss of skin ELASTICITY. Temporary swelling under the eyes due to fatigue or an allergic reaction is treated either with an appropriate sleep regimen or the approproate antiallergy medications.

The techniques used in an eye lift surgery may also be used to correct ectropion or entropion. Ectropion, from the Greek *ek*, meaning "out," and *trope*, meaning "turning," is a sagging of the lower eyelid outward, away from the eyeball. This is most commonly due to an age-related loss of muscle tone or to a facial injury or burn that heals in a way that tightens the lid and pulls it downward. The exposed eye may become dry and irritated, with heavy tearing. Artificial tears lubricate the eye and temporarily reduce irritation, but PLASTIC SURGERY to tighten the eyelid offers the only permanent relief. The opposite of ectropion is entropion, from the Greek *en*, meaning "in" and *trope*, meaning "turn, fold." Entropion is an inward folding, typically of the lower eyelid, which causes irritation as the eyelashes rub against the eye. The condition may be due to a muscle spasm or inflammation of the eyelid or weakness of the muscles controlling the lid or facial paralysis. Artificial tears or taping down the eyelid may temporarily relieve irritation, but most commonly surgery is required to eliminate the folding.

Procedure

This surgery is commonly an outpatient procedure performed with LOCAL ANESTHETIC plus oral or intravenous sedatives.

To tighten an upper eyelid, the surgeon makes an incision following the natural lines in the creases of the upper lid. He then separates the skin from the fatty tissue and muscle underneath, removes excess fat, cuts away excess muscle and skin, pulls the skin up, and anchors it smoothly in place with very fine sutures.

To tighten a lower eyelid, the surgeon makes an incision just below the lashes in the lower lid, then separates the skin of the lid from the underlying fatty tissue and muscle, removes excess fat, and trims sagging skin and muscle. He then closes the incision with very fine sutures.

To remove a pocket of fat ("bag") under the eye, the surgeon makes an incision inside the lower lid, separates the lining of the eyelid from the underlying tissue, pulls out the fat deposit, and closes the incision with very fine sutures. This procedure, transconjunctival blepheroplasty, leaves no visible scar.

To correct ectropion or entropion, the plastic surgeon performs tarsoplasty, surgery to loosen or tighten the tarsus, the tough fibrous tissue at the edge of the upper or lower eyelid.

Risks and Complications

Common side effects include bruising, discomfort, swelling and tightness, dryness or excessive tearing, gumminess, itching, or burning. There may be temporary sensitivity to light or double vision or blurred vision, and patients may be unable to wear contact lenses for at least two weeks. Sensitivity to sunlight, wind, and irritants such as perfume may occur, as well as difficulty closing eyes completely. Keeping the head elevated for several days and applying cold compresses may help reduce the swelling and bruising; eye drops may relieve dryness and/or gumminess; dark glasses will protect against bright light and/or irritants in the air.

When the stitches are removed within two days to a week, a tiny whitehead may form at the site of a stitch; the surgeon removes these with a very fine needle.

If more than one eyelid is tightened, one may heal faster than the other(s) or the scars may be asymmetrical. Rare complications include severe pain, a permanent inability to close the eyes completely, and/or ectropion (outward folding of the lower lid); these may require surgical correction.

Note: This surgery may not be appropriate for people with certain medical problems such as hypothyroidism (abnormally low secretion of thyroid hormones), Graves' disease (thyroid disorder associated with bulging eyes), dry eye, high blood pressure or heart disease, diabetes, a detached retina, or glaucoma.

Outlook and Lifestyle Modifications

The scars on the eyelids are likely to be visibly pink for six months or more after surgery, eventually fading to a thin white line. The cosmetic improvement may last for several years, depending on the patient's age and the condition of his/her skin.

Occasionally, the surgeon may inadvertently leave excess fatty tissue ("residual fat") in place on one or both eyelids. If this occurs, a second surgery may be required to remove the tissue.

Because puffy eyelids are so common, many people use simple home remedies. Some have a basis in science. One example is the application of a cold wet teabag to reduce puffiness around the eyes. Tea leaves contain tannin, an astringent that makes skin swell slightly so that it temporarily appears less puffy. Caution: tannins are irritating if they get into the eye. On the other hand, another folk remedy, applying slices of raw cucumbers as a cool, moist dressing, might feel soothing, but there is no evidence that cucumbers, which are 90 percent water, contain anything special to help with puffiness or bags under the eyes.

See also CANTHUS.

face-lift Rhytidectomy; PLASTIC SURGERY to lift and reduce the facial skin and fat so as to correct age-related sagging of the facial skin. Note: The term *midface lift* refers to the surgical repositioning of the fat pads under the cheek.

Procedures

Plastic surgeons commonly employ one of two basic techniques when performing a face-lift. The subcutaneous face-lift, or "skin only" face-lift, is a procedure most commonly used for a thin person with good skin tone and bone structure, one whose primary defect is excess facial skin, or one who has previously had a face-lift and now requires a touch-up procedure. The SMAS (superficial musculoaponeurotic system) face-lift and the deep-plane face-lift (composite face-lift) are procedures designed for a person with significant sagging of the underlying facial muscles. Note: A midface lift is a simple repositioning of the fat pads under the skin of the cheek.

Subcutaneous face-lift The surgeon injects a local anesthetic, then makes an incision behind the ears and continues down into the neck, reaching in through the incisions to lift the skin away from the underlying tissue. She pulls the loose skin tightly in a lateral direction, that is, toward the sides of the face so that the skin originally at the tragus (the piece of cartilage in front of the opening to the ear canal) reaches the outer cartilage rim of the ear. The surgeon temporarily tacks the lifted skin in place, cuts away the excess, and then closes the edge of the incision. A skin-only face-lift can be performed either as an outpatient procedure or with an overnight stay. Similarly, either intravenous (IV) sedation or general anesthesic can be used.

SMAS (superficial musculoaponeurotic system) face-lift The surgeon begins with an incision at the hairline running from the side of the forehead down to the back of the ear and curving back into the hairline at the side of the ear. Through the incision, the surgeon lifts the skin and underlying tissue, folds the muscle, and repositions the fat pad under the cheek. She then removes excess skin and fatty tissue as required to produce a smooth surface, repositions the facial skin, and sutures the skin and underlying tissues in place using both absorbable and nonabsorbable sutures to guarantee a tight closure. The surgery is usually done in a hospital, under general anesthetic.

Deep-plane/composite face-lift The surgeon makes a deep-plane incision in the lower part of the face, commonly under the eye, to lift the skin, muscle, and underlying fat of the neck and face and free the fat pad under the skin of the cheek. This produces a large composite flap, a piece of skin, including skin, muscle, and fat. The procedure allows the surgeon to pull up the facial skin, reposition the fat pad under the cheek, tighten the facial muscles, and trim away excess tissue. The result is a smoother, more youthful facial contour with reduced deep lines around the nose and mouth. This surgery is usually done in a hospital under general anesthesic.

Regardless of the surgical technique, after closing the incision, the surgeon usually applies protective ointment, covered with a nonstick dressing and a light pressure bandage. Some surgeons place drains to allow the flow of excess fluid; if so, the drains are removed within 24 hours.

Risks and Complications

Bleeding, blood clots (immediately after surgery or several days later), bruising, swelling, pain, and nerve damage are potential hazards for all types of face-lifts. To reduce the risk of complications, patients are examined frequently during the first six months after surgery.

Cosmetic complications after a face-lift may include unnatural tightness due to the surgeon's having removed too much skin; a deformed ear-lobe caused due to the lobe's being pulled down by the way the skin has been positioned; and an irregular hairline due to excess tension on hair-bearing skin or destruction of hair follicles during surgery. For men, trimming excess facial skin may reduce the size of the sideburn; to prevent this, the surgeon may remove and then reimplant the piece of hair-bearing skin in front of the ear.

Outlook and Lifestyle Modifications

A successful face-lift produces a natural-looking face. Although many surgeons believe that SMAS surgery produces longer-lasting results than a sub-cutaneous face-lift, there is no conclusive scientific proof that this is true.

See also CHEEK AUGMENTATION; CHIN RECONSTRUC-TION; EYE LIFT; FAT GRAFTING; FOREHEAD LIFT; JAW; LIP AUGMENTATION; NECK LIFT.

face transplant   Graft of the facial skin and under-lying tissue from a cadaver onto the bone structure of a living person whose face has been destroyed by disease or a burn. The transplanted tissue is expected to fit itself onto the bone structure of the recipient so that the face no longer resembles either the donor or the original face of the recipient. Another possibility is to transplant cadaver skin plus bone; this, too, would create a new face unlike that of either the donor or the recipient.

In 2005, French surgeons performed the world's first partial face transplant, grafting lips, nose, and chin tissue to replace and reconstruct facial features for a woman who had been mauled by a dog. Other such partial surgeries have followed. Two other face transplants have been performed—one in China, and a second in France. In 2006, an Ethics Board at the British National Health Service granted approval to a team of surgeons to carry out the world's first full facial transplant when a suitable candidate is identified. In the United States, surgical teams at the Cleveland Clinic in Ohio and Brigham and Women's Hospital in Boston were granted approval in 2007 to proceed with similar surgeries, again, when suitable canidates are identified.

Procedure

Once a candidate for full or partial face transplant surgery is selected, the surgery itself is basically a three-step procedure.

Step 1: As with all transplant surgery, a recently deceased donor is selected and the required tissue removed. For a face transplant, the plastic surgeon peels back the donor's facial skin from the hairline to the chin, including eyelids, lips, and underlying blood vessels, a procedure known as DEGLOVING. The tissue is removed and stored for transplant, which must take place within 15 hours, after which time the tissue will die without a continuing blood supply.

Step 2: After the surgical recipient is anesthetized, surgeons again use the degloving technique to remove the facial skin and tissue to be replaced, again being careful to clamp and preserve the underlying blood vessels.

Step 3: The surgeons place the donor skin over the recipient's facial bones, aligning the features (eyes, nose, and mouth) and connecting the patient's blood vessels to the blood vessels in the donor's facial tissue.

Risks and Complications

As with all surgery, the patient may experience swelling and bruising and a risk of infection. A transplant patient has the added risk of the body's rejecting the new tissue; to prevent this, the patient must continue to take antirejection drugs for the remainder of life.

Outlook and Lifestyle Modifications

Successful facial surgery gives the patient a normal appearance. The patient should also be able to feel sensation in the transplanted tissue and to use the facial muscles to speak and create normal expressions such as a smile. The procedure is so new that guidelines for long-term success have not yet been established, but two years after the first French surgery, the patient was reported to be experiencing sensation in the transplanted tissue and was able to move the facial tissue to form normal expressions.

Before the first transplant surgery in France, there was concern about the psychological effect of a patient's having a "new" face that looks like the donor rather than the recipient. The concern has not been resolved, but it has been somewhat alleviated because, as expected, the transplanted skin does adjust to the patient's own bone structure, making the "new" face look like the recipient's "old" one.

facial aging   Changes in the appearance of facial skin normally associated with aging. These may include

- the appearance of pigmented spots
- fine lines and WRINKLES
- loss of skin ELASTICITY
- deep wrinkles, such as those in the nasolabial fold (deep crease of facial tissue running from the outer edge of the nostril down to the outer edge of the mouth)
- loss of fatty tissue, such as the fat pad over the cheekbone
- loss of facial bone resulting in a more prominent forehead and chin

As a general rule, facial aging proceeds along a more or less regular timeline. In the 30s, skin folds begin to form on the eyelids, and fine lines appear at the side of the eyes. In the 40s, the folds between nose and mouth deepen, and vertical and horizontal folds appear on the forehead. In the 50s, the neck wrinkles, the skin around the jaw sags, and the tip of the nose droops forward. After 60, the layer of fat under the skin on the face begins to shrink, leading to more wrinkles and sagging.

How quickly these changes actually occur depends to some extent on genetics (puffy eyes and jowls may run in families), as well as a person's general health (some illnesses speed the loss of fatty tissue) and exposure to environmental factors (sunlight and smoking accelerate wrinkling).

Facial aging in younger people due to health problems or exposure to environmental factors is called premature facial aging.

The common plastic surgeries to address the changes wrought by facial aging include CHEEK AUG-MENTATION, CHEMICAL SKIN PEELS, chin reduction, DERMABRASION, EYE LIFT, FACE-LIFT, FOREHEAD LIFT, and NECK LIFT. An unproven technique called *facial stimulation* uses devices said to reverse the signs of facial aging by stimulating and tightening facial muscles. Two studies reported in the *Archives of Facial Plastic Surgery* showed no noticeable effects.

See also ULTRAVIOLET LIGHT; WRINKLES.

facial animation   See FACIAL REANIMATION.

facial block   Injection of anesthetic to numb specific areas of the face. The type of block is chosen to reflect the area on which the plastic surgeon will be working.

An infraorbital nerve block numbs the upper lip, the cheek, the side of the nose, and the lower eyelid on one side of the face. A mental nerve block numbs the lower lip and the skin below it. A supraorbital nerve block numbs the upper eyelid and forehead above it on the same side of the face. A supratrochlear nerve block numbs the upper eyelid, upper nose, and forehead on one side of the face.

facial bones   The bones around the mouth, nose, and eyes that shape the face. Repositioning or reshaping these bones is an important part of cosmetic plastic surgeries such as RHINOPLASTY, chin augmentation or reduction, and reconstructive plastic surgery, such as repairing a cleft palate.

Starting at the top of the face and moving downward, the facial bones are

- *ethmoid bone*: the floor of the front part of the skull and the roof of the nose
- *temporal bone*: front of the skull, above the eyes
- *orbit:* socket around the eye
- *lacrimal bone*: irregular thin bone of the round socket
- *nasal bone:* bone forming the structure of nose
- *palatine bone*: bone behind the upper jaw, forming part of the nasal cavity and the socket around the eye

- *omer*: triangular bone at the center of the nostrils
- *zygoma*: cheekbone
- *maxilla*: upper jaw
- *mandible*: lower jaw
- *hyoid bone*: U-shape bone between the lower jaw and larynx

facial cleft Category of birth defects; any congenital abnormal separation in the bones and/or other tissues of the face arising from the failure of the bone plates in the fetal head to fuse normally during pregnancy.

Facial clefts may be named either for their orientation on the skull or for the part of the face they affect. For example:

- A lateral facial cleft (prosoposchisis, from the Greek *prosopo*, meaning "face," *ano*, meaning "up," and *schisis*, meaning "fissure") is a cleft that stretches up from the corner of the mouth toward the ear.
- A midline facial cleft is a cleft in the center of the face that may produce various deformities including a bifid nose (cleft nose) and eyes set abnormally wide apart.
- An oblique facial cleft (macrostomia, from the Greek *macro*, meaning "large," and *stoma*, meaning "mouth") is a cleft that extends up one side of the face from the outer corner of the mouth to the inner edge of the eye.
- A cleft cheek is a congenital separation in the cheek due to the failure of the bones of the embryo's maxilla (upper jaw) to fuse properly with the forehead and nose bones.
- A cleft palate is the failure of the bones at the top of the mouth (palate) to meet.

Each of these deformities may be repaired or alleviated by appropriate PLASTIC SURGERY procedures.

The opposite condition, premature closure of the bones in the fetal skull, produces its own distinct set of deformities. An example is *harlequin deformity,* an up-tilt of the orbit (the bone surrounding the eye) due to a premature fusing of the sphenoid bone (the butterfly-shape bone at the base of the skull). This deformity, like facial clefts, may be repaired with craniofacial (skull/face) plastic surgery.

See also CLEFT LIP AND/OR PALATE.

facial contouring Surgical removal of part of the fat pad, the fatty deposit that creates the curve of the cheek; performed most commonly in persons older than 23 to 27, an age at which the fat pad begins to shrink naturally; rarely performed in people older than 50. Facial contouring is generally done for cosmetic reasons.

Procedure

The fatty tissue is removed through two incisions inside the mouth between the upper molars and the mucous membrane of the cheek. The surgeon then closes the incisions.

Risks and Complications

After surgery, soreness, swelling, and numbness are common. The stitches are removed within a week, but it may take up to four months for the swelling to subside completely. Other possible complications include infection, a starved appearance if too much tissue is removed, unequally sized cheeks, scarring, or nerve damage.

Outlook and Lifestyle Modifications

Successful surgery produces a more finely sculpted face.

See also FILLER.

facial expression Movement or positioning of facial features to transmit nonverbal messages, such as a smile to signal happiness or a frown to signal displeasure.

Several facial expressions appear to be universal among human beings. For example, tightly compressed lips are almost interpreted as anger or frustration; pursed lips as disagreement; baring the teeth and curling the lip as disgust; raised brows and/or widened eyes as surprise or skepticism; and eyes turned down or away as deception or submission. Conversely, the absence of expression—a "blank face" with the eyes open, the lips closed, and the facial muscles relaxed—suggests calmness or simply an intention not to interact with others.

The facial muscles used to form these expressions are *orbicularis oculi* (around the eye), *zygomaticus major, zygomaticus minor, masseter, sternocleidomastoid* (cheek), *nasalis* (nose), *risorius* (cheek and mouth), *levator labil superiorus* (upper lip), *depressor labil inforioris* and *depressor anguli oris* (lower lip and jaw). The muscles of the scalp are *epicranus* (front, middle, and back of the scalp), *auriculus superior, auricular anterior,* temporalis, and *temporoparietalis* (sides of the scalp).

If these muscles or the nerves that power them are damaged due to a developmental or neurological disorder, a disease (such as a tumor), an infection, an injury (including injury during surgery), or an adverse reaction to a medicine, the patient may lose the ability to form facial expressions, a major bar to normal communication.

The plastic surgeries to restore functioning of the facial muscles are known collectively as FACIAL REANIMATION.

facial grading system   See TORONTO FACIAL GRADING SYSTEM.

Facial Harmony™   See NONSURGICAL FACE-LIFT.

facial implant   See CHEEK AUGMENTATION; JAW; LIP AUGMENTATION.

facial landmarks   Ideal, imaginary structural characteristics of the forehead, eyes, ears, nose, mouth (lips), and chin; used as a guide by plastic surgeons in evaluating a patient's facial appearance and planning cosmetic or reconstructive surgery.

In this ideal, imaginary diagram the forehead slants (or rounds) slightly forward from the hairline toward the bony ridge above the eyebrows. The eyes are no less than 1.2 inches and no more than 1.4 inches apart with the highest point of the upper eyelid between the center of the eye and the corner nearest the nose and the lowest point of the upper lower eyelid nearer the outer edge of the eye. The top of the ear is level with the outer edge of the eyebrow; the external opening into the ear is midway between the outer corner of the eye and the bottom of the nose; and the ear is about half as wide as it is long.

In profile, the tip of the nose projects in front of the lips and chin; when viewed from below, the tip and the nostrils form a triangle with three equal sides. The outer edges of the mouth (lips) are on a straight line down from the center of the iris (the dark circle in the middle of each eye); the lower lip is slightly fuller than the upper. When smiling, the lips do not open so far as to reveal the gum line above the teeth, and in profile the lips line up with the chin. Currently, the features widely but not universally accepted as beautiful include

- facial symmetry (similarly sized features placed evenly on either side of the face)
- smooth, evenly colored, unblemished skin
- evenly spaced eyes (a man's eyebrows usually are straight and lie flat on the bone above the eyes, while a woman's eyebrows sit slightly above the bone and arch in the middle)
- prominent cheekbones
- straight nose with narrow nostrils and an elevated tip
- full lips
- a firm chin that lines up with the lips when seen in profile

However, these standards must be considered arbitrary. Some characteristics associated with beauty, such as facial shape, vary from one culture to another, and some vary according to gender. For example, Western societies consider an oval face ideal, while Eastern societies value a rounded face. Overall, clean-cut, strong features are considered attractive for a man's face; more rounded features are considered attractive for a woman's.

facial reanimation   Surgical, medical, and/or physical therapy to reverse or ameliorate the effects of facial paralysis, such as uncontrolled drooling due to an inability to control the lip muscles, eye irritation or drooping eyelids due to an inability to control the muscles that close the eye, and emotional depression due to an inability to speak clearly or express emotion. The aim of all facial reanimation procedures is to enable the patient to control the facial muscles so as to form facial expression, as well as to open and close the eyes and mouth.

Procedure

The surgical options include (but are not limited to) repairing damaged nerve fibers, transplanting healthy nerve and/or muscle tissue to the affected area, and/or building mechanical support for specific muscles, most commonly those affecting the eyelid. Nonsurgical options include medicines to relieve irritated eyes, tape to close the eyelids at night, and physical therapy to strengthen existing muscles.

Repairing nerve fibers   Microsurgery to rejoin fibers in a damaged nerve may enable the patient to form some facial expressions. Recovery, which begins with a pins-and-needles sensation, may take from six months to two years to complete. Some residual muscle weakness and involuntary movement are inevitable.

A nerve that has been severed straight through should be repaired as soon as possible. Three to four weeks after the injury, the nerve begins to deteriorate, the severed ends contract, new nerve fibers appear, and the muscle around the nerve thickens. Therefore, repairing the nerves as quickly as possible enables the surgeon to identify the injured ends of the nerve and align them properly, reducing the risk of nerve scarring. Note: A nerve that has been only partially severed may, in some cases, be successfully repaired up to 24 months after the injury.

Transplanting nerve tissue   If a damaged nerve cannot be repaired, nerve tissue from another part of the face or body may be grafted in place to provide some relief. An ipsilateral (from the Latin *ipse,* meaning "same," and *latus,* meaning "side") nerve graft joins branches of healthy nerves to injured nerves on the same side of the face. The advantage of this procedure is that the injury heals quickly; the disadvantage is that the procedure is only effective for branches of the facial nerve, not for the main trunk of the nerve.

The facio-facial crossover technique connects branches of the facial nerves on the unaffected side of the face to the paralyzed side of the face. The drawback is that only 20 to 50 percent of the nerve fibers from the healthy side of the face are likely to grow all the way across to the affected side, so the new nerve may not provide sufficient power to move the paralyzed muscles.

The hypoglossal-to-facial crossover technique connects nerves under the tongue (from the Greek *hypo,* meaning "under," and *glossa,* meaning "tongue") to the paralyzed side of the face, enabling the patient to move the face by pressing the tongue against the teeth. The advantages of this procedure are quick healing with little discomfort, one scar, and the ability to move the face relatively normally while eating or talking. The disadvantage is reducing the effectiveness of the donor nerve, plus abnormal tension in the facial muscle on the paralyzed side of the face due to constant stimulation as the tongue moves in the mouth.

Another possibility is to transplant nerve tissue, such as a section of the auricular nerve (from the lower jaw) or a section of the sural nerve (from the lower leg) to the paralyzed area of the face in the hope that the new nerve will generate power to control the local muscles.

Transplanting muscle tissue   If too much time passes after the injury, the original nerve will atrophy, necessitating a graft of muscle and nerve tissue from another part of the face or body. The temporalis muscle (lower jaw) is commonly used to repair the mouth, middle of the face, and eyelids; the masseter (back of the cheek), for the mouth. Other sources for grafts to repair the face are the lattissimus dorsi muscle (lower back), the gracilus muscle (thigh), the trapezius muscle (shoulder), and the pectoralis muscle (chest).

The advantages of these grafts are quick recovery from relatively simple surgery, good (though not normal) movement of the face, and a normal appearance when the muscles are at rest. As with any tissue graft, the disadvantages are possible failure of the transplanted tissue to attach properly, damage to the donor site, and the failure of the two sides of the face to move in tandem.

Creating mechanical support   The surgeon may attach very thin wire springs or gold weights to the upper eyelid. The virtue of the spring is that it allows the patient to blink; the weights, which help keep the lid down, do not.

Risks and Complications
As with all surgery, bruising and swelling are common. The more serious complications are failure of the nerve to regenerate or to transmit impulses properly to existing or transplanted muscle tissue.

Outlook and Lifestyle Modifications
Successful surgery restores to the patient the ability to move the facial muscles and form natural facial expressions.

facial scrub   See EXFOLIATION.

facial stimulation   See FACIAL AGING.

facial triangle   See TWEED'S FACIAL TRIANGLE.

fanny tuck   See BUTTOCK LIFT.

fat   See ADIPOSE TISSUE; DIETARY FAT.

fat depot   See ADIPOSE TISSUE.

fat grafting   Also known as microlipoinjection; transfer of fat cells from one part of a patient's body to another, to fill in defects such as acne scars, deep lines between nose and mouth, or forehead wrinkles; to enlarge the lips; or to restore tissue lost to an illness such as cancer. Fat grafting may also be used to make hands look younger by reducing age-related fat loss around the finger bones.

Note: This technique is not used for BREAST AUGMENTATION, because the extra fat makes it more difficult to detect breast cancers and because the fat is eventually absorbed by the patient's body, necessitating repeat procedures.

Procedure
The surgery is done on an outpatient basis, often in the doctor's office. The surgeon cleans and numbs both the site from which the fat will be extracted (commonly the abdomen) and the site to which it will be transferred. She then withdraws fat tissue with a syringe, or a cannula (hollow tube), similar to that used for LIPOSUCTION, separates fat cells from the other tissue, and injects the cells into the appropriate site, repeating the process to produce the desired contour.

Because the injected fat will eventually be absorbed by the patient's body, the surgeon will "overfill" or inject more fat than actually needed to fill the area.

Risks and Complications
If not enough material is injected, a second procedure may be required, but not sooner than three months after the original surgery.

If too much material is injected, new blood vessels may not grow as needed, leading to lumps caused by the death of transplanted tissue.

Other possible complications include infection, excess bleeding, scarring, and nerve or blood vessel damage during surgery. Ice compresses help reduce temporary redness, bruising, and swelling, but discoloration and swelling may last for several days or weeks, depending on the size of the filled area.

Outlook and Lifestyle Modifications
Because the graft comes from the patient's own body, the body will not reject the tissue. However, the fat will eventually be absorbed, necessitating additional grafts to maintain the original fullness. How long it takes for the body to absorb the fat varies from one person to another. For some people, the fatty tissue may remain plump for as long as a year, but, on average, up to 65 percent of the added fullness disappears after six months.

See also FACE-LIFT; FILLER; SKIN GRAFT.

fat injection   See FAT GRAFTING.

fat liquefication   See under LIPOSUCTION.

fat pad   See ADIPOSE TISSUE.

fat removal   See LIPOSUCTION.

fat transfer   See FAT GRAFTING.

fat transplant   See FAT GRAFTING.

fatty tissue   See ADIPOSE TISSUE.

feathering   Various techniques used make an area of the body look natural after a surgical procedure.

Procedure

After closing an incision, the surgeon smooths the edges so as to leave a rounded border rather than a sharp depression in the skin.

When doing liposuction, the surgeon removes fatty tissue in a pattern that leaves a smooth surface, rather than an indentation under the skin.

When performing hair replacement with grafts containing multiple hair follicles, the surgeon inserts grafts of single hairs to create a natural-looking hairline.

Risks and Complications

Feathering adds no specific risks or complications to the original procedure.

Outlook and Lifestyle Modifications

Successful feathering improves the appearance of the incision, fat removal, or hair transplant.

See also HAIR REPLACEMENT SURGERY.

fever   An abnormally high body temperature; in adults, generally a reading above 100.4°F/38°C by mouth; 100.5°F/38.1°C by rectum; a natural response of the immune system to an infection. The microorganisms that cause disease usually reproduce most efficiently at the normal body temperature; an increase in temperature inhibits their growth.

Other health conditions that may trigger an elevated temperature are an allergic reaction; an autoimmune disease such as arthritis; some forms of cancer; certain medicines such as antibiotics, antihistamines, barbiturates, and drugs for high blood pressure; and an injury, including PLASTIC SURGERY.

Note: An FUO is fever of undetermined origin that lasts for several days, weeks, or months with no known cause.

Symptoms and Diagnostic Path

The internal temperature of the body, as measured by mouth, by rectum, or under the armpit. The normal average is 98.6°F/37°C, but that may vary by person, age, activity, and time of day. For example, among children younger than two years old, the daily variation is about one degree, increasing to two degrees per day by age six, then stabilizing among adults, except for women of child-bearing age when the menstrual cycle can elevate temperature by one degree or more.

Body temperature is usually highest in the evening; it rises during physical activity, when one is eating or experiencing strong emotion or taking certain medications, or exposed to high external temperatures and/or high humidity.

Treatment Options and Outlook

The simplest way to lower a fever is to cool the body by removing excess clothing and covering, sponging or bathing in lukewarm water, and drinking cool liquids. Very cold baths or alcohol rubs cool the skin but induce shivering, which raises the core temperature (the temperature at the center of the body).

Acetaminophen and nonsteroidal anti-inflammatories such as aspirin and ibuprofen also help reduce fever. Fevers due to an infection, including postsurgical infection, are treated with antibiotics.

WARNING: Ibuprofen is not approved for children younger than six months of age. In children with fever, aspirin has been linked to the development of Reye's Syndrome, a condition characterized by brain damage, liver failure, and possible death. As a result, since 1986, all aspirin products sold in the United States must carry a warning not to give aspirin to children for colds, chicken pox, and flu. The National Reye's Syndrome Foundation recommends against giving aspirin to children younger than 19 with a fever-producing illness.

Risk Factors and Preventive Measures

Immediate medical attention for a fever is required in the following cases

- when an infant younger than three months has a rectal temperature of 100.2°F/37.9°C or higher
- an infant three to six months old has a fever of 101°F/38.3°C or higher
- a baby six months to a year old has a fever of 103°F/39.4°C or higher
- a child younger than two has a fever that lasts longer than 24 to 48 hours
- an older child or an adult has a fever lasting longer than 48 to 72 hours
- any person of any age has a fever higher than 105°F/40.5°C that does not respond immediately to treatment
- any case when a person with a fever is confused or irritated, has difficulty breathing, cannot move an arm, leg, or neck, or suffers a (first-time) seizure

fibrin foam   See FOAM WOUND DRESSING.

fillers   Material used by plastic surgeons to fill an abnormal space on the patient's face, such as age-related WRINKLES, or the deeper furrows between the eyebrows, or the hollow left by the age-related shrinkage of the natural fat pad in the cheek area. Fillers may also be used to erase depressed scars such as those caused by ACNE or chicken pox. The material used as filler may be natural or synthetic.

Natural Fillers

Natural fillers are made from fatty tissue and collagen, the connective tissue in skin. The tissue for the filler may be taken from the patient's own body, a process known as an autologous transplant (from the Greek word *auto,* meaning "self") or it may be harvested from a human cadaver or an animal. Tissues taken from these other sources are called allografts (from the Greek word *allo,* meaning "other").

Fatty tissue   The simplest form of natural filler is fatty tissue taken from one site on the patient's body (for example, the abdomen) via LIPOSUCTION, cleaned, and then injected into wrinkles on the face to plump up the depression left by the wrinkle. Because the body absorbs the injected material, the results are temporary, lasting anywhere from a few weeks to a few months. To maintain the new contours, the injections must be repeated.

Collagen   The connective tissue used as a filler may be taken from the patient's own body or from a cadaver or from an animal.

The U.S. Food and Drug Administration (FDA) approved the use of bovine collagen (collagen from cows) as filler in the 1970s, and for two decades therafter it was the material of choice for smoothing facial wrinkles. However, bovine collagen may trigger allergic reactions or tissue rejection in human beings; before using it, the plastic surgeon must test the patient for sensitivity to the collagen. As a result, products such as Zyderm® and Zyplast® are no longer commonly used in the United States.

Collagen fillers may also be made from collagen cells lifted from the patient's own body and then cultured (grown) in a laboratory until there is suffcient tissue for the procedure. Isolagen® is a brand name version of this kind of product. Cosmoderm® and Cosmoplast® are injectible liquids containing collagen cells. Dermolagen™ is filler made from collagen taken from cadaver skin. Unlike bovine collagen, these products do not require presurgical testing.

Fibril   A third kind of natural filler, fibril, is a powder made from fibrils, a small fiber that occurs naturally in both connective tissue and muscle tissue. The powder is mixed with the patient's own blood and then injected.

Like fatty tissue, injected collagen is eventually absorbed by the body. To maintain a smooth, rounded appearance, the patient must have repeat treatments every two to six months.

Synthetic Fillers

Synthetic fillers are man-made substances created specifically for use as fillers.

Synthetic hyaluronic acid This is a man-made version of hyaluronic acid, a natural substance in the body that holds water in the skin so that the skin looks smooth and young. Restylane™ and Juvederm™ are products containing synthetic hyaluronic acid. Juverderm is available in three formulations. The lightest-weight version, Juvederm 18™, is used for fine wrinkles such as crow's feet around the eyes or lines around the mouth. The mid-weight version, Juvederm 24™, is used to reduce moderate creases or lines in the forehead or between the eyes or from the nose to the mouth or on the cheek. The heaviest version, Juvederm 30™, is used for deep folds between nose and mouth or to augment the lips or cheeks.

More than one round of injections may be required to attain the desired result; after that, additional injections may be needed every few months to maintain the result. Hyaluronic acid should not used on patients with immune system disorders. Because it crosses the placenta and passes into breast milk, it should not be used for women who are pregnant or nursing.

Calcium hydroxylapatite This is a form of calcium found in bone, including human bone. Radiesse™, formerly known as Radiance™, is an injectible water-based gel containing microscopic particles of calcium hydroxylapatite. The product is being reviewed by the FDA as a facial filler.

Polymers A polymer (from the Greek words *poly,* meaning "many," and *meros,* meaning "part") is a natural or synthetic material made of very large molecules, some containing as many as several million units linked together. Proteins are natural polymers; plastics are synthetic polymers.

Poly-L-lactic acid This synthetic compound similar to the alpha hydroxy acids found naturally in fruits and vegetables, this material is administered in a series of injections (brand name, Sculptra®) over several months. The injections of particles of poly-L-lactic acid in solution are used to fill in the hollow left by the loss of the natural fat pad on the cheek. Sculptra™ is FDA-approved to counter tissue loss due to HIV/AIDS.

Polymethyleneacrylate (PMMA) This filler (brand name Artefill® in the United States; Artecoll® elsewhere) is a supension of miniature beads of the polymer suspended in bovine collagen. The filling is permanent, and the PMMA beads are believed to stimulate the patient's own natural production of collagen, but follow-up injections may be needed as wrinkles deepen with age. As with other products derived from bovine collagen, the patient may be tested for sensitivity before the treatment begins.

Polytetrafluorethylene (ePTFE) The proper scientific name for this material is "expanded polytetrafluorethylene," but it is best known under its brand name Gore-Tex®. For use as a filler (actually a support for the facial tissue), it is formed in sheets and rolled into a small tube inserted under the skin. The material is completely nonreactive; it does not cause any allergic or rejection reactions, but it may feel stiff rather than pliant under the skin.

Procedure

If required, the surgeon first runs a sensitivity test to determine if the patient is allergic to the filler.

During the procedure itself, the plastic surgeon cleans the patient's face with alcohol and marks the skin with a sterile marking pen to indicate the site of the filler injections. Then she may apply ice or administer a local anesthetic to numb the area (some filler solutions include a local anesthetic). She injects the filler into the area of the wrinkle, crease, or furrow. When the injections are complete, she will clean the markings off the patient's face and apply ice to soothe any temporary discomfort.

Risks and Complications

General reactions to filler injections may include redness and swelling; mild bruising; or itching, pain, or tenderness at the site of the injections. Reactions to bovine collagen products may include redness, swelling, and (rarely) acnelike eruptions.

Outlook and Lifetsyle Modifications

As a rule, fillers are eventually absorbed by the patient's body, necessitating repeat injections to maintain a level of plumpness.

finasteride Propecia™, Proscar™; prostate cancer drug whose side effects include retention of hair or increased hair growth in men. It is sometimes used to treat male pattern baldness in adult men. It must be taken for at least three months before effects are apparent and then continued indefinitely (if treatment stops, so does hair growth). Caution: Men using finasteride are less likely to develop prostate cancer, but if they do, the cancer is more likely to be aggressive and treatment resistant. Because finasteride can be absorbed through the skin, to avoid any possible damage to the genitals of a developing fetus, women who are or may become pregnant should not handle finasteride tablets.

See also HAIR LOSS; HAIR REPLACEMENT SURGERY; MINOXIDIL.

fingers and toes, congenital structural defects The most common congenital defects of fingers and toes are abnormally long or short digits or digits with abnormally curved joints. In many cases, PLASTIC SURGERY may repair or ameliorate defects such as those described here.

Boutonniere deformity From the French *boutonniere,* meaning "buttonhole," this describes a finger that bends downward at the middle joint and backward at the end joint, due to a button-hole-shape tear in the tendon holding the joint that allows the joint to slip through. This may be caused by a congenital defect, although it may result from an injury or an inflammatory condition such as rheumatoid ARTHRITIS.

Brachydactyly Shorter-than-normal fingers and/or toes, frequently associated with DOWN SYNDROME and other multidefect congenital conditions. A related condition is *brachiosyndactyly,* shorter-than-normal fingers and/or toes, with connecting tissue webbing between two or more fingers and/or toes. Poland syndrome is a related group of birth defects that includes missing hand muscles and/or webbed fingers and/or missing fingers. It was identified by British surgeon Alfred Poland (1822–72).

Camptodactyly A defect commonly affecting the fifth (little) finger or the fourth (ring) finger, which are permanently bent in toward the palm of the hand.

Clinodactyly A defect causing the fifth ("little") finger to curve in toward the fourth ("ring") finger.

Club fingers Also called Hippocratic nails, this is an hereditary defect linked to a dominant gene,

more common in boys than in girls. It is characterized by excessive growth of soft tissue that widens the tips of the fingers and/or toes so that the nails are virtually hidden under the extra tissue.

Hyperdactyly This birth defect results in more than the normal number of fingers or toes.

Windblown hand Birth defect due to a dominant gene. The fingers are bent back toward the wrist, and the thumb is webbed to the palm. The condition may be corrected with surgery early in life, commonly before the child is two years old, to remove the webbing and reposition the fingers.

Symptoms and Diagnostic Path
Structural defects of the fingers and toes are visible upon examination. X-rays may be used to document the specific internal abnormality.

Treatment Options and Outlook
Brachiosyndactyly may be treated with reconstructive surgery to separate and repair the digits. Camptodactyly and clinodactyly do not require teatment unless the curve of the finger interferes with normal hand function. If that is the case, the plastic surgeon can break and reposition the finger bones to straighten the finger(s).

Risk Factors and Preventive Measures
There are no known risk factors and/or preventive measures for these birth defects.

See also MACRODACTYLY; POLYDACTYLY.

fingers, fused See POLYDACTYLY.

fingertip repair Plastic surgery to rebuild or repair the part of the finger that includes the nail on top and the fat pad on the underside. The nerves, blood vessels, and skin must be protected during surgery to preserve the sense of touch, keep the adjacent joints intact and mobile, and make the finger look normal.

Procedures
To repair or reconstruct the fingertip, the surgeon may use one of four basic surgeries: open technique, closure and amputation, skin grafts, and skin flaps.

Open technique The surgeon cleans the wound and allows it to heal on its own. This procedure is used for small injuries (less than 1 cm/0.4 in) in length with no bone or a minimal amount of bone showing through the skin. It is used most commonly in children, who grow new soft tissue more quickly than do adults. Note: If there is bone showing through the skin, the bone is scraped clean before the wound is allowed to heal.

Closure and amputation The surgeon cleans the wound and pulls a small piece of adjacent soft tissue over the wound to close it. If necessary, the surgeon may cut away a small piece of bone so that the soft tissue closes smoothly, with no unusual tension that might interrupt healing. In a similar procedure, the cap technique, the surgeon reattaches a severed fingertip by removing excess soft tissue at the end of the finger and using the severed tip to cover ("cap") the exposed and cleaned bone. The technique, created by American plastic surgeon Elliott H. Rose, successfully maintains the finger's appearance and function.

Skin flap If the wound exposes bone and/or tendons at the tip, the surgeon cleans the wound and closes it with a piece of skin (with blood vessels attached) lifted from a site close to the fingertip, such as a healthy area on the same finger, the next finger (cross-finger flap), or the palm (thenar flap). The choice of donor site is determined by the size, shape, and site of the wound. Commonly, the flap may be left attached to the original donor site until the blood vessels and skin grow into place over the injury.

Skin graft The surgeon cleans the wound and closes it with tissue lifted from a distant site on the body, such as the wrist, arm, or groin. The graft may be skin alone or skin plus underlying fatty tissue or skin plus fatty tissue, bone, and nail tissue. The last two are used to cover an injury requiring amputation of the tip; a graft with bone and nail tissue is used only for young children who are able to integrate the tissue. Major injuries to the thumb may be repaired with a graft lifted from the large toe or the webbing between the toes.

The plastic surgery to reconstruct an undeveloped, entirely missing, or amputated thumb by transferring part of the index finger to the place on the hand where the thumb normally sits is called pollicization.

Risks and Complications

Regardless of the repair method, the common complications of fingertip repair include swelling, scarring, infection, and loss of sensation or, conversely, increased sensitivity, specifically to cold temperatures. Loss of sensation due to nerve damage is permanent; increased sensitivity usually lessens within two years after surgery.

The complication specific to open healing is shrinkage of tissue in the pad on the underside of the tip. Complications specific to amputation include deformed nails and sensitivity at the stump of the fingertip. To reduce the risk of the former, the surgeon usually removes the entire nail bed (the tissue from which nails grow). To reduce the risk of the latter, the surgeon preserves as much connective tissue as possible and closes the wound as smoothly as possible at the tip. Complications specific to skin flaps and skin grafts is the failure of the transplanted skin to thrive or joint stiffness in patients with ARTHRITIS. Cosmetic complications include the transfer of hair-bearing skin to previously hair-free surfaces such as the underside of the finger or a mismatch of skin color (for example, when skin from the lighter underside of the finger is transferred to the normally darker upper side).

Outlook and Lifestyle Modifications

Successful surgery gives the patient use of the injured finger.

See also HAND SURGERY; NAIL; SKIN FLAP; SKIN GRAFT.

Fitzpatrick Skin Type Classification Scale created in 1975 by Harvard University dermatologist Thomas B. Fitzpatrick to describe skin color from Type 1 (lightest) to Type 6 (darkest) according to the skin's reaction to sunlight.

Types 1, 2, and 3, the light skin colors, may burn before tanning, although Type 3 tans more easily than Type 2, which tans more easily than Type 1. Type 4 is light brown; Type 5 is dark brown; both tan slightly. Type 6 (black) does not tan.

Fitzpatrick Skin Typing is used to predict the potential success of a CHEMICAL SKIN PEEL. Types 1, 2, and 3 are least likely to experience discoloration and/or scarring after the peel. Types 4 and 5 are more likely to develop discoloration and/or KELOIDS (heavy scarring).

See also GLOGAU PHOTOAGING CLASSIFICATION.

fixator See under LIMB-LENGTH DISCREPANCY.

flashlamp See INTENSE PULSED LIGHT.

fleur-de-lis abdominoplasty See ABDOMINOPLASTY.

foam wound dressing Highly absorbent dressing used to control bleeding during surgery or as a dressing to promote wound healing by keeping a wound moist. One example is fibrin foam, a sterile spongelike product made from human fibrin, a natural protein fiber formed when damaged blood vessels release fibrinogen, a protein in blood that thickens into stringlike threads to form a network at the site of the injury that catches red blood cells and blood platelets. This creates a clot that stops blood flow, then dries and hardens into a protective scab.

forehead lift Foreheadplasty; PLASTIC SURGERY to elevate sagging eyebrows and smooth out lines and WRINKLES in the forehead repair—a drooping brow (eyebrow ptosis) caused by age-related loss of skin ELASTICITY or a facial injury that allows skin around the eye to fold down, giving the eye a hooded appearance.

Forehead wrinkles and furrows may be due to normal aging or a natural facial feature such as deep grooves between the eyes or low, heavy eyebrows. Characteristically, the thicker skin in the area over and to the sides of the eyes wrinkles horizontally; the thinner skin between the eyes wrinkles vertically.

Note: The forehead is part of the face from the eyebrows to the hairline, which includes the main forehead in front, the temporal area on either side, the supra eyebrow area directly over the eyebrows, and the glabella, the area between the eyes. The forehead-brow complex is the forehead and the eyebrows.

Procedures

The two basic techniques for a forehead lift are the conventional (or classic) forehead lift and the endoscopic forehead (endoforehead) lift. Both surgeries may be performed as an outpatient procedure with local anesthesic and a mild sedative, although some surgeons prefer general anesthesic, and patients who suffer from frequent headaches may be given additional local anesthetic during surgery to prevent headache afterward.

Prior to surgery, patients with short hair may wish to let the hair grow so as to cover healing incisions/scars.

Conventional/classic forehead lift Patients may be told to shampoo with an antibacterial soap on the night or morning before surgery. Right before surgery, the hair is tied with rubber bands to keep it away from the proposed incision line, and hair growing directly in front of the line may be trimmed. The surgery is performed via a coronal incision, an incision just behind the hairline that frames the forehead, beginning at ear level on one side of the face, running up and across the forehead and down the other side so that the scar will not be visible once the incision heals and the hair grows back. If the hairline is naturally high or receding, the incision is done right at the hairline. For patients who are bald, the incision is at midscalp, following the line formed by the natural fusion of the skull bones.

In either case, the surgeon lifts the skin of the forehead to separate it from the tissues underneath. He then tightens or loosens the muscles needed to produce a smooth appearance, removes excess tissue along the line of the incision, and closes the incision with sutures or surgical clips or staples. Finally, he removes the rubber bands holding the hair back and washes the area. Some physicians leave the incision uncovered; others cover it with gauze and an elastic bandage to reduce swelling.

Endoscopic forehead lift The surgeon makes several short incisions, each less than an inch long, just behind the hairline framing the forehead, and inserts an endoscope, a thin flexible tube with a camera that transmits a clear view of the tissue under the skin to a television monitor. The surgeon inserts a thin tube called a cannula through one of the other incisions, lifts the skin away from the underlying tissues, and tightens or loosens muscles as required to smooth the surface. At the same time, the eyebrows may be lifted and fixed in position with sutures or temporary or "permanent" screws. The temporary screws are removed after two weeks; "permanent" screws eventually absorbed into the body. The incisions along the hairline are closed, the area is washed, and a bandage may be applied.

Alternatively, the surgeon may perform a thread lift, inserting special surgical thread through the incisions at the hairline, pulling the threads tight and securing them to tiny hooklike anchors to lift the brow. This procedure is done with local anesthetic; the patient is awake and able to observe the change in appearance as the threads are tightened.

Risks and Complications

Swelling, bruising, and mild discomfort are commonly less severe after an endoscopic forehead lift than after a conventional/classic forehead lift. Bandages are removed within two days after surgery; sutures/staples, at the end of a week; temporary screws, after two weeks. Swelling usually disappears within two weeks, but as the incision heals, the skin may begin to itch; the itching may last as long several months until the wound is completely healed.

Numbness along the incision is also common. Occasionally the loss of sensation may be permanent due to nerve damage during surgery. Damage to the nerves controlling movement of the eyebrows may interfere with the ability to lift the eyebrows or wrinkle the forehead.

Outlook and Lifestyle Modifications

Patients may resume showering and shampooing a day or so after surgery (or when the bandage is removed). Vigorous physical work such as bending, jogging, lifting heavy objects, or any activity that raises blood pressure should be limited for several weeks or as directed by the physician. Prolonged exposure to heat or direct sunlight should be limited for several months.

Hair around the incision may be temporarily thinner for several weeks, but normal hair growth soon resumes. Rarely, a patient may require fol-

low-up surgery to repair nerve tissue or reduce a wider-than-normal scar that may be corrected with additional surgery.

See also FACIAL REANIMATION; SCAR REVISION.

foreskin replacement Circumcision reversal; creation of a substitute glans (the skin covering the tip of the penis) that is removed at circumcision.

Procedures

There are two basic methods for recreating the foreskin, surgical and nonsurgical.

Surgical re-creation of the foreskin The surgeon makes an incision around the base of the penis, degloves the penis (pulls the skin down to cover the tip), then covers the area of the penis from which the skin has been taken with a skin graft, most commonly from the scrotum.

A second option is to use a flap of skin from the scrotal sac as a second layer to create a "folded," natural-looking foreskin. This surgery is performed in several stages. First, the flap of penile skin is pulled down and placed over the tip of the penis, as described above. At the same time, a flap of scrotal skin is lifted from the scrotum and wrapped around the penis; the scrotal skin is left attached to the scrotum by two stalks (pedicles) that maintain a blood supply to the flap. After several months, when this first surgery has healed and the flaps have grown into place at the tip of the penis, the stalks of the scrotal flap are cut loose from the scrotum, and the ends of the scrotal flap are stitched in place at the end of the penis. When this second surgery has healed and the new foreskin is anchored in place with its own new blood supply, any apparent cosmetic defects will be corrected to ensure a natural look.

Nonsurgical re-creation of the foreskin The physician attaches weights and straps to the skin of the penis to tug on the skin and stretch it sufficiently to form a fold large enough to cover the tip of the penis. The procedure is painless; the patient can remove the devices as necessary (as for sexual intercourse) and replace them afterward. The stretched skin is permanently lengthened; it will not shrink back when the devices are finally removed.

Risks and Complications

Surgery to re-create the foreskin may cause temporary discomfort and swelling, as well as a slight difference in the color and texture of the natural skin versus the replacement. Like any surgery, this also carries a risk of infection and scars.

Stretching the penile skin is a slow, gradual procedure that may take as long as a year to complete, during which time many patients experience skin irritation and mild discomfort.

Outlook and Lifestyle Modifications

The benefit of foreskin replacement is that covering the tip of the penis keeps it moist, which may improve sexual stimulation, and, by reducing direct contact at the tip, may lessen the incidence of premature ejaculation. However, unlike the original foreskin, the new one does not have the specialized nerve endings, muscles, and blood vessels that transmit sensation during sexual intercourse.

forked tongue   See TONGUE SPLITTING.

freckle   See KERATOSIS.

free nipple graft   A plastic surgery technique used in surgical reduction of very large breasts.

Procedure

The surgeon lifts the nipple and areola free of the breast, trims away excess skin and underlying tissue, reconfigures the breast, and sutures the nipple and areola tissue into the appropriate place.

Risks and Complications

Transplanted tissue may fail to grow properly into place.

Outlook and Lifestyle Modifications

Successful surgery results in smaller breasts with normal nipple/areola.

See also BREAST REDUCTION.

free tissue transfer   See SKIN FLAPS.

freeze-dried graft   See BONE REPLACEMENT; SKIN GRAFT.

frost   See CHEMICAL SKIN PEEL.

frostbite   Skin damage caused by exposure to extreme cold, most commonly on the face (nose, ears, chin), the fingers, and the toes. In severe cases, PLASTIC SURGERY may be required to repair skin damage and/or loss of fingers and/or toes.

Symptoms and Diagnostic Path

Extreme cold causes ice crystals to form in the skin tissue and constricts blood vessels, reducing the flow of blood to the area. The skin reddens, then pales to a gray-blue color. The affected area is cold, tingling, painful, and then goes numb.

If blood flow is not restored, the chilled tissue dies. In severe cases, gangrene (death of skin and underlying tissues) requires removal of the frostbitten area/part in order to preserve the adjacent healthy tissue.

The condition is clearly visible on physical examination.

Treatment Options and Outlook

The first aim of treatment for frostbite is to warm the victim and the affected parts in order to prevent tissue death that may lead to the loss of the exposed areas or body parts. Safe warming is accomplished by either applying warm dressings or by immersing body parts such as hands and feet, fingers and toes, in warm water until the skin feels soft and the victim has regained sensation. The temperature of the water and/or the dressing should not exceed 108°F or 60°C.

If the frostbite cannot be reversed, the affected skin and/or body part must be removed to prevent infection and/or gangrene's spreading to healthy tissue. Plastic surgery may be required to repair skin damage and/or loss of fingers and/or toes.

full abdominoplasty   See ABDOMINOPLASTY.

full circumference liposuction   See BUTTOCK LIFT; LIPOSUCTION; THIGH LIFT.

full thickness   Describing a piece of skin or an injury that includes the entire epidermis (top layer of skin cells) and the entire dermis (layer of skin cells immediately under the epidermis). For example, a full thickness (third-degree) burn is an injury that destroys the entire epidermis and dermis. A full thickness skin flap and a full thickness skin graft are pieces of skin that include the entire epidermis and dermis. Full thickness skin necrosis is the destruction (death) of both the epidermal and dermal layers of skin, a possible complication of a LIPOSUCTION during which blood vessels supplying the area are damaged.

See also BURNS AND BURN RECONSTRUCTION; SKIN FLAP; SKIN GRAFT.

fused fingers   See POLYDACTYLY.

Galvanic current Direct current (DC), a form of electricity named for Italian physician/biologist/anatomist Luigi Galvani (1737–98), who discovered that stimulation with an electrical current causes muscles to contract. Galvanic current is used in electrolysis, a procedure to obliterate hair follicles so as to prevent hair growth. It is also used in a cosmetic procedure known as a nonsurgical or noninvasive face-lift, during which the facial muscles are stimulated with a mild electrical current in an attempt to exercise and tighten the muscles so as to lift sagging skin and/or erase wrinkles. While electrolysis is an effective method of hair removal, there is no evidence that the noninvasive face-lift produces any measurable, valuable change in appearance.

See also ELECTROLYSIS; NONSURGICAL FACE-LIFT.

gel-filled implant See BREAST RECONSTRUCTION.

genetics The scientific discipline that deals with heredity and the transmission of inherited characteristics via chromosomes and genes. Genetics determines "family history," the characteristics shared by closely related individuals. A family medical history or medical family tree is a record of illnesses among family members that documents the relationship between each member of your family. Understanding this can help you and your doctor spot patterns of specific conditions and diseases among family members.

The study of genetics is important to PLASTIC SURGERY because many of the defects corrected by plastic surgery are inherited, such as the shape of the face and body, as well as specific birth defects such as CLEFT LIP AND/OR PALATE that are repaired by plastic surgery.

These defects can be determined by a single gene with the power to transmit an inherited trait, known as a dominant trait. A dominant gene and a dominant trait are the opposites of a recessive gene and a recessive trait. To inherit a recessive trait, an individual must receive two affected genes, one from each parent. Clubbing of the fingers and toes is an example of a dominant trait. Albinism (the absence of normal pigmented cells in skin and hair) and DUPUYTREN'S CONTRACTURE are examples of recessive traits.

The terms *X-linked condition* and *Y-linked condition* describe a trait or an inherited medical condition associated either with a gene on the Y (male) or X (female) chromosome, or with a change in the structure of the X or Y chromosome, or with the presence of an extra X or Y chromosome. Rarely, the effects of some of these traits or conditions can be ameliorated by plastic surgery; most commonly, they cannot.

genioplasty See CHIN RECONSTRUCTION.

glabellar furrows See WRINKLES.

glansplasty PLASTIC SURGERY on the tip (glans) of the penis, most commonly to repair a congenital defect in which the external opening of the urethra is on top (epispadias) or on the bottom (hypospadias) of the penis rather than at the tip. The surgery constructs a more natural penis with the urethral opening at the tip so that the patient can urinate while standing.

Procedure

Once the patient is anesthetized, the surgeon lifts the skin from the top or bottom of the penis and cuts away any fibrous tissue that holds the penis in a curved position. He then extends the urethra to the tip of the penis either by stretching the urethra or by extending the urethra with tubular flaps or grafts of scrotal tissue. Next, the surgeon reconfigures the tip of the penis to create a natural cone shape. When the procedure is done, the surgeon inserts a drainage tube into the bladder to allow urine to flow as the incisions heal.

Risks and Complications

Common complications such as local swelling and minor bleeding are usually controlled with cold and/or compressive dressings. More serious complications may require surgical correction. These complications include, but may not be limited to

- a fistula, an abnormal opening in the skin
- a urethral stricture, a narrowing of the urethra that obstructs the flow of urine and leads to the creation of diverticula (pouches) in the wall of the urethra
- the accidental inclusion of irritating hair-bearing skin in the tissues used to lengthen the urethra

Outlook and Lifestyle Modifications

Successful glansplasty creates a fully functioning penis.

Glogau Photoaging Classification   A system created by San Francisco dermatopathologist Richard Glogau to categorize the amount of damage caused to facial skin by exposure to ULTRAVIOLET LIGHT, such as sunlight.

Glogau Type I describes a person with early light-related damage such as mild changes in pigment but no KERATOSIS (a wartlike growth caused by sunlight) or WRINKLES. The skin looks healthy and attractive with little or no makeup.

Glogau Type II describes a person whose skin wrinkles when he moves the muscles of the face to produce expressions such as a smile or a frown. Women with Glogau Type II skin are likely to use some foundation makeup to enhance the color and tone of the skin.

Glogau Type III describes a person whose skin is wrinkled even in repose. There are obvious changes in pigment, visible keratoses. Women with Glogau Type III skin usually use a heavy foundation makeup.

Glogau Type IV is heavily wrinkled skin, with yellow-gray discoloration, and (often) a history of skin cancers. When a woman with Glogau Type IV skin uses makeup, the makeup cakes in the wrinkles of the skin.

Plastic surgeons use the Glogau system as one guide when deciding which type of CHEMICAL SKIN PEEL will most effectively repair a patient's skin. For example, a superficial peel is considered sufficient for a patient with Glogau Type I skin; a deep peel may do more damage than good. Patients with Glogau Type II or Type III skin do well with a superficial or a medium peel. A patient with Glogau Type IV skin is a candidate for a deep peel.

See also FITZPATRICK SKIN TYPE CLASSIFICATION.

glutealplasty   See BUTTOCK LIFT.

gluteus muscles   Three-layer muscle stretching from the top of the pelvic bone to the femur, the long bone in the thigh. The top layer (gluteus maximus) stretches all the way from the pelvis to the femur; it is used to extend the hip and move the thigh backward. The second layer of the muscle (gluteus medius) and third layer of the muscle (gluteus minimus) also start at the top of the pelvic bone but stretch to the side of the femur; their function is to move the leg to the side, away from the body. Preserving the function and integrity of these muscles is important during PLASTIC SURGERY to reconfigure the buttocks.

See BUTTOCK LIFT.

glycolic acid peel   See CHEMICAL SKIN PEEL.

Gore-Tex™   See FILLERS.

graft   See BONE REPLACEMENT; NEUROPLASTY; SKIN GRAFT.

Gram-negative bacteria See GRAM STAIN.

Gram-positive bacteria See GRAM STAIN.

Gram stain Four-step laboratory procedure used to determine which antibiotics to use to treat infections, including an infection that may occur after PLASTIC SURGERY.

The test categorizes bacteria as Gram positive or Gram negative according to their reactions to a laboratory stain. The test was created by Danish physician Hans Christian Joachim Gram (1853–1938). The test is valuable because the two groups of bacteria react differently to specific antibiotics, enabling doctors to choose the drug most effective in treating a bacterial infection after surgery, including plastic surgery.

To run the test, first, the technician places a bacteria specimen on a slide and covers the slide completely with crystal violet, a purple pigment; after 60 seconds, the technician washes the slide with water, leaving a bluish purple sample on the slide. Second, the technician covers the slide with an iodine solution, lets it stand for 60 seconds, and again rinses the slide with water, leaving a specimen still bluish purple in color. Third, the technician adds ethanol (alcohol), one drop at a time, until the specimen is no longer bluish purple, and then rinses the slide with water. Fourth, the technician applies a safranin (a red dye) and lets the slide stand for one minute. At this point, positive bacteria are still bluish violet; Gram-negative bacteria turn pink.

growth factor(s) Protein(s) in the blood that stimulate cells to divide and reproduce. Growth factors are important in PLASTIC SURGERY because they play an important role in the proliferative stage of wound healing when the body builds new tissue after the injury of an incision. Transforming growth factor (TGF) stimulates the growth of keratin cells; epidermal growth factor (EGF), insulinlike growth factor (IGF), and platelet-derived growth factor (PDGF) stimulate the growth of connective tissue (collagen).

See also HEALING PROCESS.

gum reshaping Oral surgery to remove excess or infected gum tissue. It reduces the size of infected pockets around the teeth, thus lowering the risk of recurring infection that destroys bone around the teeth. It may also improve the patient's appearance by reducing a gummy smile, a condition in which the gums cover part of the teeth, making the teeth look shorter than normal.

Procedure

The surgery is commonly performed under local anesthesic by a periodontist (a dentist specializing in diseases of the gums). Depending on the condition and the amount of tissue to be cut away, the reshaping may be done as conventional surgery using a scalpel or with a laser. The latter removes excess tissue with minimum trauma and loss of blood.

Risks and Complications

Bleeding is common; infection is rare.

Outlook and Lifestyle Modifications

The cosmetic benefit of this surgery is a more attractive smile; the medical benefits include a tighter gum line, which is easier for the patient to keep clean and more resistant to infection. If periodontal disease progresses, the procedure may be repeated.

gynecomastia Nonmalignant enlargement of the male breast. True gynecomastia is enlargement due to an increase in glandular breast tissue triggered by an imbalance in the body's natural production of male and female hormones; pseudogynecomastia is enlargement due to an increase in fatty tissue; i.e., obesity.

Symptoms and Diagnostic Path

The identifying sign of gynecomastia is an enlarged male breast. A patient with weight-related breast enlargement is clearly overweight; a patient with hormone-related breast enlargement may show signs of feminization such as small/shrunken testicles, loss/lack of male pattern body hair, or feminine pattern of body fat (breast and hips) rather than the male pattern (shoulders and abdomen).

To determine whether the breast enlargement is hormone-related, the physician may order blood tests to show male and female hormone levels. If the hormone levels are abnormal and a clinical examination of the testicles and/or breast is inconclusive in identifying a tumor, the physician may order an ultrasound examination of the testicles and/or a mammogram and/or a chest/abdomen/pelvic X-ray or a CT-SCAN to locate a tumor in those areas.

Treatment Options and Outlook

The standard medical treatment for hormone-related gynecomastia in adults is testosterone replacement or estrogen suppression therapy; among adolescents, gynecomastia usually disappears on its own as hormone levels settle into a normal male pattern. The standard medical treatment for weight-related gynecomastia is weight loss.

Liposuction to remove fatty tissue or breast reduction surgery to remove fat, glandular tissue, and excess skin so as to firm and flatten the chest are options for patients whose gynecomastia is a family trait or does not resolve completely after hormone treatment or weight loss. Both procedures are most successful in younger men with firm skin. Neither is advised as a first step for men who are overweight and/or obese and have not yet tried exercise and/or weight loss diets.

Risk Factors and Preventive Measures

Pseudogynecomastia may run in families among members of the group whose body type is prone to overweight; controlling weight reduces the risk of breast enlargement.

Many cases of hormone-related gynecomastia occur without an identifiable trigger. However, the condition is most common among teenage boys or among older men taking hormones to suppress prostate cancer, or among men using steroids. Other risk factors for hormone-related gynecomastia include mumps (which damages the testicles), testicle injury, prescription estrogen drugs or beverage alcohol or phytoestrogens (estrogenlike substances in plant food, such as soy products) that increase the body's natural synthesis of the female hormone, or medicines that inhibit the body's natural synthesis of testosterone. Medical drugs that affect these hormone levels include, but are not limited to, some antifungal agents, antacids, anticancer drugs, antidepressants, blood pressure medication, and the recreational drugs heroin and marijuana.

See also BREAST REDUCTION; LIPOSUCTION.

hair Threadlike decorative protein (keratin) structures. Modern standards of beauty require fairly precise amounts of hair, making the presence of excess amounts of hair or the absence of sufficient quantities a factor in determining the necessity for a number of PLASTIC SURGERY procedures such as hair removal and hair transplants.

Human beings have three types of body hair. Lanugo, very fine hair covering the fetal body, is entirely shed right before or right after birth. Vellus hair is the short fine body hair found over most of the body with the exception of the lips, nipples, palms, soles of feet, external genital areas such as the membrane covering of the outer vaginal area, the navel, and scar tissue. Terminal hair is the thicker, darker body hair that appears under the arms and in the pubic area at puberty in response to the secretion of male hormones. Men, who secrete significantly more male hormones than do women, also develop terminal hair on chest, abdomen, legs, and arms.

Regardless of its site or type, each hair on the body arises from a hair follicle, a tube that opens on the skin and widens underneath into a bulb-shape matrix containing the blood vessels and nerves that nourish hair. Cells produced in the matrix continually divide and multiply, pushing older cells up toward the surface of the skin. In the process, the older cells die, hardening into a hair shaft composed of a cortex (outside of the shaft) made of overlapping flat colorless cells and a cuticle (inside of the shaft) made of protein and pigment cells whose color is an hereditary trait. Note: Coarse scalp hair has a second inner core called the medulla.

Hair growth occurs in a cycle with three distinct stages. The first stage is *anagen,* a period of active growth that starts as soon as a new hair begins to form and lasts from three to seven years. The second stage is *catagen,* a resting period of two to four weeks during which the follicle stops producing new hair cells. The third stage is *telogen,* a period of three to four months during which an old hair is shed and a new hair begins to grow in the hair follicle.

Hair growth is a continuous process. As human beings age, the cycle slows, leading naturally to excess hair loss and/or baldness. Other factors affecting the hair-growth cycle include some medical drugs, some illnesses, and some physical and emotional trauma. The list of medicines that affect hair growth includes (but is not limited to) anticoagulants (blood thinners), antidepressants, gout remedies, oral contraceptives, and drugs used in cancer chemotherapy, all of which interrupt the activity of all rapidly dividing cells, including healthy hair cells. Physical and emotional factors that affect hair growth include (but are not limited to) alopecia, serious injury or illness, an hormonal imbalance, diabetes, lupus, thyroid disease, or a fungal infection. Each of these factors may cause temporary excessive hair loss, presumably by interrupting the telogen phase of the hair-growth cycle.

See also HAIR LOSS; HAIR REMOVAL; HAIR REPLACEMENT SURGERY.

hairline incision See FACE-LIFT.

hair loss Alopecia; an autoimmune disorder in which the body's immune system attacks the hair follicles, the small pits in the skin from which hair grows, resulting in hair loss.

Symptoms and Diagnostic Path
Alopecia is diagnosed by its appearance and/or its link to a specific medical condition or medication.

Alopecia areata is the loss of hair in small, round areas of the scalp. *Alopecia capitis totalis, alopecia totalis,* or *alopecia universalis* is the complete loss of hair on scalp and face. *Alopecia congenitalis* is the absence of all hair at birth. *Alopecia hereditaria* (male-pattern baldness) is an inherited condition, caused by one dominant gene in men or two recessive genes in women. *Alopecia areata marginalis* is the loss of hair at the hairline. *Alopecia mediamentosa* is hair loss caused by a medicine such as those for cancer chemotherapy. *Alopecia senilis* is normal, age-related hair thinning or loss. *Scarring alopecia (cicatricial alopecia)* is hair loss due to scarring after an injury, commonly a burn.

Treatment Options and Outlook

Hair lost to *alopecia areata* may grow back and fall out several times; corticosteroids reduce the immune response and may encourage regrowth. Hair loss linked to a medicine or a medical condition may disappear when the patient is cured or stops using the medicine. Male-pattern baldness may be slowed by MINOXIDIL (Rogaine®) or FINASTERIDE (Propecia®), drugs that stimulate new hair growth.

Risk Factors and Preventive Measures

About 4 million Americans have alopecia. There is no link to gender, race, or ethnicity, but one in five people with *alopecia areata* have a close relative with the condition. On the other hand, most children with alopecia do not have a parent with alopecia; most parents with alopecia do not pass it on to their children. If one identical twin has alopecia, the odds that the other twin will have it are only slightly higher than 50 percent. Therefore, if alopecia is inherited, the culprit is likely to be a group of genes rather than just one.

See also HAIR.

hair plugs   See HAIR REPLACEMENT SURGERY.

hair removal   Nonmedical procedures or cosmetic surgery to remove excess, unwanted hair on body surfaces. Nonmedical over-the-counter hair-removal products produce temporary results.

PLASTIC SURGERY hair-removal techniques usually produce longer-lasting results; some remove hair permanently.

Nonmedical methods of depilation (removing the hair above the surface of the skin)   Shaving cuts hair right at the surface of the skin; it works best on the face, arms, underarms, and legs. Chemical depilatories dissolve the bonds that hold the cells in a hair together so that the hair can simply be washed away. Depilatory products are usually labeled for use on a specific part of the body. For example, a depilatory that is safe to use on the arms or legs may not be safe to use on the face or in the pubic area.

Nonmedical methods of epilation (removing the entire hair, including the root in the hair follicle beneath the skin)   Plucking is pulling out hair with a tweezer, one strand at a time. It is best used in areas where only a few hairs must be removed, as on the eyebrows or, for a woman, on the chin. Hot waxing, like plucking, pulls out excess hair, but from relatively large areas such as the leg. The benefit of hot waxing is that results last longer than shaving or chemical depilation; the downside is a risk of infection and the possibility that the process may leave stray hairs behind.

Brazilian waxing is a procedure performed by dermatologists or aestheticians to remove hair from the entire female genital area. The hair is clipped short, hot melted wax is applied, allowed to cool and harden, and then peeled away, pulling the hair with it. Possible adverse effects include redness, irritation (including later irritation caused by tight clothing), infection, sensitivity to heat, and permanent darkening of skin exposed to sunlight too soon after waxing.

Plastic surgery methods of hair removal   Exposure to high-intensity light such as a laser destroys hair down to the root, producing a relatively long-lasting smooth surface. The process may require more than one treatment, but it is safe to use on most areas of the body. Electrolysis, which can be used on all areas of the body, delivers a mild electrical charge that destroys the hair follicle so that the hair cannot grow back.

In 2000, the Food and Drug Administration (FDA) approved the sale of a nonprescription skin cream (Vaniqa®/eflornithine hydrochloride) that penetrates into the hair follicle, where it reduces the production of an enzyme that normally stimulates the growth of hair cells. Vaniqa does not remove hair; it is used along with a hair removal method to slow regrowth.

See also ELECTROLYSIS; GALVANIC CURRENT; HAIR; LASER.

hair replacement surgery PLASTIC SURGERY to reduce a bald area of the scalp and replace it with hair-bearing skin.

Procedures

There are three basic surgical methods used to remedy baldness. In order of increasing complexity, they are skin grafts, scalp expansion with SKIN FLAPS, and scalp reduction (scalp lift).

Skin grafts Hair replacement with SKIN GRAFTS is commonly done in a doctor's office or an outpatient surgery center, with LOCAL ANESTHESIC. The surgeon cuts the hair short on the area of the scalp from which the grafts will be taken and injects small amounts of a saline (saltwater) solution to keep the skin taut as the grafts are lifted with a small round punch or a scalpel. The number of grafts depends to some extent on their size. For example, on average the surgeon transplants from about 50 punch grafts to 700 mini- or micro-grafts per surgical session. The grafts are placed about one-eighth of an inch apart in the bald area of the scalp, positioned so that the new hair will grow in a natural pattern. Once the original grafts have healed, the open spaces will be filled in with additional grafts over a period of several months. When the enough grafts have been transplanted, the surgeon cleans the scalp and may cover it with gauze; occasionally a pressure bandage is used to reduce possible swelling. Note: The skin grafts used in hair replacement are usually named for their size and/or shape and/or number of individual hairs they provide. For example, micro-grafts have one to two hairs; mini-grafts have two to four hairs; punch grafts (hair plugs) are circular pieces of skin with 10 to 15 hairs. Linear slot grafts or slit grafts, with one to 10 hairs, are straight-edge pieces of skin sized to fit into small slits in the skin of the scalp. Strip grafts are relatively long straight pieces

of skin with 30 to 40 hairs. A linear slot graft is a strip of hair-bearing skin with a linear punch and cut to the graft size needed, usually one hair at the hairline, two to four hairs right behind that, and up to six hairs for fill-in.

Scalp expansion with skin flaps This multipart procedure is usually done in a hospital under general or local anesthesic. The first step is to implant a balloonlike tissue expander under hair-bearing skin on the scalp next to a bald area. Over a period of weeks, the expander is inflated with increasing amount of a saline (saltwater) solution to stretch and grow new skin. When enough new skin has formed, a second surgery is performed to remove the skin from a bald spot at the front of the scalp, lift a hair-bearing piece of skin from farther back on the scalp without completely detaching it, move the flap forward, and suture it into place at the front of the scalp. Because the flap is not completely detached from the scalp when moved forward, it maintains its original blood supply, increasing the possibility that it will settle successfully into the new site. The surgeon closes the incision; if bandages are used, they typically come off the following day; stitches are commonly removed after seven to 10 days. Note: The skin flap used in this surgery may carry as many hairs as nearly 400 punch grafts or 2,000 mini- or micro-grafts. A Dardour flap is one type of skin flap used in this procedure, introduced by French dermatologist/plastic surgeon Jean-Claude Dardour.

Scalp reduction This procedure, which is done in a hospital under general anesthesic, is used only for men or women with a sufficient amount of loose skin on the scalp. The surgeon begins by separating the bald area in the front of the scalp from the underlying tissues, lifting the bald skin and cutting it away. Then he loosens the hair-bearing skin farther back on the scalp and gently stretches the skin, along with its underlying tissue, forward to join hair-bearing areas on the top and side of the scalp, and closes the incisions. If bandages are used, they typically come off the following day; stitches are commonly removed after seven to 10 days.

Risks and Complications

Bruising, bleeding, and mild pain are possible. Complications specific to skin flaps and grafts include failure of the skin to implant successfully at its new location. Scalp reduction may cause a sensation of tightness at the incision; pain lasting several months; visible scarring due to tension on the incision; or nerve damage when the skin is lifted from the scalp and pulled forward.

In the first few weeks after hair replacement surgery with skin grafts, hairs growing on the grafted skin may fall out. If the graft has implanted successfully, new hair growth generally begins within two months, and the hair grows back at an average rate of about half an inch per month. If one or more grafts fail to implant and the skin dies, additional surgery is required to fill in the space. Small bumps at the site of surgical incisions for grafts and/or flaps can be removed surgically.

Occasionally, as the newly positioned scalp settles into place after scalp reduction, the skin may stretch and the bald area may grow bigger again, or there may be a line of hair-free skin on either side of the incision, or the hair may grow in an unusual direction.

Outlook and Lifestyle Modifications

After successful surgery, the patient should have a hairline that looks normal.

hair transplant   See HAIR REPLACEMENT SURGERY, SKIN GRAFTS.

hairy nevus   See MOLE.

halo nevus   See MELANOMA.

Halsted procedure   See MASTECTOMY.

hammer nose   See ROSACEA.

hand surgery   Reconstructive PLASTIC SURGERY to repair a congenital structural defect such as syndactyly (fused fingers) or to replace skin and underlying tissue damaged by an injury such as a burn or a fracture or to relieve discomfort due to a medical condition such as arthritis.

Procedure

Among the procedures used by plastic surgeons during hand surgery are tissue grafting to move healthy tissue (skin, bone, muscles, tendons, or nerves) from another part of the body to the site of an injury or defect; skin flaps to replace damaged skin with healthy skin from an adjacent area; and microsurgery to reattach an accidentally amputated finger or hand or replace an amputated finger with a toe. In some cases, such as severe burns, more than one surgery may be required.

Risks and Complications

As with other surgery, the possible complications include reactions to the anesthesic, bruising, swelling, bleeding and blood clots, infection, and nerve damage leading to loss of sensation or free hand movement.

Outlook and Lifestyle Modifications

Successful hand surgery, followed by a structured period of physical therapy, usually relieves pain and/or restores feeling and free movement to injured or defective hands.

See also ARTHRITIS; CARPAL TUNNEL SYNDROME; DUPUYTREN'S CONTRACTURE; FINGERS AND TOES, CONGENITAL STRUCTURAL DEFECTS; MICROSURGERY; REPLANTATION; SKIN FLAPS; SKIN GRAFTS.

hanging skin   When a person becomes severely obese, skin expands to accommodate large amounts of fat and underlying tissue. During years of obesity, the skin loses its natural ELASTICITY, and if the patient loses massive amounts of weight, he/she will be left with large areas of loose, sagging skin, most commonly on the abdomen, upper arms, buttocks, and thighs. The term used to describe this excess tissue is *hanging skin.*

Symptoms and Diagnostic Path

Hanging skin is clearly visible when the patient is examined.

Treatment Options and Outlook

The preparation for this surgery includes serious weight loss, which may be preceded by bariatric (weight loss) surgery to reduce the size of the stomach itself. Once the patient has lost a sufficient amount of weight, the surgeon may begin to schedule one or more surgeries to remove the hanging skin. These procedures, known collectively as *excess skin removal*, include (but are not limited to) such common cosmetic procedures such as ABDOMINOPLASTY, ARM LIFT, BUTTOCK LIFT, NECK LIFT, and THIGH LIFT.

In each case, once the patient is anesthetized, the surgeon makes an incision around the affected area and separates the excess skin and underlying tissue from the body, being careful to maintain and reconnect the blood vessels supplying the remaining tissue. When the surgery is finished, the wound is bandaged, usually with a COMPRESSION GARMENT to reduce the risk of blood clots and improve the final contour in the area, which will not be visible for several weeks or months.

Risk Factors and Preventive Measures

The only preventive measure is to maintain a normal weight and avoid obesity.

Hapsburg jaw Also called mandibular prognathism, this condition occurs with an extremely prominent lower jaw (mandible) and overdeveloped lower lip (Hapsburg lip), whose size increases with age. Occasionally the jaw is positioned so far forward that normal speech and eating are difficult. The inherited trait, due to one or more gene defects, is named for the Hapsburg family prominent in Spanish and Austrian/German royalty after the Renaissance and has been traced back to a Polish princess who married an Austrian Hapsburg early in the 15th century. The family trait, which may be ameliorated with chin reduction surgery via PLASTIC SURGERY to reduce the size of the chin/jaw, is gender neutral, occurring among both males and females in the family group.

See also CHIN RECONSTRUCTION.

harlequin deformity See FACIAL CLEFT.

healing process Multistage process by which the body repairs an injury by controlling bleeding, cleansing the wound, making new cells, and rebuilding tissue structures. This process applies to all injury, both accidental and deliberate; i.e., a surgical injury such as the incisions created during PLASTIC SURGERY.

First, the body releases vasoactive amines, natural chemicals that automatically constrict blood vessels so as to slow the loss of blood.

Next, small particles in blood called platelets clump together to form a clot that closes the wound. The platelets also release growth factors, natural chemicals that attract fibroblasts, the cells that produce fibrin, the threads that form a network to support the now-hardened clot (scab) over the wound. Under the scab, white blood cells called leukocytes flood into the site. The leukocytes engulf and clear away debris such as dead cells; at the same time, they release healing compounds such as growth factors and cytokines (the group of natural substances that includes interleukin-1). This continuing activity produces the characteristic redness, swelling, and heat of inflammation. At the same time, the fibrin network produces and supports new connective tissue, and the wound site fills with proteins such as keratin that are needed to form new skin cells. Nearby blood vessels sprout new branches to nourish the growing cells, a part of the healing process that may continue for up to a month.

The final phase of healing is remodeling, a series of changes that may go on for years. As collagen is created and degraded, the area of the wound becomes smaller. The body begins to produce specialized "connecting" cells called myofibroblasts that pull the edges of the wound together.

An injury such as a deep cut or burn or sore or a surgical incision that penetrates below the top layer of skin and damages the layers of connective tissue underneath leaves a permanent scar. The mark, red at first, eventually fades to white. If cells that produce skin color and hair have been destroyed, the scar will stay colorless and hairless. The severity of the scarring depends on the extent and site of the injury and individual characteristics such as the patient's skin color, the thickness of the skin, and the amount of connecting cells the body produces naturally. People who produce normal amounts of connecting cells develop flat scars at the level of the surrounding skin. People who produce less than normal amounts of connecting cells may develop an atrophic scar, flat tissue slightly below the level of the skin around it. People who produce excessive amounts of connecting cells may develop a hypertrophic scar, thickened tissue raised above the level of the surrounding skin. A raised, thickened scar that grows beyond the edges of the original wound is called a keloid.

See also BOTOX; CONNECTIVE TISSUE; INFLAMMATION; KELOID; SCAR REVISION; SKIN.

hemangioma An unusual grouping of dilated small blood vessels. A hemangioma on or near the surface of the skin is called a superficial hemangioma. A hemangioma in the deeper layers of the skin or in or on an internal organ is called a cavernous hemangioma. An angioma in channels of the lymph system is called lymphangioma. Hemangiomas on or in the skin may be present at birth or appear within a few months afterward. Examples of hemangiomas are the *naevus flammus neonatorum* (sometimes called an angel's kiss), a red birthmark that fades quickly, usually within a year after birth; and the *cherry hemangioma*, a bright red benign tumor composed of bunched blood vessels, ranging in size from a dot to a large raised bump. Cherry hemangiomas are also known as De Morgan's spots after Campbell De Morgan (1811–76), the British physician who identified them.

Cyrano nose, a nose reddened and swollen by a hemangioma, is a birth defect named for Savinien de Cyrano de Bergerac, the 17th-century French soldier, satirist, scholar, and dramatist whose skill with a sword and large nose were immortalized in Edmund Rostand's romantic drama *Cyrano de Bergerac* (1897).

Symptoms and Diagnostic Path

Superficial hemangiomas are diagnosed by simple physical examination. An internal cavernous hemangioma is diagnosed via a CT SCAN or an MRI, usually to determine the cause of unexplained internal bleeding.

Treatment Options and Outlook

Most hemangiomas are small, with no effect on a person's health. However, a hemangioma on the eyelid may interfere with the development of normal vision; a hemangioma near the nose or mouth makes it difficult for an infant to eat or breathe normally; and a large cavernous hemangioma, particularly an internal one, may bleed heavily or become infected.

Small superficial hemangiomas (sometimes called "strawberry spots") are usually left untreated and often fade or disappear naturally. If the hemangioma bleeds or is infected, irritated, or unattractive, it may be shaved off the skin with a surgical blade or destroyed with electrodesiccation, green light LASER, or cryotherapy. Slightly larger superficial hemangiomas may be removed with a laser. Injected steroids or yellow light lasers or a combination of the two may be used to shrink large hemangiomas on the eyelid to as to allow normal vision.

Risk Factors and Preventive Measures

Hemangiomas are birth defects; there is no known way to prevent them. The condition is equally common among men and women of all races, most frequently shows up in the 20s and 30s, and then becomes increasingly frequent with age.

hemifacial atrophy Progressive shrinking of the skin, underlying fat, muscle, connective tissue, and bone on one side of the face, most commonly on the left side. In rare cases, this condition spreads down the body to the tissues of the torso, including the internal organs, plus the arm and leg on the affected side. It may be accompanied by darkening of the skin, loss of facial hair, facial nerve pain, and/or seizures.

The disorder usually appears before age 10 and progresses over a period ranging from two to 10 years before stabilizing. Its course is uncertain; some patients have minimal damage; others suffer significant loss of appearance, strength, and sensitivity.

Symptoms and Diagnostic Path

The most common early sign of hemifacial atrophy is a painless cleft (opening) at or near the imaginary centerline dividing the two sides of the face or, more commonly, the forehead, along with a bluish tint to the skin on the affected side.

The damage due to hemifacial atrophy is evaluated via simple physical examination as well as radiological studies (CT-SCAN), which are also useful in establishing a treatment regimen.

Treatment Options and Outlook

There is no known cure for hemifacial atrophy; treatment focuses on reconstructive PLASTIC SURGERY and DENTISTRY to improve the facial structure and make it possible for the patient to speak clearly and eat easily. The techniques that may be used to rebuild the face include, but are not limited to, grafts of skin, fat, and bone from the patient's own body; and/or injections of body fat or liquid plastics (silicone); and/or prosthetic implants.

Risk Factors and Preventive Measures

Hemifacial atrophy, which occurs more frequently in females than in males, is a rare condition with no known cause. There is no known prevention.

hemifacial microsomia   Also called HM, OMENS syndrome; congenital defect characterized by underdevelopment of one side of the face, commonly one side of the lower half of the face. The severity of the condition is described by the OMENS classification, a system that measures the presence or absence of five specific defects

- *o*rbital asymmetry (unevenly placed eyes)
- *m*andibular hypoplasia (underdeveloped lower jaw)
- *e*ar deformity
- *n*erve involvement
- *s*oft tissue deficiency (lack of supporting tissue under the facial skin)

About one-third of children born with HM have problems on both sides of the face; in a significant minority of cases, the child also has other physical defects, a condition known as OMENS-Plus syndrome.

Symptoms and Diagnostic Path

As the child grows, the effects of HM are clearly visible, ranging from minor asymmetry such as one side of the lip higher than the other to severe underdevelopment such as a deformed or absent ear with damaged nerves and impaired hearing.

Treatment Options and Outlook

The most common PLASTIC SURGERY to repair the face is a single operation during which the surgeon rebuilds the lower jaw with bone taken from the patient's own body and repositions the chin toward the center of the face, thus repositioning the lip as well. Some surgeons prefer a technique called distraction, separating the bone of the lower jaw so as to stimulate the patient's body to produce new bone cells to fill the space. The drawback to this technique is that additional surgeries are required if the body does not produce enough new bone to fill the gap. Patients with additional defects, such as a partially or completely missing ear, will require additional reconstructive surgery.

Risk Factors and Preventive Measures

Hemifacial microsomia occurs in approximately one in every 3,000 to 5,000 live births, more frequently among boys than girls, and most commonly on the right side of the face. Parents with HM have a 3 percent chance of having a child with the condition. There are no known preventive measures.

See also OMENS.

h-flap incision   See SKIN FLAPS.

high-lateral-tension abdominoplasty   See ABDOMINOPLASTY; BUTTOCK LIFT; THIGH LIFT.

Hippocratic nails   See FINGERS AND TOES, CONGENITAL STRUCTURAL DEFECTS.

Hippocratic oath   At graduation, all American doctors, including plastic surgeons, recite some form of the oath commonly attributed to the ancient Greek physician Hippocrates, outlining a physician's responsibility to patients and the profession:

> I swear by Apollo Physician and Asclepius and Hygieia and Panaceia and all the gods and goddesses, making them my witnesses, that I will fulfill according to my ability and judgment this oath and this covenant:
>
> To hold him who has taught me this art as equal to my parents and to live my life in partnership with him, and if he is in need of money to give him a share of mine, and to regard his offspring as equal to my brothers in male lineage and to teach them this art—if they desire to learn it—without fee and covenant; to give a share of precepts and oral instruction and all the other learning to my sons and to the sons of him who has instructed me and to pupils who have signed the covenant and have taken an oath according to the medical law, but no one else.
>
> I will apply dietetic measures for the benefit of the sick according to my ability and judgment; I will keep them from harm and injustice. I will neither give a deadly drug to anybody who asked for it, nor will I make a suggestion to this effect. Similarly I will not give to a woman an abortive remedy. In purity and holiness I will guard my life and my art. I will not use the knife, not even on sufferers from stone, but will withdraw in favor of such men as are engaged in this work.
>
> Whatever houses I may visit, I will come for the benefit of the sick, remaining free of all intentional injustice, of all mischief and in particular of sexual relations with both female and male persons, be they free or slaves.
>
> What I may see or hear in the course of the treatment or even outside of the treatment in regard to the life of men, which on no account one must spread abroad, I will keep to myself, holding such things shameful to be spoken about.
>
> If I fulfill this oath and do not violate it, may it be granted to me to enjoy life and art, being honored with fame among all men for all time to come; if I transgress it and swear falsely, may the opposite of all this be my lot.
>
> (Source: Ludwig Edelstein, *The Hippocratic Oath: Text, Translation, and Interpretation.* Baltimore: Johns Hopkins Press, 1943.)

As the practice of medicine changed, so did the Hippocratic Oath. In 1948, following the Nuremberg Trials in which German doctors were found guilty of violating medical ethics in the Nazi concentration camps, the World Medical Association adopted the Declaration of Geneva.

The declaration lays out guidelines for ethical medical research and reemphasizes the physician's humanitarian responsibility to patients:

> I will remember that I do not treat a fever chart, a cancerous growth, but a sick human being, whose illness may affect the person's family and economic stability. My responsibility includes these related problems, if I am to care adequately for the sick.

Sixteen years later, Louis Lasagna (1923–2003), then academic dean of the School of Medicine at Tufts University, once again rewrote the oath, this time to counter what he described as a new tendency to treat diseases rather than patients. Today, Lasagna's oath is the one most commonly used in American medical schools:

> I swear to fulfill, to the best of my ability and judgment, this covenant:
>
> I will respect the hard-won scientific gains of those physicians in whose steps I walk, and gladly share such knowledge as is mine with those who are to follow.
>
> I will apply, for the benefit of the sick, all measures which are required, avoiding those twin traps of overtreatment and therapeutic nihilism.
>
> I will remember that there is art to medicine as well as science, and that warmth, sympathy, and understanding may outweigh the surgeon's knife or the chemist's drug.
>
> I will not be ashamed to say "I know not," nor will I fail to call in my colleagues when the skills of another are needed for a patient's recovery.
>
> I will respect the privacy of my patients, for their problems are not disclosed to me that the world may know. Most especially must I tread with care in matters of life and death. If it is given me to save a life, all thanks. But it may also be within my power to take a life; this awesome responsibility must be faced with great humbleness and awareness of my own frailty. Above all, I must not play at God.
>
> I will remember that I do not treat a fever chart, a cancerous growth, but a sick human being, whose illness may affect the person's family and economic stability. My responsibility includes these related problems, if I am to care adequately for the sick.
>
> I will prevent disease whenever I can, for prevention is preferable to cure.
>
> I will remember that I remain a member of society, with special obligations to all my fellow

human beings, those sound of mind and body as well as the infirm.

If I do not violate this oath, may I enjoy life and art, respected while I live and remembered with affection thereafter. May I always act so as to preserve the finest traditions of my calling and may I long experience the joy of healing those who seek my help.

hirsutism Hypertrichosis; growth of hair on face, chest, abdomen, back, and around the nipples in women, most commonly due to an excess production of the male hormone testosterone or to an inherited family trait.

Symptoms and Diagnostic Path

Hirsutism due to an inherited family trait usually appears naturally at puberty. Hirsutism due to a medical condition or drug appears abruptly later in life and may be accompanied by symptoms such as failure to menstruate, ACNE, deepening voice, male-pattern balding, an increase in muscle tissue, and an enlarged clitoris. The latter form of hirsutism is diagnosed via tests to determine blood levels of male hormones; very high levels of testosterone may indicate the presence of an ovarian or adrenal tumor that can be conclusively diagnosed via imaging studies such as a CT-SCAN.

Treatment Options and Outlook

Treatment depends on the cause. Hypertrichosis is treated with simple hair removal methods ranging from tweezing and shaving to chemical depilation to electrolysis and/or laser hair removal. Hormone-dependent hirsutism may respond to simple methods such as diet to reduce weight and lower hormone production, or it may require surgery to remove a tumor and/or antiandrogens or steroid drugs to reduce the secretion of male hormones or block their action.

Risk Factors and Preventive Measures

Hypertrichosis, a severe nonhormone-dependent form of hirsutism also known as "werewolf syndrome," may run in families, an inherited trait most common among white persons with dark skin, less common among African Americans, and least common among Asian and Native Americans.

The risk factors for hormone-dependent hirsutism in women include ovarian cancer, or cancer of the adrenal gland that increases the production of male hormones, or medicines that alter the body's natural hormonal balance, or the natural decrease in the secretion of estrogen at menopause.

hollow foot See CLUB FOOT.

holmium laser See LASER.

hound dog eyes See EYE LIFT.

HO:YAG laser See LASER.

Huger blood supply zones Areas of blood vessels in the abdomen, which must be taken into account when planning any abdominal plastic surgery to avoid damaging a patient's circulatory system. *Zone I*, directly over the rectus abdominus, the large muscle that controls the tilt of the pelvis, the curve of the spine, includes major arteries in the chest and abdomen. *Zone II*, on the back of the abdominal wall, includes arteries that supply the abdomen, the groin, and the legs. *Zone 3*, over the oblique muscles that sit on either side of the rectus abdominis, includes the arteries that supply the lower back. Because this area provides the skin for the flap most commonly used in abdominoplasty, plastic surgery in this area requires care to avoid damaging the blood supply.

See also ABDOMINOPLASTY.

Hutchinson freckle See MOLE.

hydrocolloid dressing Gel-based, nonstick material spread into a wound or imbedded in a wound cover that creates or maintains a moist environment and encourages the healing process by liquefying and removing dead tissue on the wound surface. Hydrogel sheets are gels in sheet form, some with an adhesive border. Gel filler is changed daily as are sheets without an adhesive border are changed; dressings with an adhesive border may be changed up to three times a week. They may be used in cosmetic or plastic surgery as in any other kind of medical treatment.

Hydroflex penile implant   See PENILE IMPLANTS.

hydroquinone   See SKIN BLEACHES/LIGHTENERS.

hyperhydrosis   Hyperhidrosis; excessive perspiration due either to oversensitive sweat glands or to a malfunction of the nerves producing excessive amounts of a chemical that triggers perspiration; the condition may be treated with Botox® injections similar to those used by plastic surgeons.

Symptoms and Diagnostic Path

The identifying sign of hyperhydrosis is excessive sweating, most commonly on the palms (palmar hyperhydrosis); other common sites are the armpits (axillary hyperhydrosis), the soles of the feet (plantar hyperhydrosis), and the face/head (craniofacial hyperhydrosis). Rarely, the entire body may be involved.

Blood tests may be used to rule out medical conditions such as thyroid disorders or diabetes sometimes linked to heavy sweating. If these are negative, a thermoregulatory sweat test is administered. The physician applies a moisture-sensitive powder to the skin. At room temperature, the powder changes color from yellow to dark purple on areas where the patient perspires. The patient then enters a cabinet where heat and humidity trigger sweating all over the body; patients with hyperhydrosis will produce even more sweat on the palms. Patients without hyperhydrosis do not sweat on the palms.

Treatment Options and Outlook

Medical treatment for moderate hyperhydrosis includes topical over-the-counter or stronger prescription aluminum hexahydrate, tannic acid, or formalin antiperspirants, oral antiperspirants, and antianxiety or antidepressant medications for those whose sweating is triggered by emotions. Surgery to remove some sweat glands or to sever the nerve pathways to the glands is the only permanent cure for severe hyperhydrosis.

In 2004 the U.S. Food and Drug Administration (FDA) approved the use of Botox injections to reduce excess underarm sweating by blocking the nerves that trigger the sweat glands. The treatment, which may require several injections, is not permanent, but in two large (600-patient) double-blind clinical trials, 91 percent of those given Botox had 50 percent less underarm sweating four weeks after the injections versus 36 percent of those who got placebo injections; another study showed the results lasting up to six months. As of this writing, the FDA has not approved the use of Botox injections to treat hyperhydrosis on other parts of the body.

Risk Factors and Preventive Measures

Hyperhydrosis, which is believed to affect as many as 8 million Americans, sometimes runs in families. There are no known specific risk factors or preventive measures.

See also BOTOX; HYPERPIGMENTATION/HYPOPIGMENTATION.

hyperpigmentation/hypopigmentation   Inherited or acquired darkening of the skin, usually in a small area, due to stimulation of melanocytes, cells in the skin that make melanin, a brown skin pigment. In PLASTIC SURGERY, temporary or permanent darkening may follow a chemical face peel, which can leave skin overly sensitive to sunlight. To prevent this, plastic surgeons usually recommend the use of sun blockers for a period of time after a peel.

The opposite condition, hypopigmentation is an inherited or acquired lack of pigment in the skin. The three most common types of hypopigmentation are albinism (an inherited recessive disorder), vitiligo (a skin condition caused by the destruction of pigment-producing skin cells), and postinflammatory hypopigmentation (loss of pigment due to an inflammatory skin disorder, an infection, or an injury such as a burn or a scar). Loss of pigmentation after some forms of plastic surgery, such as a CHEMICAL SKIN PEEL, may be permanent.

Symptoms and Diagnostic Path

To determine the cause of unexplained darkening (or lightening) of the skin, the doctor may perform a BIOPSY to examine skin cells or examine the skin with a Wood's lamp (an ULTRAVIOLET LIGHT that can detect fungal infections).

Treatment Options and Outlook

If the darkening is due to a disease, the doctor will treat the disease. If the darkening is benign, with no disease present, a nonprescrption skin bleach may be used to lighten the skin.

Risk Factors and Preventive Measures

Exposure to sunlight is a common trigger, as are fungal infections or an endocrine disorder such as Addison's disease. Certain medications such as antibiotics that increase sensitivity to sunlight can also cause hyperpigmentation. To avoid darkening after plastic surgery, patients are advised to avoid prolonged exposure to sunlight and to use sunscreens.

See also SKIN BLEACHES.

hypertrophic scar See KELOID.

hypospadias See GLANSPLASTY.

ice pack   See COLD PACK.

ice pick scar   Small, deep indentations, commonly on the cheeks, resembling the impression made by a thin pointed object such as an ice pick; the characteristic scar left by acne or chicken pox.

Ice pick scars are difficult to remove. Common techniques used to smooth the skin, such as a dermabrasion, may actually make these scars more visible. If the scars are highly visible, the surgeon may choose to remove them with a surgical punch, an instrument that cuts out a small, deep cylinder of tissue; the resulting wound is closed with stitches or a small skin graft. The wound cutomarily heals with no visible scar.

See also ACNE; DERMABRASION.

IL   See under IMMUNOTHERAPY.

iliac bone   Ilium; flat, flaring part of the hip bone, above the hip joint. The ilium is used as a donor site for grafts of the patient's own bone because it is easy to reach surgically and has a large amount of bone tissue available from either the front (anterior) or the back (posterior) side of the bone.

Tissue from the thinner anterior iliac bone is commonly used in surgery to reconstruct the curved bone of the lower jaw; if larger amounts of tissue are required, the graft is usually taken from the thicker posterior iliac bone.

Taking tissue from the front of the bone shortens the time required for surgery because the patient does not have to be turned during the operation and the bone graft can be removed from the hip as the recipient site is being prepared.

The iliac crest is the curved, thick top of the iliac bone, visible as the bulge of the pelvic bone just below the waist. An iliac crest bone flap is bone and tissue taken from the curved top of the hip bone. It is used most commonly to reconstruct the mandible, the curved bone of the lower jaw.

Harvesting iliac bone may cause bleeding, difficulty in walking, and/or paresthesia (unusual sensation) in the area around the hip, all of which become more likely the more muscle tissue is removed.

Ilizarov technique   See LIMB-LENGTH DISCREPANCY (LLD).

imaging   Noninvasive diagnostic techniques such as computerized axial tomography (CT), MAGNETIC RESONANCE IMAGING (MRI), pet-scan, ultrasound, and X-ray used to create a picture of internal structures. These images of bones, organs, and blood vessels are used to facilitate diagnosis and to plan treatments. In PLASTIC SURGERY, imaging gives the surgeon a blueprint for complicated procedures such as separating CONJOINED TWINS or repairing FACIAL CLEFTS.

The process of using diagnostic imaging to show sections of the body is called laminography. CT-SCANS and magnetic resonance imaging are examples of modern laminographic examinations.

See also X-RAY EXAMINATION.

immune system   Collective name for a group of organs, a circulatory system and specialized blood cells whose purpose is to identify, isolate, and destroy foreign organisms and substances in order to protect the body from infection and/or disease. A healthy immune system is vital to wound healing and thus vital to the success of any surgery, including PLASTIC SURGERY.

Cytokines are a key part of the immune system. These are proteins that manage immune responses, enable cells to send messages back and forth, and play a role in the production, growth, and development of new cells, as in wound healing.

Immunodeficiency is the failure of the immune system. Primary immunodeficiency is a condition arising from a defect in the immune system itself, for example, an inability to form specific disease-fighting cells. Secondary immunodeficiency is the condition arising from an illness (such as kidney disease) that damages a previously healthy immune system. An autoimmune disease is a condition characterized by tissue damage or loss of body function due to the action of cells from the body's own immune system.

A person whose immune system is not functioning properly is immunocompromised; for example, a viral infection such as HIV/AIDS may overwhelm the immune system, leaving a person immunocompromised, without the natural resources necessary to fight infection.

A substance that interferes with the function of the immune system is an immunosuppressant. For example, after an organ transplant, patients are given medications designed to depress the immune system and prevent the body from rejecting the new organ. These medicines may also be used to treat autoimmune conditions such as certain types of hair loss *(alopecia areata)*, Crohn's disease (chronic inflammation of the digestive tract), psoriasis, or rheumatoid ARTHRITIS, in which the body mistakenly attacks its own tissues. Some common immunosuppressants are azathioprine (Imuran®), cyclosporine (Neoral®, Sandimmune®, SangCya®, Thymoglobulin®), and tacrolimus (Prograf®). The primary complication associated with taking one of these drugs is an increased susceptibility to infection.

See also LYMPHATIC SYSTEM.

immunotherapy   Medical treatment that aims to alter the IMMUNE SYSTEM either to suppress its function so as to allow the body to accept foreign material such as tissue (bone or skin graft) transplanted during PLASTIC SURGERY or to increase its activity so as to ameliorate the effects of allergens, disable disease-causing microorganisms, or destroy malignant tumors.

Immunotherapy for allergies consists of injections of very small amounts of allergens that sensitize the patient's body, enabling it to produce protective antibodies. Immunotherapy for bacterial or viral infections exposes the patient to vaccines containing small amounts of live or dead microorganisms, such as the polio virus, enabling the body to produce antibodies to attack the microbe. Among nonmedical persons, the term *immunotherapy* is most commonly associated with a variety of proposed treatments for cancer, including cytokines (interferon and interleukin); monoclonal antibodies; and cancer vaccines.

Cytokines are proteins made naturally by white blood cells in response to infection or inflammation. The cytokine, interferon-alpha (IFN-alpha), was the first to demonstrate an ability to activate the immune system and slow the growth of malignant tumors. It is approved by the Food and Drug Administration (FDA) for treating several cancers, including the skin cancer melanoma and the blood cell cancers chronic myelogenous leukemia (CML), hairy cell leukemia, and multiple myeloma.

Another cytokine, interleukin-2 (IL-2) is used to treat kidney cancer and melanoma. Interleukins are groups of compounds synthesized and released by the immune system that enhance proliferation and response of immune system cells. For example, interleukin-2 (IL-2) also increases the production of T-cells and B-cells, immune system cells that fight infection.

Other cytokines, such as interferon-beta, are currently under investigation for their value as cancer treatments. The side effects of treatment with interferons and interleukins include a feeling of weakness and illness, with flulike symptoms. The severity of the reaction depends on the size of the dose.

Monoclonal antibodies (mABs) are artificial antibodies manufactured to target a specific biological substance such as a cancer cell or a cell associated with the production and/or growth of cancer cells, used in cancer diagnosis as well as treatment. Cells containing monoclonal antibodies can be injected to help treat certain cancers. For example, rituximab (Rituxan®) is used in treating non-Hodgkin's lymphoma, and trastuzumab (Herceptin®) is used for some breast cancers. Enhanced monoclonal antibodies linked to cytotoxic (cell-killing) drugs can be used to deliver the drug to specific cells. Until the monoclonal antibody reaches the cancer cell, its parts remain bound together. Once inside the cancer cell, the cytotoxic drug separates from the antibody and attacks the cancer cell. As a result, the cancer drug does not harm healthy tissue, thus reducing the incidence of the side effects of traditional chemotherapy.

Cancer vaccines are similar to other vaccines; they contain an antigen (in this case, cancer-related material) designed to stimulate the immune system to produce antibodies to attack body cells containing the antigen. Most cancer vaccines are still being tested in animals; one, targeting MELANOMA, appears to be the first one proven effective in stimulating a human immune system response to a specific cancer.

incision placement guidelines   Suggested patterns for surgical incisions, including the incisions made during PLASTIC SURGERY so as to minimize scarring. The three best-known systems are the Langer lines, the Kraissl lines, and the Borges lines.

The Langer incision lines, developed by Austrian anatomist Carl von Langer (1819–97), follow the anatomy of structures under the skin. The Kraissl lines, developed by Cornelius J. Kraissl (1902–99), parallel the lines of greatest tension in the skin. The Borges lines, developed by Alberto Facundo Borges (1919–), follow relaxed skin tension lines, the grooves in relaxed skin.

The Langer lines were created based on research with cadavers. The Borges lines and the Kraissl lines are based on research with living patients. Modern surgeons generally consider the Borges lines the best guide to surgery on the face and the Kraissl lines best for elective surgery on the body, because these two systems produce incisions that usually heal faster and form smaller scars.

Indian rhinoplasty   See PLASTIC SURGERY; RHINOPLASTY.

Indian rubber skin   See ELASTICITY.

inflammation   Normal body response to an infection or a sudden interruption in the flow of blood to tissues, as occurs during PLASTIC SURGERY when the skin is cut by an incision or tissue if transplanted from one part of the body to another.

The signs of inflammation are redness, swelling, heat, and pain. These reactions are triggered by the release of chemicals from leukocytes, immune system cells that attack infectious agents, clean up injured tissue, and start the healing process.

Untreated inflammation may damage or destroy healthy tissues. To prevent this, antibiotic medicines are used to relieve inflammation due to infection. Corticosteroids or nonsteroidal anti-inflammatories such as aspirin, ibuprofen (Advil®, et al.), or naproxyn (Naprosyn®) are used to relieve inflammation due to an autoimmune response, a condition such as rheumatoid ARTHRITIS in which a person's immune system mistakenly attacks his/her own body.

inflatable implant   See PENILE IMPLANT.

Integra® artificial skin   See under BURNS AND BURN RECONSTRUCTION.

intense pulsed light (IPL)   A tool similar to a LASER; the IPL instrument emits energy in the form of high-intensity light that is absorbed into chromophores (pigmented cells), where it is transformed into heat that erases coloring agents such as hemoglobin, the red pigment in red blood cells, and melanin, the brownish pigment in dark spots on the skin.

IPL, which does not damage cells in the top layers of the skin, is used by plastic surgeons to lighten or erase vascular irregularities such as very small VARICOSE VEINS ("spider veins") and PORT WINE

STAINS, as well as to lighten flat, pigmented birth-marks, freckles, hormone-related changes in skin color such as CHLOASMA ("mask of pregnancy"), and age-related "liver spots."

See also LASER SKIN RESURFACING.

intercostal nerve block   See ANESTHESIOLOGY.

interleukin   See IMMUNOTHERAPY.

intersex   Intersex conditions are disorders in which an individual may have the chromosomes of one gender and either incomplete internal organs and/or external genitals of that gender, or internal reproductive organs and/or external genitals of both genders.

True gender is determined by the presence of the sex chromosomes (two X chromosomes in a female or one X and one Y in a male), usually accompanied by fully formed characteristic external female or male genitalia (vagina or penis and scrotum) and internal reproductive organs (ovaries or testes). PLASTIC SURGERY procedures may be used to repair or construct the appropriate genitals.

The term *ambiguous genitals* describes external sexual organs whose gender is not readily apparent at birth. For example, a genetic female may be born with a clitoris large enough to resemble a penis, while a genetic male may be born with a penis small enough to be mistaken for a clitoris. Other forms of ambiguous genitals include the presence of both ovaries and testicles with external genitals that are neither clearly male nor female, or the presence of undescended testes with external female genitals.

Symptoms and Diagnostic Path
There are four basic categories of intersex conditions:

1. An individual with *46, XX Intersex* has female chromosomes but external genitals that appear male.
2. An individual with *46, XY Intersex* has male chromosomes but incompletely formed exter-nal male genitals that may appear female and incomplete, and abnormal or absent internal male reproductive organs (testes).
3. An individual with *true gonadal intersex* has either female chromosomes or male chromo-somes (or both) and both ovarian tissue and testicular tissue, either as one ovary and one testis or a single gland (ovotestis) with both kinds of tissue. (The word *hermaphrodite*, the classical term for an individual born with both male and female reproductive organs, is derived from Hermes, the Greek god of male sexuality, and Aphrodite, the goddess of female sexuality and love.)
4. An individual with *complex or undetermined inter-sex* has one of a variety of combinations of male and female chromosomes or a missing X chro-mosome or an extra copy of either the X or Y chromosome.

The most obvious symptoms of intersex con-ditions in newborns are ambiguous genitals, for example:

- a very small penis that looks like a clitoris
- an enlarged clitoris that looks like a penis
- an apparent scrotum that is really a partial fusion of the lips of the vagina
- undescended testes that are actually ovaries

Symptoms that appear later in life include the absence of puberty, delayed puberty, the appear-ance of male characteristics in a presumed female, or the appearance of female characteristics in a presumed male.

Laboratory tests to diagnose intersex condi-tions include an evaluation of the levels of male or female sex hormones and a definitive chromosome analysis to determine whether the individual is XX (female) or XY (male).

Physical examination, endoscopy, ultrasound, or an MRI may be used to determine the presence or absence of internal reproductive organs.

Treatment Options and Outlook
Previously, newborns with ambiguous genitals were assigned a gender as quickly as possible based

on external physical appearance. Because the male-to-female surgery was easier, most intersex newborns were surgically altered to female.

The introduction of tests to identify true chromosomal gender and the recognition that intersex conditions affect an individual's psychological health as well as his/her physical appearance and function have changed the treatment options. Today, surgery for intersex children is preceded by appropriate physical testing to ascertain gender and most commonly postponed until the child is old enough to participate in the surgical decisions.

Once the decision is made, any inappropriate internal reproductive organs are removed and reconstructive plastic surgery creates the appropriate external genitals.

Risk Factors and Preventive Measures

Both males and females produce male and female sex hormones; the difference between the genders lies in the ratio. A female produces more female sex hormones; a male, more male sex hormones. Therefore, while the risk factors for intersex conditions vary with the condition, a common cause is something that upsets the natural hormone balance.

46, XX intersex may be due to a female fetus's being exposed to excess amounts of male hormones during pregnancy, most commonly due to a congenital defect in the fetal adrenal gland, or to a pregnant woman's having a male hormone secreting tumor (usually an ovarian tumor). If the condition becomes obvious later in life, around puberty, it may be due to an insufficient production of aromatase, an enzyme required to convert male hormones to female hormones in a female body.

46, XY intersex may be due to a failure of the male fetus's adrenal glands to produce sufficient testosterone so that the testes fail to develop during pregnancy or because the fetus is deficient in enzymes required to make testosterone. Later in life, males born with normal testes may have insufficient amounts of 5-alpha-reductase, an enzyme required to convert testosterone to dihydrotestosterone (DHT), the form of the hormone required to sustain male sexual organs and function. Or the male body may produce a normal amount of male

sex hormones, but the hormones may not function properly.

The causes of true gonadal intersex and complex or undetermined intersex are unknown, although some animal studies suggest that the former may be linked to exposure to environmental chemicals such as pesticides.

See also GLANSPLASTY; PHALLOPLASTY; VAGINOPLASTY.

interval image   See POSTSURGICAL DEPRESSION.

intestinal substitution vaginoplasty   See VAGINOPLASTY.

intradermal nevus   See MOLES.

intraoral approach   Surgery on the cheek, chin (jaw), or nose performed through an incision inside the mouth, rather than through an incision in the skin of the face. For example, during PLASTIC SURGERY to round the cheek or enlarge the chin, the surgeon may insert an implant through an incision inside the mouth, thus avoiding a scar on the face. During surgery to straighten or enlarge or reduce the size of the nose, the surgeon may also work with an incision inside the mouth, again to reduce the external scarring.

See also CHEEK AUGMENTATION; CHIN RECONSTRUCTION; RHINOPLASTY.

intubation   In medicine, placing a tube into one of the body openings; most commonly into the nose or mouth, down through the larynx, and into the trachea (throat) to maintain a flow of air for a person who is anesthetized or unconscious and unable to breathe or cough on one's own.

If the patient is unconscious or under anesthesia during surgery, including PLASTIC SURGERY, the physician will use a laryngoscope, a viewing tube inserted into the larynx that separates the vocal cords and allows an easy entrance for the oxygen tube.

Rapid Sequence Induction (RSI) is an emergency procedure during which the doctor administers a short-acting narcotic and a drug such as succhinylcholine to paralyze and relax the muscles in the throat so that the tube can be inserted into a patient who is awake. An alternative for a conscious patient is the use of LOCAL ANESTHETIC plus a flexible endoscope (tube), a procedure that allows patients to breathe on their own while the breathing tube is inserted.

Tracheotomy is surgery to create an opening through the skin of the neck into the throat in order to insert a breathing tube for long-term use.

Needle cricothyrotomy (from the Greek *krikos*, meaning "ring," and *tome*, meaning "incision") is the insertion of a hollow needle through the skin of the neck and into the throat (in males, just below the Adam's apple) to maintain airflow in an emergency; later, when the patient reaches the hospital, a tracheotomy is performed if necessary.

involuntary nervous system   See under NERVOUS SYSTEM.

iodine (I)   Nonmetallic element; nutrient essential for thyroid function. In medicine, an iodine antiseptic solution such as alcohol-based tincture of iodine or water-based povidone-iodine is used as an antimicrobial agent effective to prevent infection from an injury. It is used in PLASTIC SURGERY when an incision is made to protect against a wide variety of organisms, including bacteria, fungi, protozoas (one-cell organisms), and viruses. Finally, iodine-123 is a component of radioactive compounds such used in diagnostic IMAGING.

Isolagen®   See FILLERS.

Italian rhinoplasty   See PLASTIC SURGERY; RHINOPLASTY.

J

janiceps CONJOINED TWINS attached at the head with their faces pointed in different directions, similar to the head of the Roman god Janus. *Janiceps asymmetros* is a set of conjoined twins with one full face and one only partially formed.

Other terms for twins joined at the head, a category accounting for approximately 2 percent of all conjoined twins, are syncephaly (from the Greek *syn*, meaning "together," and *cephalos*, meaning "head") and craniopagus (from the Greek *kranion*, meaning "skull," and *pagos*, meaning "joined"). If the twins are born with two fully formed heads and separate brains, neurosurgeons may be able to separate the twins; plastic surgeons must then repair and reconstruct the skulls.

To date, surgeries to separate twins joined at the head have produced mixed results, including the death of both twins, the death of one twin, or the suvival of both but with brain damage ranging from minor to disabling.

jaw Jaws; the maxilla (upper jaw) and the mandible (lower jaw); two large, curved bones that frame the mouth and serve as the base in to which the teeth are set.

The maxilla is a pair of bones (maxillae), one on each side of the face that fuse as the fetus develops, forming the bottom of the orbits (the circular bone around the eyes), the sides and bottom of the nasal cavity, the bone roof of the mouth, and the upper jaw. In the human skull, the maxillae abut the following eight separate cranial and facial bones:

- the frontal (forehead) bone
- the ethmoid bone (top of the orbit, side and top of the nasal cavity)
- the nasal bone (bridge of the nose)
- the lacrimal bone (side of the nose next to the eye)
- the cheekbone
- the inferior nasal concha (bone at the back of the nasal cavity)
- the palatine (palate) bone
- the vomer (small triangle at the base of the nose)

Like the maxilla, the mandible is composed of two bones that fuse during fetal development. Unlike the maxilla, which is fixed to the other bones of the skull, the mandible moves up and down and side to side powered by muscles connected to joints at each side of the face that connect the jawbone to the skull.

Plastic surgery on the jaw, also known as maxillofacial surgery, can repair defects such as a cleft lip and/or palate or a misalignment of the jaws that impedes chewing or speech or breathing. Plastic surgeons can also improve appearance, for example, by augmenting or reducing the size of the chin (the front edge of the lower jaw) or by reconstructing a jaw damaged by injury. Orthognathic ("straight jaw") surgery combines orthodontic treatment with jaw surgery.

See also CHIN LIFT; CHIN RECONSTRUCTION; CLEFT LIP/PALATE.

Jennings, Hal Bruce, Jr. (1915–) Pioneering American plastic surgeon whose career was spent in the U.S. Armed Services. Jennings worked in plastic and reconstructive surgery on casualties of World War II, trained with Vilray Papin Blair and James Barrett Brown, and served as the chief of the plastic surgery service at Walter Reed Army Hospital and as consultant to the U.S. surgeon general on plastic surgery. He left military service in Vietnam to be sworn in as U.S. deputy surgeon general in July 1969. The following October he became the first plastic surgeon to be named U.S. surgeon general (1969–73).

jersey finger Painful swelling coupled with an inability to flex the first joint of a finger caused by an injury to the tendon that occurs when trying to catch or grab something, such as a door handle. Jersey finger is a common sports injury that occurs when one player grabs another's jersey and the fingers are yanked and overextended. If no bones are broken, the treatment may be simple splinting of the finger. A broken bone or torn tendon is repaired surgically; if the skin is damaged or lost, PLASTIC SURGERY with SKIN GRAFTS or SKIN FLAPS may be required.

See also HAND SURGERY.

Jessner's peel An alcohol-based solution of salicylic acid (14 percent), lactic acid (14 percent), and resorcinol (14 percent) used alone or with trichloroacetic acid (TCA) for a medium-depth chemical skin peel to smooth skin damaged by the sun and/or to remove superficial ACNE scars or benign lesions such as actinic keratoses. Created by German-born American dermatologist Max Jessner (1887–1978) in 1950.

See also CHEMICAL SKIN PEEL.

Joseph, Jacques (Jakob Lewin Joseph) (1865–1934) Prussian-born Berlin-trained physician and the leading European plastic surgeon of his time, Joseph is commonly regarded as a founder of modern PLASTIC SURGERY and widely known for promoting the psychological benefits of cosmetic surgery. He coined the label *anti-dysplasia* for the desire for "normal" features. His first surgery, an ear pinning (see EAR PINBACK) (1896) on a boy who had refused to attend school because he was a subject of ridicule, won him praise from the Berlin Medical Society but cost him his job as assistant to a leading orthopedic surgeon who believed Joseph had put the practice

at risk with an unproven operation. He performed his first nose reduction surgery in 1898. He served as director of the Division of Facial Plastic Surgery of the Charite Hospital in Berlin during World War I and authored the classic textbook *Rhinoplasty and Other Facial Plastic Surgery.*

jowls Sagging pads of fat and fibrous tissue under the skin beneath the jaw, often associated with a sagging chin ("witch's chin"), most commonly due to age-related loss of skin ELASTICITY and/or stretching of facial ligaments and connective tissue.

Symptoms and Diagnostic Path

The fat pads are clearly visible, often along with creases running from the corner of the mouth down to the lower jaw.

Treatment Options and Outlook

Nonsurgical options such as exercise to tone the facial muscles rarely produce any noticeable result. Surgical options include LIPOSUCTION to remove some of the excess fat and/or injections to insert FILLER that smooths the creases. Alternatively, the plastic surgeon may tighten the skin with multiple small tucks along the jaw line or with a traditional face-lift. The face-lift gives a longer-lasting but not permanent remedy; eventually, the fat may return or the connective tissue will sag. Note: Removing too much tissue when correcting the jowls causes a caved-in appearance. If the error is caught while the surgery is under way, the surgeon will correct it immediately with a graft of tissue from the neck. If the error is not caught until the patient heals, a second surgery may be required.

Risk Factors and Preventive Measures

Jowls are a feature that may run in families. There are no preventive measures.

See also FACE-LIFT.

junctional nevus Benign, evenly pigmented brown-to-black spot located at the level of skin where the epidermis (top layers of skin cells) joins the dermis (lower layers of skin cells); occasional found inside the mouth, on the palate, or the gum tissue. Because a junctional nevus may convert to a MELANOMA (potentially fatal skin cancer), if the spot changes color or begins to grow, the surgeon may excise the tissue and send it for a BIOPSY.

Once removed, the junctional nevus will not grow back.

See also MOLES.

Juvederm™   See FILLERS.

Kazanjian, Varaztad Hovhannes (1879–1974) American plastic surgeon born in Armenia; known for his service as a reconstructive surgeon during World War I and subsequent development of techniques to repair facial injuries and deformities. A graduate of Harvard Dental School and Harvard Medical School, Kazanjian was the first professor of plastic surgery at the medical school and later the chief of the dental school's department of prosthetic dentistry. He authored more than 150 articles on plastic and reconstructive surgery of the face and jaws and coauthored *The Surgical Treatment of Facial Injuries,* a standard reference. One-time president of the American Association of Plastic Surgeons, the American Society of Maxillofacial Surgery, and the New England Society of Plastic and Reconstructive Surgery, he was also an honorary member of the British Association of Plastic Surgeons in London, the Royal College of Physicians and Surgeons in Glasgow, the Massachusetts Dental Society, the American Society of Plastic and Reconstructive Surgery, and the Academy of Oral Surgery.

keloid Thick, raised scar at the site of an injury, caused by an error in the normal healing process leading to the production of an excessive amount of connective tissue (collagen fibers), plentiful blood vessels, and a thickened top layer of skin. Keloids may be round, oval, or oblong with smooth edges or have clawlike fingers extending beyond the edges of the original wound.

An abnormal scar that does not extend beyond the edges of the original wound is known simply as a hypertrophic scar. A hypertrophic scar may develop after medium and deep chemical skin peels and is most common in people with dark skin (Fitzpatrick skin Types 5 and 6) but can develop in

patients with light skin (Fitzpatrick skin Types 1, 2, 3, and 4).

Symptoms and Diagnostic Path

Keloids are commonly diagnosed by their appearance: first red, then brownish, then pale. A BIOPSY may be used to confirm the characteristic pattern of collagen fibers and blood vessels.

Treatment Options and Outlook

Most keloids are simply a cosmetic problem. Some are painful or itchy. Large facial keloids may be disfiguring, and keloids over a joint may restrict movement.

The most common treatments for any keloid are specialized dressings, surgery, postsurgical medical therapies, and postsurgical radiation. The choice of treatment is determined by the size and location of the keloid, the patient's age and medical condition, and his/her response to previous treatment. Because keloids are likely to recur, the effectiveness of any therapy cannot be judged until a sufficient period of time (usually a year) has passed.

Specialized dressings An occlusive dressing is a bandage made of silicone or nonsilicone sheets to cover the keloid and keep it moist. Before the bandage is applied, the surgeon may apply Scarguard, a cream containing silicone, hydrocortisone (a steroid), and vitamin E, which may reduce existing scar tissue and prevent the formation of new scars. A pressure dressing is a device or garment (i.e., leggings) made of an adhesive or nonadhesive elastic fabric that compresses the scarred area, making it more difficult for collagen fibers to cling together, thus thinning the scar. As many as 70 percent of patients using an occlusive dressing show some improvement; as many as 60 percent using pressure dressing show up to 75 to 100 percent reduction in scarring.

Surgery Excisional surgery (cutting out the keloid) rarely prevents a new scar from forming at the site, but the surgeon can lower the risk of recurrence by adding postsurgical therapies such as a pressure dressing or injections of corticosteroids or interferon, or follow-up radiation therapy. LASER surgery is used to shrink blood vessels in the area of the keloid to reduce redness, thin the scar, and make the skin softer and more pliable. The most effective laser surgery is a procedure done with a pulsed dye laser (recurrence rate as low as 25 percent). The least effective is the ND:YAG laser (recurrence rate 53–100 percent). The most effective surgical treatment appears to be cryosurgery (*cryo*, meaning "cold") to freeze the keloid with liquid nitrogen, destroy skin cells, and reduce the scar. Its recurrence rate goes as low as 25 percent.

Postsurgical medical therapies Injecting corticosteroids into the lesion after cutting out a keloid lessens inflammation and reduces the production of the collagen fibers, thus lowering the risk of recurrence. Recent studies suggest that postsurgical injections of the immune system stimulator interferon or application of a skin cream containing the IMMUNE SYSTEM stimulator imiquimod may be even more successful at reducing tissue proliferation leading to thick scars. The possible side effects of corticosteroid injections include skin shrinkage at the site of the injection and/or a change in skin color; imiquimod may cause mild irritation and darkening of the skin.

Various laboratory studies suggest that the following drugs may also prove useful in blocking the formation of excess tissue leading to thick postsurgical scars:

- bleomycin and 5-FU (cancer drugs that inhibit with unregulated cell growth)
- retinoic acid (Retin-A), a form of vitamin A commonly used to flake off the top layers of skin
- tacrolimus and rapamycin (immune system modulators that inhibit the growth of connective tissue)
- verapamil (an antihypertensive that blocks the formation of collagen)

Postsurgical radiation Irradiating the site after surgical removal of a keloid strongly reduces the incidence of recurrence; however, the treatment remains controversial due to its potential to damage the skin.

Risk Factors and Preventive Measures

Keloids are most common among people with dark skin, least common among those with very light skin. They occur most frequently in people younger than 30; more commonly among young women than among young men, possibly due to a higher number of cosmetic surgical procedures such as ear piercing among females.

A tendency to forming keloids may be inherited as a dominant or a recessive trait, most commonly among people with BLOOD TYPE A and certain types of HLA/human leukocyte antigen.

Because the primary cause of keloids is a skin injury, people known to form keloids should avoid nonessential surgical procedures, such as skin piercing, tattoos, or unnecessary cosmetic plastic surgery, and should seek medical treatment for injurious skin conditions such as severe acne.

See also BLOOD TRANSFUSION; FITZPATRICK SKIN TYPE CLASSIFICATION; SCAR FORMATION; SCAR REVISION.

keratosis Small wartlike growth composed of skin cells containing keratin, the primary protein in skin cells. Seborrheic keratoses ("barnacles of aging") are benign slightly raised light brown spots that may turn thick, dark, and rough; they appear in adulthood. Actinic keratoses (also known as *Keratosis actinica, keratosis solaris, solar keratosis, keratosis senilis,* or *keratoma senile*) are small tan, pink, or red raised spots on the skin.

Keratoses, which are triggered by exposure to ultraviolet light, are the most common type of precancerous skin lesion. Up to 20 percent of all actinic keratoses progress to squamous skin cell cancers. Of these, those on the skin rarely spread to internal organs, but those on the lips (actinic cheilitis) are more likely to spread to other parts of the body. Early treatment with a variety of PLASTIC SURGERY techniques is used to remove both kinds of keratoses.

A mild form of keratosis is a freckle. This is a yellow or brown spot, usually on fair skin, commonly linked to exposure to sunlight. The number of freckles commonly increases as a person ages.

Symptoms and Diagnostic Path

Keratoses may itch, crust, peel, or bleed. They are diagnosed by their appearance; suspected malignancy in an actinic keratosis is diagnosed by BIOPSY.

Treatment Options and Outlook

The usual treatments for keratoses are surgery, topical medications, and photodynamic (light) therapy. The choice of treatment depends on the site and nature of the keratosis as well as the patient's age and general health.

Surgery Cryosurgery is the most common treatment for actinic keratosis. The surgeon sprays or paints on liquid nitrogen, freezing the lesion so that it shrinks, crusts, and eventually falls off. Cyosurgery may cause some temporary swelling at the site; dark-skinned patients may experience a permanent lightening at the site.

A second form of surgery is curettage and desiccation; the surgeon injects a LOCAL ANESTHETIC, shaves or scrapes a sample off the top of the lesion for a biopsy, removes the entire lesion with a sharp instrument, and cauterizes the site to dry it and stop the bleeding. This surgery may leave a scar.

A third form of surgery is laser surgery, using a carbon dioxide or erbium YAG laser to remove the epidermis (top layers of skin) and (if needed) reach into the dermis (underlying layers). Lasers are useful for removing lesions in hard-to-reach or narrow places, as well as on the face, scalp, and lips. Laser surgery may require a local anesthetic; it may scar or lighten the skin.

Topical preparations These medical and nonmedical creams, solutions, or gels are most commonly used to remove early lesions on the face, ears, and neck. Medications used in topical products include the anticancer drug 5-fluorouracil (5-FU) or the immune system stimulator imiquimod or hyaluronic acid (a lubricant that occurs naturally in joints) plus diclofenac (an anti-inflammatory drug). 5-FU may cause mild redness, swelling, and crusting to occur; all topical treatments may cause some temporary damage to the skin, but scarring is rare. Note: In very mild cases, the surgeon may simply apply trichloroacetic acid/TCA, the nonmedical agent used for CHEMICAL SKIN PEELS.

Photodynamic Therapy (PDT) The surgeon applies 5-aminolevulinic acid/5-ALA (a naturally occurring photosensitizer), then exposes the site to ultraviolet light, activating 5-ALA, which selectively destroys cells in the lesion without damaging the surrounding normal skin, although some temporary redness and swelling may occur.

Risk Factors and Preventive Measures

A tendency to form seborrheic keratoses may be inherited, but the single most important risk factor for developing actinic keratoses is repeated exposure to the sunlight. Other triggers include the ultraviolet light in artificial tanning devices, extensive exposure to X-rays, and exposure to certain industrial chemicals.

People with fair skin, light hair, and light-colored eyes are at highest risk for actinic keratoses, but even people with dark skin can develop actinic keratoses from unprotected exposure to the sun. People whose immune system has been compromised (perhaps by cancer chemotherapy, organ transplant, or AIDS) are also at higher risk. Because the damage due to sun exposure is cumulative, the incidence of actinic keratosis generally increases with age.

The best protection against ultraviolet light damage is to wear sunscreen and protective clothing during outdoor exposure in all weather: the ultraviolet rays in sunlight reach the ground through clouds and reflect off sand, snow, and water.

See also ULTRAVIOLET LIGHT.

KTP laser   See LASER.

K-wire   Kirschner wire; named for Martin Kirschner (1879–1942), the German surgeon who, in 1901, introduced the first minimally invasive surgery designed to anchor a broken bone, commonly in the spine or hand, so as preserve joints/limbs. K-wire is used in reconstructive plastic surgeries to hold broken bones in place; the use of the K-wire for this purpose is called K-wire fixation.

kyphosis   Also called buffalo hump, dowager hump, and humpback kyphosis. Curve in the spine, due to the vertebrae (bones of the spine) leaning forward, usually in the upper part of the back, forming a hump.

Symptoms and Diagnostic Path

Some mild curvature of the back is common, beginning in adolescence and affecting boys more often than girls. It is noted only if it changes the body's appearance, rounding the shoulders and bending the back. Mild kyphosis that does not produce symptoms may be detected in routine examination and confirmed by an X-ray showing the deformed vertebrae.

Treatment Options and Outlook

Treatment most often consists of wearing a spinal brace or sleeping on a rigid bed. In mild kyphosis, the spine may straighten slightly with treatment, but whether the treatment prevents the curve from worsening remains unclear. When the curvature is more severe, treatment may improve symptoms and prevent worsening. Rarely, despite treatment, the curvature progresses to the point where surgery is needed to straighten the spine.

Risk Factors and Preventive Measures

There are no risks associated with a spinal brace. If the condition must be treated with surgery, then the normal risks of undergoing a surgical procedure apply.

labiaplasty (labioplasty) PLASTIC SURGERY to reduce pain or discomfort during sexual intercourse, improve sexual function, and enhance appearance by reshaping the external female genitalia, the labia minora, the smaller inner lips of the vagina, and/or the labia majora, the larger outer lips.

The term *vaginal rejuvenation* is used to describe labiaplasty plus plastic surgery to tighten the muscles in the vaginal passage that have been stretched, most commonly by childbirth, and re-creation of the hymen (the thin membrane covering the vaginal opening of a woman who has not had sexual intercourse).

Procedures

The three basic types of labiaplasty are reduction labiaplasty, augmentation labiaplasty, and liposuction labioplasty. The surgery, performed on an outpatient basis with local anesthesic, usually takes from one to two hours.

Reduction labiaplasty This is surgery to trim excess tissue from labia minora stretched by child-bearing or natural aging. The procedure may be done via a standard surgery with an Iris scissors (an instrument that leaves an edge similar to the natural edge of the labia minora) or with a laser scalpel. The surgeon cuts away part of the top layer of the labia minora, retaining the underlying tissue, and closes the incisions.

Augmentation labiaplasty This two-step procedure is designed to rejuvenate aging labia. In step one, the surgeon uses LIPOSUCTION to remove and process fatty tissue from an area of the patient's body. In step two, the surgeon transplants the fatty tissue into the labia.

Liposuction labiaplasty This is surgery to remove excess fatty tissue from the labia majora and the pubic area so as to create a smoother, younger-looking appearance.

Risks and Complications

Swelling, bruising, bleeding, mild discomfort, and infection may occur. Regardless of the procedure, scarring is minimal because the incisions are hidden in the natural creases of the vaginal or pubic area. Bleeding is less common after laser surgery because the laser cauterizes (seals) blood vessels as it cuts.

Outlook and Lifestyle Modifications

Patients are commonly advised to avoid vaginal penetration for up to six weeks, but once the tissues have healed completely, intercourse is likely to be more comfortable than it was before the surgery. As the tissue swelling recedes, the difference in the labia will be apparent, but the final results will not be visible for several months.

laminography See CT-SCAN; IMAGING; MAGNETIC RESONANCE IMAGING (MRI).

laparoscopy A form of endoscopy; a minimally invasive diagnostic or surgical procedure originally used only by gastrointestinal, urological, or gynecological surgeons to view the organs in the abdominal cavity through a small incision in the skin and underlying tissue. Today, it is also used in PLASTIC SURGERY; for example, to see an abdominal surgical field or to harvest tissue, such as tissue from the omentum (a layer of fatty tissue under the skin of the abdomen) for grafting.

Procedure

Diagnostic laparoscopy identifies tumors, inflammation, and other medical conditions in the abdominal or pelvic organs, including the fallopian tubes, ovaries, uterus, small bowel, large bowel, appendix, liver, and gallbladder. Laparoscopic surgery remedies, repairs, or reconstructs conditions in these organs. Both are performed under general or local anesthesic in a hospital or outpatient facility.

The surgeon begins by making a small incision through the skin below the navel, introducing a gas (carbon dioxide) into the abdominal cavity to lift the wall of the abdomen so that the organs are clearly visible. The surgeon then inserts the laparoscope into the abdominal cavity through a small incision in the skin. The laparoscope is a narrow metal tube with its own light source and a channel that can accommodate a miniature television camera and instruments such as a surgical scalpel and/or scissors. If necessary, the surgeon will make additional incisions to accommodate other instruments for surgery.

When the procedure is finished, the surgeon removes the gas from the abdominal cavity; the small incisions are most commonly taped to heal without sutures.

Risks and Complications

The major risk during laparoscopy is organ puncture leading to uncontrolled bleeding or a spill of intestinal contents into the abdominal cavity. Both may require the surgeon to switch from closed (laparoscopic) surgery to open surgery through a conventional incision.

Other possible complications include infection and pain at the site of the incisions. The gas used during laparoscopy presses against the bladder; after surgery the patient may feel a repeated urge to urinate. The gas also irritates the diaphragm; the patient may feel pain there and at the shoulder, which share some nerves with the diaphragm.

Outlook and Lifestyle Modifications

Laparoscopy usually provides a clear diagnosis. As a general rule, laparoscopic surgery is less traumatic than open surgery. However, in some cases, such as surgery to remove a malignant tumor in the colon, laparoscopic surgery may take longer than an open procedure, requiring the patient to remain longer under anesthesic. For some patients, particularly the elderly, the risk of a long period of anesthesia may outweigh the advantages of minimally invasive surgery.

See also ENDOSCOPY; MINIMALLY INVASIVE SURGERY.

laser Acronym for *l*ight *a*mplification by the *s*timulated *e*mission of *r*adiation; a device that produces a powerful beam of light, releasing intense heat that can be used as a surgical instrument. The term *laser* was first used by Columbia University physics student Gordon Gould, who built the first optical laser in 1958. Hughes Research engineer Theodore A. T. Maiman created the first commercially produced laser in 1960. It drew energy from a synthetic ruby, a stone made of corundum plus chromium atoms. In cosmetic and PLASTIC SURGERY, ruby lasers have been used to remove body and facial hair and to fade explosive tattoos (marks on the skin caused by imbedded particles of material such as gunpowder) or abrasive tattoos (marks due to particles of road surfacing material imbedded when a passenger is thrown from a car during an automobile accident).

Physicist Ali Javan of the Massachusetts Institute of Technology created the first gas laser (helium and neon) in 1960. Physicists R. W. Hellwarth and F. J. McClung introduced Q-switching in 1962, and physicist C. Kumar N. Patel invented the first carbon dioxide laser while at the Massachusetts Institute of Technology in 1964.

Plastic surgeons frequently use lasers in procedures such as LASER SKIN RESURFACING (laserbrasion) to smooth the skin, lighten unusual pigmentation, or remove unwanted hair or to shrink very small VARICOSE VEINS, or as a surgical tool to shrink or remove certain tumors such as HEMANGIOMAS (tumors composed of blood vessels). Plastic surgeons may also use lasers during procedures to perform photocoagulation, a technique that seals blood vessels and stops bleeding; cancer surgeons use the same technique to treat some forms of cancer by ablating (destroying) blood vessels that would otherwise provide nourishment to a tumor.

How Lasers Work

Lasers generate energy by using light or electrical current to "excite" the molecules in a mineral or gas inside a chamber. When the chamber opens, the energy escapes as a beam of high-intensity light.

- A *continuous wave laser* releases energy as a steady beam of light.

- A *pulsed laser* releases energy as a single burst of light or a series of bursts. (Note: A computer-controlled pulsed gas laser is sometimes called an eximer laser.)

- A *Q-switched laser* releases energy in short (1,000,000,000th second) bursts of intense light that can heat tissue to a temperature over 300°F. Although the energy released by Q-switched lasers is potentially hazardous to the eyes and skin, Q-switched lasers designed to operate with light that is eye-safe are used in DENTISTRY to cut surfaces, such as those of teeth.

Energy Sources for Lasers

Solid state lasers draw their energy from minerals; gas lasers are powered by gases.

Solid state lasers This type of laser is commonly powered by gemstones or silver-colored metallic minerals known as "rare earth elements." The latter commonly occur in nature together with nonmetallic elements in compounds such as phosphates (rare earth elements plus phosphorus), carbonates (carbon), fluorides (fluorine), and silicates (silica). The list of rare earth elements includes cerium (Ce58), dysprosium (Dy), erbium (Er), europium (Eu), gadolinium (Gd), homium (Ho), lanthanum (La), lutetium (Lu), neodymium (Nd), praseodymium (Pr), promethium (Pm), samarium (Sm), scandium (Sc), terbium (Tb), thulium (Tm), ytterbium (Yb), and yttrium (Y). Common solid state lasers include:

- *Alexandrite laser* This is powered by a gemstone named in honor of the Russian czar Alexander II. Natural alexandrite is mined in Brazil, Myanmar, Rhodesia, Russia, and Sri Lanka; synthetic alexandrite is human-made. The color of both natural and synthetic alexandrite varies according to the light in which the gem is seen: red in natural light, green under a fluorescent bulb. Either way, the light is absorbed by melanin, the brown pigment in skin; alexandrite lasers are used to remove brown skin marks and/or tattoos without damaging the surrounding skin.

- *KTP laser* This is powered with potassium titanyl phosphate (KTiOPO4) crystals to produce a green light absorbed primarily by blood vessels in the skin. It is used to treat some vascular lesions and some light brown spots on the skin.

- *YAG (yttrium-aluminum-garnet) laser* This laser draws energy from a crystal containing the elements yttrium and aluminum plus garnet, a semiprecious stone. The YAG crystal may also contain one rare earth element: erbium (Er), a gray-silver metal identified by Swedish scientist Carl Mosander in 1843; holmium (Ho), a brown material discovered by Swedish chemist Per Theodor Cleve in 1879; or neodymium (Nd), a bright silvery highly reactive metal identified in 1885.

- *Er:YAG laser* This emits energy that is well absorbed by water. It penetrates very slightly into the skin where liquid in the skin cells lessens its heat, making it ideal for removing very thin layers of skin without damaging healthy tissue, erasing fine facial lines and wrinkles, light scars, and lightly pigmented spots. The ER:YAG laser is also as a drill to prepare dental cavities for filling.

- *HO:YAG laser* Also known as the "holmium laser" or the "infrared holmium YAG laser," this is used in laser thermal keratoplasty (LTK), heating the edge of the cornea to create tiny pits or depressions that shrink as they heal, reshaping the cornea (the transparent part of the outer wall of the eyeball) so as to correct mild to moderate far-sightedness or astigmatism. Because it transmits light through flexible fibers, the HO:YAG laser is frequently used in laparoscopic (minimally invasive) surgery; for example, to remove bone and CARTILAGE during arthroscopy (from the Greek *arthron*, meaning "joint," and *scopeo*, meaning "look at") for a damaged knee.

- *Nd:YAG laser* Also known as the Q-switched Nd: YAG laser, this emits two light beams, an invisible near-infrared light and a visible green light, both of which penetrate deeply enough into the body to coagulate tissue. The red light is used to remove deeply pigmented marks on the skin, including blue-black tattoos; the green light removes brown spots or red tattoos. The Nd:YAG laser is also used for hair removal and to correct cloudiness at the back of the capsule around the lens of the eye after the lens is removed during cataract surgery.

Gas lasers This type of laser produces a light beam by passing an electric current through gas; for example, a mixture of helium and neon. Common gas lasers used in plastic surgery include:

- *Argon laser* This laser is powered by argon (chemical symbol Ar), one of the "noble gases," a group of elements listed in Column VIIIA/Group 0 of the Periodic Table of the Elements. The others are helium (He), neon (Ne), krypton (Kr), xenon (Xe), radon (Rn), and ununoctium (Uuo). Argon lasers emit a blue green light easily absorbed by hemoglobin, the red pigment in red blood cells. Argon lasers are customarily used to treat blood vessel disorders such as hemangioma (tumor composed of blood vessels), rosacea (enlarged vessels on the nose and face), and spider veins (very small varicose veins).

- *CO_2 (carbon dioxide) laser* This is powered by solid CO_2. It emits a colorless light easily absorbed by water or water-bearing tissues such as skin and commonly employed to removed skin cancers, small areas of pigmented skin, or warts. Solid CO_2 is also used as a chemoexfoliant (a substance that causes the surface of the skin to peel) in a CHEMICAL SKIN PEEL.

The term *red light laser* refers to He-Ne (helium-neon) laser. The term *yellow light laser* refers to a pulsed dye laser or an argon laser, each of which emits a yellow light.

laserbrasion See LASER SKIN RESURFACING.

laser skin resurfacing Also called LASER facial resurfacing laserbrasion and facial rejuvenation; PLASTIC SURGERY that uses lasers to smooth the surface of the skin, usually facial skin. There are two types of laser skin resurfacing: ablative laser skin resurfacing and nonablative laser skin resurfacing.

Ablative laser skin resurfacing The carbon dioxide and ER:YAG (erbium: yttrium-aluminum-garnet) lasers used for this procedure damage cells on the surface of the skin, triggering the release of natural chemicals that reduce inflammation and the production of new collagen (connective tissue) and skin proteins. Ablative laser skin resurfacing is usually recommended to reduce moderate-to-severe lines in the skin and/or long-term sun damage. The treatment produces clear, significant changes in the skin; when the injury caused by the laser heals, the skin is usually smoother and often lighter in color. However, potential adverse effects include redness and swelling that last for several weeks, as well as temporary or permanent darkening of the skin and (infrequently) scarring.

Nonablative laser skin resurfacing The intense pulse light (IPL) and ND:YAG (neodyminium: yttrium-aluminum-garnet) lasers are nonablative; they do not damage cells on the surface of the skin. Instead, they appear to affect cells in the dermis, the second layer of skin, triggering a response similar to what occurs with ablative laser skin resurfacing. Nonablative skin resurfacing is most often recommended to repair slight changes in pigmentation or fine WRINKLES or spider veins. The procedure is less likely than ablative skin resurfacing to cause skin darkening, which means it can be used safely on patients with darker skin.

See also CHEMICAL SKIN PEEL; DERMABRASION; MICRODERMABRASION.

LASIK *Laser-Assisted In Situ Keratomileusis;* LASIK surgery corrects nearsighted, farsighted, and astigmatic vision by reshaping the cornea, a clear structure at the front of the eye that bends and focuses light to create an image on the retina at the back of the eye, a phenomenon called refraction. If the cornea and the eye are not perfectly shaped, the image they transmit is distorted. LASIK is designed to correct a medical condition, imperfectly shaped structures in the eye. However, because glasses or contact lenses can satisfactorily correct vision, some consider LASIK to be purely cosmetic surgery, done to eliminate the need to wear glasses.

Procedure

The surgeon numbs the patient's eye, cleans the surrounding area, positions an instrument called a lid speculum to hold the eyelids open, places a ring on the eye, and applies suction to lift the cornea. Using a knife called a microkeratome attached to the ring, the surgeon cuts a flap in the cornea, folds it back to expose the middle layer of the cornea (the stroma), and activates a computer-controlled pulsed gas LASER (an Eximer laser) to reshape the cornea by vaporizing part of the stroma. When sufficient tissue has been vaporized, the flap is replaced (without stitches), and the surgeon places a protective shield over the eye.

Note: In May 2006, researchers at the Mayo Clinic in Rochester, Minnesota, released data from a study comparing microkeratome LASIK with a completely bladeless procedure using lasers to cut the flap at the beginning of the surgery. The study included 20 patients, each underwent microkeratome surgery in one eye, and bladeless surgery in the other. Six months later, the results of bladeless surgery, measured by the patient's ability to read an eye chart, to distinguish bright objects from dark ones, and to see glare (as from a car's headlights), were the same as those for surgery done with the microkeratome.

Risks and Complications

During surgery, the most likely complications are failure to produce a flap long enough to allow the laser room to reach the stroma, a flap that comes free from the surface of the eye, or a "buttonhole," a small tear in the flap. In the first case, the surgeon will usually stop the surgery, wait several months, and then do the operation again. In the second case, because surgeons mark the cornea with ink prior to surgery, it may be possible to continue with the surgery and then simply put the flap in place along the guidelines; some surgeons, however, may choose to abort the surgery, let the flap heal, and then do the surgery again in several months. In the third case, the surgeon will stop the surgery, replace the flap with the "buttonhole," and allow it to heal for several months. If there is no scar-

ring, the surgeon may be able to eventually do the LASIK procedure. If there is scarring, there may be some loss of vision, and the surgeon may not be able to do the procedure.

After LASIK surgery, a patient's vision may be less acute than before, or he may have problems seeing in low light (loss of night vision), develop double vision, or see glare or halos around objects, a complication more common in people with large pupils. Other possible complications include temporary or permanent "dry eye" leading to discomfort and blurred vision; movement of the flap from its original position; and inflammation and/or infection.

LASIK was first approved for eye surgery in 1998; to date, no company has yet presented sufficient evidence for the Food and Drug Administration (FDA) to issue formal conclusions about the long-range safety or effectiveness of the procedure. As of this writing, LASIK is not approved for persons younger than 18, because the surgery is not considered advisable for individuals whose eyesight is changing; i.e., those requiring a new prescription for contact lenses or glasses in the past 12 months. LASIK may also not be a good choice for people with a history of "dry eye" (inability to produce sufficient amount of tears to moisten the eye), glaucoma, herpes infection in or around the eye, hypertension affecting the eye, keratoconus (thinning of the surface of the eye), an inflammation of the eye, or a previous eye injury or surgery.

Outlook and Lifestyle Modifications

To reduce the risk of infection, the patient may be advised to wait several weeks before applying makeup around the eye, at least a month or more before resuming strenuous sports activity, and several months before swimming or using hot tubs.

Immediately after LASIK, the clarity of vision may fluctuate; the results of LASIK may not be final for three to six months after surgery. Even after LASIK, farsighted individuals may continue to lose visual acuity as they grow older.

See also RADIAL KERATOTOMY.

Le Fort fracture classification See LE FORT PROCEDURE.

Le Fort procedure PLASTIC SURGERY to repair facial defects due to APERT'S SYNDROME, a congenital defect in which the bones in the top of the face (forehead and mideye) and those at the bottom of the face (jaws and chin) grow at a normal rate while those in the center (nose and cheeks) do not, creating a "dished in" face.

The procedure is named for French surgeon Rene Le Fort (1869–1951), whose studies on cadaver heads led to the classification of facial fractures as Le Fort Types I, II, and III. Le Fort Type I fracture goes through the top jaw above the roots of the teeth, separating the jaw and palate from the upper part of the face. Le Fort Type II fracture is similar to Type I but goes up the nose and into the bony socket around an eye. Le Fort Type III fracture completely separates the bone of the face from the cranium (the top of the skull).

Procedure

To correct this, the surgeon detaches the top facial bones from the bottom and fills in the area with bone grafts to create a more normal facial structure.

Risks and Complications

Common surgical complications include swelling, discomfort, and pain, and the risk of infection. More serious complications include damage to nerves and blood vessels, including damage to those of the eye, resulting in impaired vision or blindness.

Outlook and Lifestyle Modifications

A successful procedure gives the patient a normal appearance.

leg reshaping See BUTTOCK AUGMENTATION; BUTTOCK LIFT; CALF AUGMENTATION.

Lejour breast reduction See BREAST REDUCTION.

lentigo (lentigines) Freckle; benign, small, naturally occurring pigmented spot whose emergence may be triggered by exposure to ULTRAVIOLET LIGHT or as a consequence of a multisymptom genetic disorder.

Lentigo simplex (simple lentigo, juvenile lentigo), the most common form of lentigo, is a benign round or oval spot with jagged or smooth margins and evenly distributed brown or black pigmentation. It may be present at birth or appear later in childhood.

Solar lentigo (actinic lentigo, senile lentigo, sun spot, liver spot) is a benign, flat, wrinkled or depressed, tan-to-black spot triggered by exposure to natural ultraviolet light (sunlight). Tanning-bed lentigo is a benign spot triggered by exposure to artificial ultraviolet light; i.e., in tanning salons. Ink spot lentigo (reticulated black solar lentigo) is a benign, irregularly shaped, darkly pigmented spot occurring most commonly on sun-exposed skin among people of Celtic ancestry. PUVA lentigo is a pale brown spot triggered by exposure to ultraviolet light during long-term (up to five years) treatment for psoriasis. Radiation lentigo may follow exposure to extraordinarily high doses of radiation, as during the nuclear accident at Chernobyl.

Symptoms and Diagnostic Path

Lentigines are diagnosed by their appearance. If necessary, a BIOPSY can distinguish lentigines from malignant pigmented lesions such as melanoma. Lentigines linked to genetic conditions are diagnosed by identifying the underlying medical problem.

Treatment Options and Outlook

Skin bleaches may lighten the spots. Cryosurgery (freezing the lentigo with liquid nitrogen) and laser surgery are also effective, but continuing exposure to sunlight may lead to the appearance of new lentigines. For people with lentigines associated with genetic abnormalities, the outlook depends on the severity of the underlying condition.

Risk Factors and Preventive Measures

The single most important cause of lentigines is exposure to natural or artificial ultraviolet light, especially for people with light skin. Sunscreens and protective clothing can decrease the incidence and/or darkening of solar lentigines, tanning-bed lentigines, and ink-spot lentigines.

See also KERATOSIS; LASER; MELANOMA; PUVA; RADIATION.

Lewis blood type   See BLOOD TYPE.

limb-length discrepancy (LLD)   Condition in which one arm or leg is significantly shorter than the other due either to a normal variation between the two sides of the body, a birth defect, or a medical condition such as bone lost to a malignant tumor, or from an infection that develops after an injury such as a broken bone that destroys bone tissue.

Symptoms and Diagnostic Path
The variation in limb length is clear; X-ray pictures are used to show the exact nature of the discrepancy and enable the surgeon to plan reconstructive surgery.

Treatment Options and Outlook
Small differences in leg length (less than an inch) may be resolved with a prosthetic (an artificial extension for the limb) or an orthotic ("lift") in the shoe on the shorter leg. If the difference in limb length is more severe, LLD may be treated with reconstructive surgery to make the shorter limb longer (limb lengthening) or to make the longer limb shorter (limb shortening).

Limb lengthening   This is a reconstructive procedure usually reserved for cases in which the difference in limb length is greater than an inch. Cosmetic limb lengthening simply to increase height is rare due to the difficulty and possible complications of the surgery.

Immediate lengthening, also known as acute lengthening, is surgery to lengthen the bone in one step. Once the patient is anesthetized, the surgeon cuts the bone, moves the ends apart, inserts a bone transplant, and fixes the ends in place with a surgical screw or metal plate. She then inserts a bone-shape biodegradable structure (bioscaffold) to which new bones cells can cling as they fill in the space between the ends of the natural bone. Because the tissues (muscles, nerves, blood vessels) around the bone do not stretch very far, this

surgery is used only to achieve a small increase in bone length, for example in the bone in the lower arm from the elbow to the wrist.

Gradual lengthening increases the length of a bone slowly over a period of weeks or months. The original procedure for lengthening limbs is the Ilizarov technique created by Russian orthopedic surgeon Gavril Abramovitch Ilizarov (1921–92). This process requires a protective, supporting frame called the Ilizarov distractive device, also known as an external fixator. The surgeon builds the device by inserting thin wires through the skin into a bone, tying the protruding ends of the wires to metal rings circling the limb, and connecting these rings to other rings along the line of the bone. Once the frame is in place, the bone is surgically divided, preserving the outer layer with its nerves and blood vessels. Then the frame is gradually adjusted over a period of months, pulling the ends of the bone apart to encourage the growth of new bone tissue that will lengthen the affected bone, along with new soft tissue (skin, muscle, blood vessels).

In some cases, the surgeon may insert a metal rod into the bone. The rod reduces the risk of the new bone's breaking or bending when the external support is removed, but it increases the risk of bone infection. Ideally, the bone will grow one inch every 2.5 to three months, faster in children, slower in adults. Once the desired length is achieved and the surgeon determines that the bone has healed, the frame is removed. If necessary, the process can be repeated in several years. Note: An alternative to the use of the Ilizarov device is surgery to insert an expandable metal rod into either the femur (thighbone) or tibia (shin bone) and then make a small crack in the bone. As the patient moves his leg, the rod expands.

Limb shortening   The surgical steps in this procedure vary with the age of the patient. For adults, the surgeon makes an incision in the limb and removes a section of the bone to be shortened. She then joins the ends of the bone with a metal plate and surgical screws or inserts a surgical rod into the bone to hold it in place as it heals. For growing children, the aim is to stop or slow the activity at growth centers on the longer leg so that the shorter leg can catch up by the time the bones have reached adult length, usually in the middle of the teen years. Growth in the lower legs occurs primarily in the "growth plates" at each end of the long bones. To stop the growth, the surgeon makes multiple small incisions to drill into the bone and reposition a block of bone in the area to tie down the growth plate, a procedure called epiphyseodesis.

Common complications of surgery may include swelling, bruising, infection, and/or a reaction to the anesthesic. Complications specific to limb lengthening with an external fixator are infection, joint stiffness, and healing too fast or too slow. To reduce the risk of infection, the surgeon will instruct the patient in how to clean the wires and pins leading from the frame into the bone. Severe joint stiffness may interrupt the lengthening process; however, physical therapy can minimize the incidence of stiffness in the hip, knee, ankle, shoulder, elbow, and wrist. If the bone heals too quickly, the surgeon may need to break it again to continue the lengthening. On the other hand, if healing is too slow, the fixator may have to remain in place for a longer period of time or the surgeon may have to perform additional surgery to insert a bone graft.

Risk Factors and Preventive Measures

For some time after limb lengthening, the new bone is less dense and sturdy than the original bone, so the patient must adjust physical activity to reduce the risk of fracture. After limb shortening, the muscles in the limb may be weakened, requiring physical therapy. Limb shortening via epiphyseodesis is an irreversible procedure; the resulting adult height may be less than if the shorter leg had been lengthened rather than the longer leg shortened, and the adult body may appear too long for the legs.

limb lengthening   See LIMB-LENGTH DISCREPANCY (LLD).

limb shortening   See LIMB-LENGTH DISCREPANCY (LLD).

linear slot graft   See HAIR REPLACEMENT SURGERY.

lip augmentation   PLASTIC SURGERY to make the lips fuller and reduce age-related fine lines around the mouth by injecting or inserting a natural or synthetic biocompatible FILLER or synthetic implant, or with laser surgery.

Note: Before scheduling this procedure, the surgeon will test the patient for an allergic reaction to the various fillers. People with a history of allergic reactions, with a skin infection, or an inflammatory condition such as severe ACNE, are usually advised to postpone the augmentation.

Procedures

The surgeon cleans the area around the lips and numbs it with a LOCAL ANESTHETIC (commonly lidocaine).

Injections   The surgeon injects filler material into the lip. The products used for this procedure include an autologous transplant (fat or collagen harvested from the patient's own body); collagen processed from donated human cadaver or animal skin (e.g., Alloderm®, Autologen®, Dermalogen®, Fascian®, Zyderm®, Zyplast®); synthetic injectable gels (e.g., HylaForm®, Perlane®, Restylane®); and powdered calcium plus bone tissue (Radiance®).

Implants   The surgeon inserts the implant material through small incisions at the corners of the mouth, tunnels it through under the surface of the lip, trims the implant to fit the lip, and closes the incisions. The implants used for this procedure (Advanta®, Gore-Tex®, SoftForm®) are threads or tubes or solid structures made of expanded polytetrafluoro-ethylene (ePTFE). Depending on its construction, the implant ranges from very soft to slightly firm.

Laser surgery   The surgeon exposes the lip and/or surrounding area to a laser in order to stimulate collagen and elastic tissues under the skin; as the skin heals, the collagen and elastic tissues tighten. The result is a smoother, fuller lip.

Risks and Complications

General risks include temporary swelling, bruising, bleeding, and difficulty in chewing or brushing the teeth. An allergic reaction to the local anesthetic may occur with any procedure.

Complications specific to injected fillers may include an uneven lip, larger on one side than the other, or an allergic reaction to a synthetic material, or rejection of filler from human or animal donors. Complications specific to an implant may include an infection around the implant, an allergic reaction to the implant, or the implant's slipping out of place. Laser surgery may redden the skin, but the color fades within a few weeks.

Outlook and Lifestyle Modifications

For the first few days, the patient may be advised to sleep with his/her head elevated on two pillows. In most cases, the patient can return to normal activities within a day, and recovery is complete within a week, but to reduce the risk of injury to the lip, the surgeon may advise avoiding contact sports for up to two months.

Collagen injections feel and look natural, as do fat injections (occasionally injected fat may clump and look lumpy). Both collagen and fat are eventually absorbed into the body, collagen more quickly than fat. To maintain lip fullness, these injections must be repeated periodically.

Implants are considered semipermanent, meaning that they will remain in place unless surgically removed. Laser surgery is permanent.

See also LASER; LIP LIFT; LIP PLUMPER.

lipectomy See LIPOSUCTION.

lip lift PLASTIC SURGERY to make the upper lip look fuller by decreasing the distance between the bottom of the nose and the top of the lip.

Procedure

The one- to two-hour operation may be done under general anesthesic or local anesthesic plus sedation, usually at an outpatient surgery center. After administering the anesthesic, the surgeon makes an incision at one of three sites: at the base of the nose (subnasale or bullhorn incision), along the edge of the top of the upper lip (gull-wing incision), or inside the nose (lip suspension).

Incision at the base of the nose The surgeon makes the incision along the curves under the nostrils, lifts the skin and underlying tissue between nose and upper lip, and removes a strip of skin or skin and underlying fat and muscle under the nose. She then brings the top edge of the remaining tissue up closer to the nose, and sutures it in place, being careful to maintain the two peaks of the cupid's bow at the top of the upper lip.

Incision along the top of the upper lip The surgeon makes an incision along the vermilion border, the line where the red pink-red tissue of upper lip meets the skin above the lip. The surgeon then cuts away a strip of skin or skin and underlying fat and muscle above the lip. She then lifts the upper lip and sutures the edge of the upper lip to the bottom edge of the remaining skin closer to the nose, being careful to maintain the two peaks of the cupid's bow at the top of the upper lip.

Incisions inside the nose The surgeon makes several small incisions inside the nose and threads permanent sutures through the incisions and down to the inside of the upper lip, tying the sutures so that the lift is symmetrical on both sides of the upper lip. The incisions inside the nose are sutured closed; the holes where the sutures enter the inside of the lip will heal naturally without suturing and without visible scarring.

Risks and Complications

Temporary numbness, swelling, bruising, and difficulty chewing or speaking are common. Infection, blood clot at the site of the incision, or an allergic reaction to the anesthesic are possible. More serious complications may include permanent numbness due to nerve injury during surgery, scarring, or asymmetry of the lip.

Outlook and Lifestyle Modifications

For the first few days, the patient may be advised to sleep with his/her head elevated on two pillows. The normal recuperation period is about two weeks, but to reduce the risk of injury at the incisions, the surgeon may advise avoiding contact sports for up to two months.

The lip lift produces the most visible results for a patient with a very thin upper lip. As with other forms of face-lift, the results last five to 10 years, or until the natural age-related loss of skin elasticity occurs. The suspension surgery, with its supporting sutures, tends to give longer lasting results.

See also FACE-LIFT; LIP AUGMENTATION; LIP PLUMPER.

lip lines Radial wrinkles; age-related fine lines radiating outward on the skin around the lips. They are caused by the natural loss of elastin (elastic fibers) and collagen (connective tissue) and exacerbated by exposure to sunlight. Deep lines may be reduced with collagen injections, chemical peels, and/or laser treatments. They may also sometimes be corrected by dental prosthesis or changes in tooth or bit relationships. Superficial lines may be smoothed with glycolic acid exfoliants, cosmetic lotions that slough off the rough top layer of skin cells, or simple moisturizers. Sunscreens reduce the risk of sun damage.

See also FACE-LIFT; FACIAL AGING; WRINKLES.

lipoaspiration See LIPOSUCTION.

lipocontour See LIPOSUCTION.

lipofilling Minimally invasive surgery to round and smooth the face using grafts of fatty tissue from the patient's own body.

Procedure

The surgeon begins by performing LIPOSUCTION to remove fatty tissue from the patient's abdomen or buttocks. The tissue is processed, purified, and injected into the area around the jaw, and/or along the cheekbones, and/or in the folds around the mouth to restore the oval contours of the face and smooth WRINKLES. This surgery may be done as a stand-alone procedure or along with a more extensive face-lift.

Risks and Complications

Minor bruising, swelling, and discomfort may follow the procedure.

Outlook and Lifestyle Modifications

A successful procedure results in temporarily smoother facial appearance. The fat is eventually absorbed by the body, usually within six months. To maintain the round smoothness, the procedure must be repeated.

See also FACE-LIFT; FAT GRAFTING.

lipoplasty See LIPOSUCTION.

liposculpture See LIPOSUCTION.

liposuction Also called contouring. Surgical procedure to reshape the body by removing fat deposits under the skin, commonly at the abdomen, hips, buttocks, thighs, knees, upper arms, chin, and cheeks. Microliposuction is removal of fat from the face and/or neck. Spot liposuction is removal of fat from a very small area, such as the cheek. Full circumference liposuction reduces and smooths the thighs with liposuction performed through several incisions in a circle around the entire thigh.

Liposuction in a small area is generally performed with a LOCAL ANESTHETIC. For larger areas such as the abdomen, the surgeon may use a regional anesthetic, such as an epidural block (an injection that numbs the body from the abdomen down). If the patient is having several procedures at one time, the surgeon may administer general anesthetic to put the patient to sleep.

Procedures

Modern plastic surgery commonly uses one of three basic liposuction techniques

- tumescent liposuction
- external ultrasonic assisted liposuction (UAL)
- power assisted liposuction (PAL)

Tumescent liposuction The surgeon makes a small incision in the skin and inserts a cannula (a narrow tube attached to a vacuum pump or a large syringe). Through the cannula she injects saline (salt water) fluid with local anesthetics to make the fat swollen and firm (tumescent) while causing the blood vessels in the area to contract so as to reduce blood loss as the fatty tissue is removed.

Ultrasonic Assisted Liposuction (UAL) This procedure is essentially the same as tumescent liposuction except that the surgeon uses a metal probe or paddle to transmit ultrasonic energy and heat in an attempt to break down the cells in fatty tissue. For Internal UAL, the surgeon inserts a metal probe through the skin into the fatty tissue; for External UAL, the surgeon applies the metal paddle to the outside of the skin. These techniques do not improve the outcome of liposuction, and both may cause burns. The Food and Drug Administration (FDA) has never approved the use of UAL devices for liposuction.

Power Assisted Liposuction (PAL) For this procedure, the surgeon attaches the cannula to a mechanical device that makes the cannula spin or move quickly into and out of the incision. As of this writing, there is no firm proof that this technique produces better results than simple tumescent liposuction.

Note: Dry liposuction, wet liposuction, and super wet liposuction are outmoded liposuction techniques. The first did not use any injected solution of local anesthesic; the second used a moderate amount; the third used more, but less than for modern tumescent liposuction. All three procedures required general anesthetic; all produced significant blood loss.

Risks and Complications

There are many possible adverse effects associated with liposuction: infection, blood clots, excessive loss of fluids, excessive fluid accumulation, burns from the instruments, nerve damage, organ perforation by the moving cannula, and adverse reaction to the anesthesic or other medicines.

Tumescent liposuction is usually performed as an outpatient procedure with local anesthetic alone, eliminating the risks associated with general anesthesic. In addition, this technique cuts blood loss to a level as low as 1 percent of the fluid removed from the body, reducing the need for transfusions and the risk of blood clots.

Outlook and Lifestyle Modifications

The surgery should leave no more than a tiny scar where the cannula is inserted. Six weeks later, when the swelling subsides, the skin should look tighter and smoother.

lip plumper   Over-the-counter cosmetic product containing an ingredient designed to make the lips look fuller temporarily. Longer-lasting plumpness requires PLASTIC SURGERY, such as LIP AUGMENTATION or a LIP LIFT. There are three basic types of lip plumpers.

- One type contains ingredients such as caffeine, cinnamon oil, ginger oil, menthol, or peppermint oil that irritate the lips and make them swell slightly.
- A second type of lip plumper is made with retinol, a form of vitamin A that promises to smooth the lips and/or increase the production of collagen. This effect remains unproven.
- A third type of lip plumper simply provides a base to which lipstick clings. Repeated applications of lipstick over the base build several layers that last longer and make the lips look slightly fuller.

As with all cosmetics, lip plumpers may have different effects on different users depending on individual sensitivities to various ingredients. Some women find lip plumpers extremely irritating; others experience an allergic reaction to the plumpers, particularly to those that contain herbal oils.

lip reduction   Cheiloplasty; PLASTIC SURGERY to ameliorate macrochelia, unusually large, prominent lips. It is a 15- to 30-minute procedure, usually done on an outpatient basis with regional or LOCAL ANESTHESIC, with or without sedation. In some cases, nonsurgical treatment may reduce prominent lips. For example, steroid drugs may reduce swelling due to a medical condition, while orthodontics can reduce lips pushed outward by crooked teeth.

Procedure

Once the patient is anesthetized, the surgeon cleans the face to reduce the risk of infection. She then makes an incision running the length of the lip along the inside of the mouth and removes a strip of tissue from one (or both) lips, before closing the incision with sutures.

Risks and Complications

After surgery, temporary numbness, swelling, bruising, and difficulty chewing or speaking are common, as are minor discomfort, tingling, an occasional sharp pain, or a feeling of heat or cold in the lips. Infection, a blood clot at the site of the incision, or an allergic reaction to the anesthesic are possible. More serious complications may include permanent numbness due to nerve injury during surgery, scarring, or asymmetry of the lip.

Outlook and Lifestyle Modifications

For the first few days, the patient may be advised to sleep with his/her head elevated. Nonabsorbable sutures are removed within 10 days; absorbable sutures resolve on their own. The normal recuperation period is about two weeks, but to reduce the risk of injury at the incisions, the surgeon may advise avoiding contact sports for up to two months.

lip shave   Surgery to remove precancerous tissue on the surface of the lip or a larger tumor in the lip.

Procedure

The tissue is removed from the lip either with a laser or a conventional scalpel. If there is a marked loss of tissue, the plastic surgeon may repair the defect by creating a flap or graft from the mucous membrane lining the inside of the lip to replace the lost tissue and preserve the normal appearance of the lip.

Risks and Complications

After surgery, temporary numbness, swelling, bruising, and difficulty chewing or speaking are common, as are minor discomfort, tingling, an occasional sharp pain, or a feeling of heat or cold in the lips. Infection, a blood clot at the site of the incision, or an allergic reaction to the anesthesic are possible. More serious complications may include permanent numbness due to nerve injury during surgery, scarring, or asymmetry of the lip.

Outlook and Lifestyle Modifications

Successful surgery produces a normal lip with adequate movement and sensation.

See also LASER; SKIN FLAP; SKIN GRAFT.

lip suspension   See LIP LIFT.

liquid silicone implant   See SILICONE.

liver spot   See LENTIGO.

local anesthetic   Drug commonly used in PLASTIC SURGERY and/or cosmetic DENTISTRY to alleviate pain without causing loss of consciousness. Local anesthetics may be injected or applied to the skin. Bupivacaine and novocaine are examples of injectible local anesthetics; lidocaine is an example of a local anesthetic that may be applied to skin or mucous membrane.

When given by injection, local anesthetics may interact with certain medicines such as drugs used to treat high blood pressure, heart disease, irregular heartbeat, some antidepressants, and sedatives.

Certain medical conditions such as asthma, a blood clotting disorder, heart disease, high or low blood pressure, migraine headache, kidney disease, or Type 1 (insulin dependent) diabetes may worsen if the patient is given an injected local anesthetic. When applied to the skin, local anesthetics may worsen the symptoms of certain skin conditions.

Unexpected, sometimes life-threatening adverse effects associated with injected local anesthetics include, but are not limited to

- an allergic reaction (hives; itching; swelling of the lips, tongue, or throat that interferes with breathing)
- bleeding or bruising
- chest pain and/or irregular heartbeat
- convulsions
- dizziness and/or drowsiness
- fever

- headache
- nausea and/or vomiting

Common expected and usually minor side effects associated with local anesthetics include but are not limited to

- back pain
- temporary constipation or incontinence
- difficulty in opening the mouth
- temporary impotence
- persistent or prolonged numbness
- skin rash
- tingling sensation

long bone   See BONE.

long bone reconstruction   See BONE REPLACEMENT.

loop electrosurgical excision procedure (LEEP)   See WART REMOVAL.

L-shaped implant   See RHINOPLASTY.

lunchtime peel   See MICRODERMABRASION.

Lund and Browder chart   See BURNS AND BURN RECONSTRUCTION.

Lutheran blood type   See BLOOD TYPE.

lymphatic system   Major component of the immune system; essential for healing after an injury, either an accidental injury or a deliberate injury such as the incision made during PLASTIC SURGERY.

The organs in the lymphatic system are the tonsils, adenoids, spleen, and thymus. The lymph circulatory system includes lymph vessels and lymph nodes.

The vessels, which are similar to blood vessels, transport a clear-to-white fluid called lymph around the body. Lymph is composed of chyle (fluid released by the intestines after digesting food), plus red blood cells and white blood cells, primarily lymphocytes, specialized white blood cells that circulate through lymph vessels then leave the lymphatic system, traveling through the blood stream to identify and attack foreign body matter such as bacteria, fungi, viruses, and cancer cells and/or sweep up and eliminate debris such as wornout red blood cells in the spleen.

The most important lymphocytes are B cells, which are produced in bone marrow, and T cells and helper T cells, which are made in the thymus, a gland located behind the breastbone. B cells bind to and engulf antigens (substances that trigger an immune response). The resulting antigen/protein fragment attracts and binds to helper T cells and T cells, forming a complex that releases antibodies (substances that attack the antigens). T cells can also destroy diseased cells such as cancer cells.

Lymph nodes are small bean-shape nodules clustered in areas of the body such as the neck, armpit, and groin and produce immune system cells such as lymphocytes. The nodes also serve as filters, enlarging to remove foreign matter such as microorganisms and cancer cells while producing extra white blood cells to fight infection. Lymphedema is a swelling due to the obstruction of a lymph node or vessel, such as swelling of the arm as a possible complication after breast surgery in which lymph nodes around the breast were removed.

See also IMMUNE SYSTEM.

macrochelia See LIP REDUCTION.

macrodactyly Abnormally large toes or fingers due to excessive growth of bone, skin, and fatty tissue. It is an uncommon birth defect more likely to affect fingers than toes, and it may usually be repaired with PLASTIC SURGERY.

Symptoms and Diagnostic Path

The condition is diagnosed by observation and confirmed with X-ray or MRI imaging to show the formation of bones and soft tissue.

Treatment Options and Outlook

If only one finger is affected, the hand may function despite the deformity and no treatment is required. Surgery may be required if the affected finger is very large, if more than one finger is affected, or if a patient's toe is enlarged, making it difficult to wear shoes. Treatment commonly involves more than one procedure over a period of several months. The number of surgeries depends on the extent of the deformity. For example, the surgeon may simply remove thickened skin and fatty tissue and graft new skin to cover the wound. Or he may shorten or remove bones in the fingers, hand, foot, or toes. In rare cases, the surgeon may remove an entire finger or toe and construct a new one in its place. The aim of plastic surgery is to remove sufficient bone and soft tissue to create a functioning hand and/or make it possible to walk comfortably. In most cases, significant improvement is possible.

Risk Factors and Preventive Measures

The cause of macrodactyly has not been identified. Although it sometimes occurs along with other physical problems, it is not an inherited condition.

See also FINGERS AND TOES, CONGENITAL STRUCTURAL DEFECTS; MAGNETIC RESONANCE IMAGING (MRI).

macroglossia Unusually large tongue with excess tissue. This condition is associated with certain genetic disorders such as DOWN SYNDROME, and with congenital conditions such as decreased production of thyroid hormone or HEMANGIOMA (blood vessel tumor). Medical conditions such as pellagra (niacin deficiency disease) or enlarged tonsils or adenoids and structural problems such as a malformation of the jaws that pushes the tongue forward may also be factors.

Symptoms and Diagnostic Path

An unusually large tongue may interfere with breathing, chewing, swallowing, and speaking. Simple physical examination can identify some causes; for example, a hemangioma is clearly visible. Laboratory studies are used to diagnose large tongue due to a medical condition such as a vitamin or hormone deficiency. Imaging studies such as X-rays, MAGNETIC RESONANCE IMAGING (MRI), and ultrasound clarify the size and construction of the tongue as well as the oral cavity. Family history or genetic studies may provide evidence of an inherited disorder such as Down syndrome.

Treatment Options and Outlook

An enlarged tongue due to a medical condition, such as a vitamin or hormone deficiency, or an infection or inflammation is treated medically to correct the underlying problem.

If the enlargement cannot be treated medically, PLASTIC SURGERY to remove excess tissue and reduce the tongue to normal size can open the airway and improve speech, chewing, and swallowing. Follow-up care may include speech therapy.

Risk Factors and Preventive Measures

There are no preventive measures for a large tongue associated with a genetic disorder. Preventing or alleviating medical conditions such as a nutrient deficiency reduces the risk of large tongue associated with one of these conditions.

macromastia   See BREAST RECONSTRUCTION.

macular stain   This benign flat or raised spot on a newborn's skin, colored pink, red, or blue by bunched small blood vessels, is the most common type of vascular birthmark. The macular stain may also be called a salmon patch; a macular stain on the eyelid or forehead is sometimes called "angel's kiss"; on the back of the neck, "stork bite." The former generally fade within the first two years of life; the latter may linger into later life and if dark enough to be cosmeticallty annoying may be obliterated with a laser.

See also HEMANGIOMA; LASER; PORT WINE STAIN.

magnetic resonance imaging (MRI)   This noninvasive diagnostic technique employs strong magnets and radio waves to create detailed pictures of soft tissue such as the internal organs, ligaments, and muscles that that cannot be seen with other techniques such as X-rays.

The human body is more than 60 percent water, molecules with one oxygen atom and two hydrogen atoms. The MRI machine creates an image by stimulating ("exciting") protons, electrically charged particles, in the hydrogen atoms in these water molecules. When the body is exposed to a strong magnetic field and pulses of radio waves during an MRI scan, the excited protons release a burst of energy. When the pulse ends, the protons relax; the burst of energy ends.

The signals produced by excited protons are longer than those released by relaxed protons. Based on the pattern of longer and shorter energy signals, a computer in the MRI machine translates the signals into a picture showing variations in water content that enable the radiologist to see different kinds of tissue and identify changes due to a disease. For example, the signal given off by protons in hydrogen cells in a tumor lasts longer than those produced by protons in hydrogen cells in healthy tissue.

Because the MRI machine uses no radiation, it is usually the preferred technique for examining the reproductive organs, the pelvic area, and the bladder. However, MRI scans may be avoided in the first 12 weeks of pregnancy unless there is a strong medical reason to performing them. Note: As a rule, X-rays produce better images of bone; CT-SCANS are preferred for cases where there is severe internal bleeding.

Procedure

The standard MRI is a tube with strong magnets in the walls and a table that slides in and out of the tube. The radiologist places the patient on the sliding table and leaves the room but can speak to the patient over an intercom while collecting images from the MRI scanner. During the scan, the patient must remain still for several seconds while the MRI creates its images but can relax between picture-taking sequences, and often, a relative or friend may remain in the room while the test is conducted.

The scan itself takes from 15 to 45 minutes, depending on how many images are required. When the scan is finished, the patient may be asked to wait until the images are examined to see if more pictures are needed.

Risks and Complications

For some procedures, the radiologist may inject contrast material (dye) to highlight some tissues such as blood vessels. The contrast material used during an MRI scan is less likely than the dye used during X-rays and CT-scans to produce an allergic reaction.

The strong magnetic field used for MRI will pull any substance such as iron, nickel, cobalt, and various mixtures of these materials that can be magnetized. To prevent injury during the scan, the patient must remove any clothing with metallic accessories, such as zippers and snaps, and inform the radiologist/technician about any implanted devices including (but not limited to)

- an artificial joint or heart valve
- heart pacemaker
- intrauterine device/IUD
- implanted port or catheter (tubes to allow continuous administration of medicines)
- metal plates, pins, screws, or surgical staples
- shrapnel fragments or bullets
- stents (devices made to hold a blood vessel open)
- tattoos (including permanent eyeliner) created with ink that may contain metallic dust

Dental fillings or braces are not magnetic; neither are dentures, glasses, hairpins, hearing aids, or most jewelry, but any of these may distort the MRI image. If possible, they should be removed.

Some people feel claustrophobic in the standard closed MRI machine. The newer machines are shorter and wider; "open MRIs" are wider and may be open on one or more sides. As a result, the magnets in the machine are not as closely bunched, and the quality of the images from these machines may not be as good as those from closed MRIs. During the scan, the magnets make a loud pounding noise; wearing earplugs reduces the sound.

Outlook and Lifestyle Modifications
MRI is a useful diagnostic tool. Its only drawback is that occasionally it may not distinguish between tissue and edema (fluid collected in an area).

See also CT-SCAN; RADIATION; X-RAY EXAMINATION.

makeover See EXTREME MAKEOVER.

malar implant See CHEEK AUGMENTATION.

malarplasty See CHEEK AUGMENTATION.

male pattern baldness See HAIR LOSS.

Malinac, Jacques W. (1889–1976) Polish-born plastic surgeon Jacques W. Malinac immigrated to the United States in 1923. He established the first division of PLASTIC SURGERY at a public hospital (in New York City) and became a founder of the American Society of Plastic Surgeons (ASPS)[originally the American Society of Plastic and Reconstructive Surgeons] in 1931. He created the Educational Foundation of ASPS, now the Plastic Surgery Educational Foundation (PSEF) in 1948 and served as its president until 1955.

mammoplasty See BREAST AUGMENTATION; BREAST REDUCTION.

marionette lines See FACE-LIFT; WRINKLES.

masque Natural or manufactured exfoliant cosmetic product that removes rough top skin cells, leaving behind a temporarily smoother surface.

Natural facial masques may include preparation of various fruits and vegetables such as citrus fruits and cucumbers that contain acidic compounds called alpha hydroxy acids. Manufactured facial masks may be made of wax or fake "mud" or "rubber."

Procedure
The plastic surgeon, cosmetician, or the patient himself spreads a liquid, paste, gel, or other exfoliant product on the face; allows the masque to cool, thicken, or harden; and then washes or peels it away, taking along the top layer of roughened dead skin cells.

Risks and Complications
The skin may be reddened and irritated, more so if the process is repeated too often in a short time period. Allergic reactions to natural or synthetic products may occur. To avoid these problems with natural products, avoid any fruit or vegetable to which the patient is sensitive. To avoid the reaction with manufactured products, test for a reaction in a small area first and follow the directions on the package.

Outlook and Lifestyle Modifications
A temporarily smoother skin surface.

mastectomy Removal of the breast, most commonly to remove a malignant tumor.

Procedures

There are four basic types of mastectomy: The radical mastectomy, the modified radical mastectomy, the simple mastectomy, and the quadrantectomy. Each of these surgeries is performed under general anesthetic.

A *radical mastectomy,* also known as the Halsted procedure after Baltimore surgeon William Stewart Halsted (1852–1922), who introduced the procedure in 1894, is surgery to remove the entire breast, all the axillary lymph nodes (lymph nodes under the arm), and the chest wall muscles under the breast. Currently, this procedure is used only when a cancer has metastasized to the chest muscles.

A *modified radical mastectomy,* currently the most common form of mastectomy, removes the entire breast and some of the axillary lymph nodes.

A *simple mastectomy,* also known as a total mastectomy, removes the entire breast and perhaps some lymph nodes in the breast tissue but none of the axillary lymph nodes or the muscle under the breast. Currently, this procedure is used for women with ductal carcinoma in situ (DCIS) or for mastectomy to prevent breast cancer in high-risk patients.

In a *quadrantectomy,* the surgeon removes the tumor and some surrounding tissue in the affected section (quadrant) of the breast while conserving most of the remaining breast. This is usually followed by radiation therapy.

Risks and Complications

Short-term complications may include bruising, swelling, discomfort, and bleeding or leakage from the wound. Depending on the extent of the surgery, long-term complications may include lymphadema (swelling in the arm next to the breast due to removal of lymph glands, which normally carry fluid out of the affected tissue) and/or reduced movement in the arm.

Outlook and Lifestyle Modifications

Mastectomy is often followed by PLASTIC SURGERY to repair or reconstruct the breast.

See also BREAST RECONSTRUCTION.

mastopexy See BREAST LIFT.

mastoplasty See BREAST LIFT; BREAST REDUCTION.

meatoplasty See under EAR PINBACK; EAR RECONSTRUCTION; PHALLOPLASTY.

medical leeches In 2004, the Food and Drug Administration (FDA) approved the marketing of leeches (*Hirudo medicinalis*) as a medical device for use in PLASTIC SURGERY during skin grafting and during surgery to reattach severed limbs, fingers, or toes whose injured blood vessels may be unable to carry away pooled blood that might damage tissues, leading to infection and possible loss of the graft or reattached digit. As the leeches drain excess blood, they release saliva containing a natural anticoagulant called hirudin, plus vasodilators, compounds that dilate blood vessels. Together, these encourage healing by maintaining circulation in reattached blood vessels.

Procedure

The surgeon punctures the patient's skin with a needle to start the flow of blood and applies one or more leeches to suck out pooled blood and keep blood flowing into newly attached blood vessels. The leeches feed for up to an hour, each taking in up to 30 milliliters (slightly more than one ounce) blood. When full, the leeches simply drop off; the anticoagulant in the leeches' saliva keeps blood flowing freely through the blood vessels for up to 10 hours. The treatment is painless; in addition to hirudin and compounds that dilate blood vessels, the leeches release a natural anesthetic.

Risks and Complications

Wound infection is the main risk. Leeches carry *Aeromonas hydrophila,* bacteria that keep the blood from spoiling and enable the leech to digest its meal. Some studies show that leeches transmit this organism to as many as one of five patients. Healthy patients are unlikely to experience any problems, but to reduce the risk of wound infection, the surgeon will prescribe antibiotics for patients with a weakened immune system.

Note: Medical leeches are raised in controlled sites and laboratories certified by the FDA. All batches are registered and tracked in the same way as medical drugs. Once used, leeches are disposed of as hazardous waste material.

Outlook and Lifestyle Modifications

The use of medical leeches increases the success of skin grafts and reattachment surgery.

melanoma   A malignant tumor composed of pigmented cells, most commonly on the skin but also in the eye. Malignant melanoma is the least common but most dangerous form of skin cancer; PLASTIC SURGERY is often used to repair the damage left when a malignant melanoma is surgically removed.

Symptoms and Diagnostic Path

Any change in the size or color of a MOLE; or redness and swelling beyond the mole; or pain, tenderness, or itching; or bleeding or scaling may suggest malignant melanoma. BIOPSY of the mole provides a conclusive diagnosis.

The specific signs of melanoma are described by the acronym ABCD:

A = Asymmetry (a mole larger one one side than on the other)
B = Border (irregular)
C = Color (uneven, with multiple shades of black and browns or blues and red)
D = Diameter (larger than 6 mm/.25 inch)

A halo nevus is a benign pigmented spot on the skin surrounded by a depigmented area that is sometimes confused with malignant melanoma because the latter may occasionally appear white or gray.

Treatment Options and Outlook

Melanomas of the skin are staged (classified) in five categories that describe the thickness and depth of the tumor and the possibility of its having spread. The treatment is predicated on the stage of the tumor.

Stage 0 melanoma, present only in the top layer of skin cells, is treated surgically to remove the tumor along with a slim 0.5 cm/0.2 in border of adjacent healthy skin and underlying tissue. Stage I melanoma is removed surgically with a 1 cm/0.4 in border. Stage II melanoma is removed surgically with a 3 cm/1.2 in border. Stage III primary melanoma, a skin tumor that has spread to the lymph nodes, is treated with surgery to remove the tumor and the adjacent lymph nodes to reach cells that have spread to other parts of the body. Stage IV (metastatic) melanoma is treated with chemotherapy and/or radiation.

Melanoma on the skin of a finger or toe or under the finger- or toenail may require amputation of the affected digit. Plastic surgery (skin grafts/flaps) may be required to repair the scars and/or tissue deficits and restore function left after surgery for Stage II or Stage III melanoma or any large melanoma at any stage for an amputation.

Risk Factors and Preventive Measures

In the United States, malignant melanoma is the fifth most common cancer in men and the sixth most common in women. The most important environmental trigger is exposure to excessive amounts of ultraviolet radiation, as in sunlight, during childhood, a risk that is highest among people with fair skin who burn easily rather than tan.

Familial atypical mole and melanoma syndrome (FAAM), a condition characterized by the presence of many unusually shaped or colored nonmalignant moles, is a sign of genetic tendency to develop melanoma.

Limiting exposure to sunlight and using adequate protection such as tightly woven clothing and lotions/creams/gels that block the sun's rays may reduce the risk of melanoma. A monthly self-examination of the skin may increase the chance of finding incipient melanoma. After surgery for melanoma regular follow-up appointments reduce the risk of a recurrence going unnoticed.

See also FINGERTIP REPAIR; RADIATION; SCAR REVISION; SKIN FLAPS; SKIN GRAFTS.

membrane   Thin tissue covering a body surface or the surface of an organ. Plastic surgeons often use membrane tissue to repair or reconstruct damaged or missing body parts, for example during a

LIP SHAVE (a procedure to remove a tumor from the surface of the lip) or VAGINOPLASTY. In addition, each cell in the body is covered with a semipermeable membrane (selectively permeable membrane), a tissue that allows some, but not all, molecules to pass through. As a consequence, medical drugs must be designed to pass through the membranes surrounding the cell in the organ for which the medicine is meant. For example, a drug designed to treat kidney disease must be designed so as to pass through the membrane surrounding a kidney cell.

There are three basic types of membranes covering body/organ surfaces: fibrous membranes, serous membranes, and mucous membranes. Fibrous membranes such as the dura mater (the membrane lining the skin) and the periosteum (the membrane covering a bone) are strong tissues composed of fibrous connective tissue. Serous membranes such as the peritoneum (the membrane lining the abdominal cavity) release a watery fluid to moisten the membrane and keep it from sticking to other tissues, including organs. Mucous membranes, tissues lining organs as well as passages that open out of the body such as the mouth, nose, reproductive, and alimentary canals, are protected by specialized glands that secrete mucus, a clear sticky fluid that keeps the membranes moist, even in the presence of air.

A membrane dressing is a synthetic wound covering that mimics the function of a natural membrane. Some examples are a water-based gel product such as Vigilon™, a polyurethane product such as Meshed Omiderm™, or a silicone product such as Silon II™, used in PLASTIC SURGERY to reduce discomfort and speed healing of surface wounds, typically a burn.

mentoplasty   See CHIN RECONSTRUCTION.

mermaid syndrome (Sirenomelia sequence)   This is a rare birth defect in which a child is born with a single leg or with two legs joined together. The joined legs may be linked simply by the skin covering the legs or the bones of the legs may be fused from the lower back to the ankle in a position resembling that of the mythical mermaid. It is usually associated with additional deformities such as missing fingers, abnormal internal organs, and/or missing genitals and urinary or anal openings. Mermaid syndrome, estimated to occur in one of 60,000 to 100,000 live births, is more common among girls than among boys.

Symptoms and Diagnostic Path

Once the baby is born, the condition is diagnosed by physical appearance; X-ray or sonogram picture can confirm the extent of the fusion. Mermaid syndrome may be diagnosed during pregnancy with ultrasound that shows fused or abnormally close leg bones and/or abnormal internal organs.

Treatment Options and Outlook

Mermaid syndrome is generally considered a fatal disorder. In recent years, however, two cases—one in the United States and one in Peru—have been reported in which plastic surgeons successfully separated the child's legs and repaired the genital-urinary tract.

Risk Factors and Preventive Measures

No risk factors or preventive measures have been conclusively identified.

metric system   A system of measurement used worldwide for all scientific and medical measurements, including the measurements used by plastic surgeons in planning their procedures. The metric system is the common system of measurement in all countries except England and the United States, which still use what is called the English system, whose standard measurements are the foot, the pound, and the quart.

In the metric system, all units are related by factors of 10 so that converting from one measure to another within the metric system is simply a matter of multiplying or dividing by 10 or a multiple of 10, that is, moving the decimal point one or more spaces to the left or right.

The basic metric unit of length is the meter (m); the basic unit of weight is the kilogram (kg); the basic unit of volume is the liter (l). Smaller and/or larger units are described by adding a specific prefix such as deci- (1/10th), centi- (1/100th), milli- (1/100th), and so on. For example, one meter equals 10 decimeters, 100 centimeters, 1,000 millimeters, 1,000,000 micrometers, and 1,000,000,000 nanometers.

COMMONLY USED METRIC PREFIXES

Decreasing Amounts	Increasing Amounts
Deci (tenth)	Deka (ten)
Centi (hundredth)	Hecto (hundred)
Milli (thousandth)	Kilo (thousand)
Micron (millionth)	Mega (million)
Nano (billionth)	Giga (billion)

CONVERTING FROM METRIC TO ENGLISH UNITS*

Length	Multiply by
Centimeters to inches	0.39
Meters to feet	0.32
Kilometers to miles	0.62
Weight	
Grams to ounces (dry)	28.6
Kilograms to pounds	2.2
Volume	
Milliliters to fluid ounces	28
Quarts to liters (liquid)	1.1
Quarts to liters (dry)	0.9

CONVERTING FROM ENGLISH TO METRIC UNITS*

Length	Divide by
Inches to centimeters	0.39
Feet to meters	0.32
Miles to kilometers	0.62
Weight	
Ounces to grams (dry)	28.6
Pounds to kilograms	2.2
Volume	
Fluid ounces to milliliters	28
Quarts to liters (liquid)	1.1
Quarts to liters (dry)	0.9

*Note: Conversion figures are approximate. For example, the conversion figure for grams to ounces is given here as 28, but 100 grams is commonly considered equal to 3.5 ounces, which makes the exact conversion figure 28.571428.

Mettauer, John Peter (1787–1875) A native of Virginia, Mettauer studied at Hampden-Sydney College in Hampden-Sydney, Virginia, in 1805–06, then continued his medical education and practice at the Philadelphia Dispensary before returning to Virginia. In 1827, well before PLASTIC SURGERY became a recognized medical specialty, Mettauer, a pioneering gynecologist and surgeon, performed the first cleft palate surgery in America, using instruments he designed himself and which are today on display at Hampden-Sydney College. Ten years later, in 1837, Mettauer founded a private medical school, which eventually became the first medical department at Randolph Macon College in Ashland, Virginia.

microdermabrasion Also called particle skin resurfacing, "lunchtime peel." Noninvasive, painless treatment to smooth ACNE scars, fine lines, and WRINKLES. Depending on the condition of the skin, the procedure takes less than an hour.

Procedure
The surgeon cleans, rinses, and dries the area to be treated and then uses a controlled spray of very fine aluminum oxide crystals 100 microns/0.004 inches wide to remove the top layer of skin cells without injuring the skin. For normal skin, the procedure takes up to 40 minutes and may be repeated up to five to nine times with a week or 10 days between treatments to allow the skin to recover completely.

Risks and Complications
Skin irritation or injury is possible but unlikely when the procedure is done correctly.

Outlook and Lifestyle Modifications
Improvement is visible after first treatment. The patient's skin looks smoother and shows fewer wrinkles. Further treatments and maintenance may be required every month or so to preserve the effct.

See also CHEMICAL SKIN PEEL.

micrognathia See under CHIN RECONSTRUCTION.

micrografts   See HAIR REPLACEMENT SURGERY.

microlipoinjection   See under FAT GRAFTING.

microliposuction   See LIPOSUCTION.

microsurgery   This is a surgical technique employing microscopes and miniaturized surgical instruments to repair very small body structures such as blood vessels and nerves during various procedures, including plastic surgeries such as bone grafts, REPLANTATION, and SKIN GRAFTS.

The microscopes used in this procedure may be either floor- or ceiling-mounted devices or surgical loupes (magnifying lenses mounted on an eyeglass frame) worn by the surgeon. The large microscopes, which magnify the surgical field up to 40 times, are equipped with controls that allow the surgeon to adjust the field of vision, moving closer or farther from the operating site, and they usually have a camera that sends a picture to a TV monitor visible to the entire operating team. Surgical loupes magnify the surgical field up to six times.

Plastic surgeons most commonly use microsurgery to join blood vessels and nerves when reattaching an amputated body part or transferring tissue from one part of the body to another.

See also REPLANTATION; SKIN FLAP; SKIN GRAFT.

microtia   This birth defect is a deformity of the external ear, sometimes including the middle and inner ear. Unilateral microtia affects one ear; bilateral microtia affects both ears and is more likely to involve hearing loss. The ear(s) may be repaired or reconstructed with PLASTIC SURGERY.

Symptoms and Diagnostic Path
Microtia is diagnosed by physical examination. In Grade I microtia, the entire ear is smaller than normal, but its features, such as earlobe and the CARTILAGE outer rim, are well defined. In Grade II microtia, some features of the ear, such as the outer rim, are missing. In Grade III microtia, the patient has a piece of skin and/or cartilage, atresia (no

external ear canal), and a malformed lobe at the bottom. Anotia is the complete absence of external ear tissue.

Treatment Options and Outlook
Plastic surgery can construct the frame of the external ear with cartilage taken from the patient's rib area, covering the cartilage with skin taken from the patient's own body, ideally from adjacent, non-hair-bearing skin.

This surgery is usually not performed until the patient is at least five years old so as to allow the body to grow enough rib cartilage to reconstruct the defective ear or ears, and, for a patient with only one defective ear, to allow the normal ear to grow, giving the surgeon a better chance to match the size and shape of the healthy ear. Once the surgery has healed completely, the surgeon can facilitate hearing by drilling an opening to the internal ear canal.

Risk Factors and Preventive Measures
Microtia is estimated to occur once in every 6,000 to 12,000 live births, most frequently among children of Japanese or Navaho descent, more commonly among boys than among girls. Unilateral microtia is more common than bilateral microtia, accounting for up to 90 percent of all cases, most often on the right side of the head. There is no confirmed cause for this defect, although some researchers suspect an inadequate supply of blood to the developing fetal ear.

midface lift   See FACE-LIFT.

midface reconstruction   See LE FORT PROCEDURE.

midforehead lift   See FOREHEAD LIFT.

midline facial cleft   See BIFID NOSE; FACIAL CLEFT.

midpalatal suture opening   See CLEFT LIP AND/OR PALATE.

midsection liposuction   See LIPOSUCTION.

Millard, David Ralph, Jr. (1919–) American plastic surgeon who developed and popularized various techniques now considered standard for facial plastic surgeries such as CLEFT LIP AND/OR PALATE repair, FACE-LIFT, and RHINOPLASTY. Millard authored *Cleft Craft: The Evolution of Its Surgery* (1977) and was named one of 10 Plastic Surgeons of the Millennium by the members of the American Society of Plastic Surgery in 2000.

minerals (dietary)   Minerals are a major class of nutrients required, many of which are essential for the proper healing of tissues after accidental injury and/or surgical incisions such as those required for PLASTIC SURGERY.

As opposed to vitamins, which are multipart chemical substances, minerals are elements, substances composed of only one kind of atom. Minerals occur naturally in rocks and metal ores. There are minerals in plants and animals, such as the calcium in some dark green leaves and the iron in meat, fish, and poultry, but the plants get the minerals from the soil in which they grow, and the animals get the minerals by eating the plants.

Nutritionists classify the minerals in food as either major minerals (more than five grams stored in the body; more than 100 mg required each day for a healthful diet), trace elements (less than five grams stored in the body; less than 100 mg required each day), or electrolytes (positively charged mineral particles that facilitate the transmission of impulses from cell to cell in the body). The major minerals considered vital for human beings are calcium, phosphorous, magnesium, and sulfur. The trace elements considered vital are iron, zinc, iodine, selenium, copper, manganese, fluoride, chromium, and molybdenum. The electrolytes are sodium, potassium, and chloride. Calcium, iron, copper, and zinc all play an important role in the synthesis of proteins and the production of connective tissue required for healing.

mini face-lift   See MASQUE; NONSURGICAL FACE-LIFT.

minimally invasive surgery   Procedures performed via injection or with surgery that involves the smallest possible incision or several small incisions and the insertion of a stiff or flexible tube to accommodate small specialized surgical instruments.

The instruments used in minimally invasive surgery may include (but are not limited to)

- fiber-optic lights that illuminate the internal surgical area
- a miniature, microscope-equipped camera that allows the surgeon to visualize the patient's

Age (Years)	Calcium (mg)	Phosphorus (mg)	Magnesium (mg)	Iron (mg)	Zinc (mg)	Iodine (mg)	Selenium (mg)
Males							
19–30	1,000	700	400	8	11	150	55
31–50	1,000	700	420	8	11	150	55
51–70	1,200	700	420	8	11	150	55
70+	1,200	700	420	8	11	150	55
Females							
19–30	1,000	700	310	18	8	150	55
31–50	1,000	700	320	18	8	150	55
51–70	1,000/1,500*	700	320	8	8	150	55
70+	1,000/1,500*	700	320	8	8	150	55

MAJOR MINERALS: RECOMMENDED DIETARY ALLOWANCES

*The higher figure is for women taking postmenopausal estrogen supplements. Source: National Academy of Medicine, reports, 1989–2004.

internal organs and tissues from pictures transmitted to a television screen

- miniaturized surgical instruments such as scalpels and tweezers

The general name for procedures employing these instruments and techniques is endoscopy, named for the endoscope, a tube through which the instruments are introduced into the body. Laparoscopy is endoscopy specific to the abdominal area; a laparoscope is the tube used to introduce instruments during laparoscopy.

Note: In addition to endopscopy and laparoscopy, the American Society of Plastic Surgeons includes the following procedures on its list of plastic surgeries utilizing minimally invasive techniques:

- Botox injections sclerotherapy (injections to constrict and fade small VARICOSE VEINS/spider veins)
- CHEMICAL SKIN PEELS
- MICRODERMABRASION
- LASER hair removal
- endoscopic abdominoplasty
- endoscopic FACE-LIFT/FOREHEAD LIFT
- endoscopic BREAST AUGMENTATION
- endoscopic reconstructive surgery on the breast

In each case, the benefits of minimally invasive surgery are less pain, faster recovery, fewer complications, and minimal scarring. However, in some cases, such as surgery to remove a malignant tumor in the colon, a minimally invasive procedure may take longer than an open procedure, through a longer incision, requiring the patient to remain longer under anesthesic. For some patients, particularly the elderly, the risk of a long period of anesthesia may outweigh the advantages of minimally invasive surgery.

See also ENDOSCOPY; LAPAROSCOPY.

minoxidil Marketed either as a generic product or under the name Rogaine®, this topical solution may promote hair growth in small follicles on scalp, brow, and beard area. It is approved by the U.S. Food and Drug Administration (FDA) for adults and children, to treat male pattern baldness, and it may also be useful for patients with *alopecia areata*. With regular use, new hair growth usually appears in about three months; if the treatment stops, the hair growth ceases. Possible side effects include burning, stinging, or redness when first applied to the skin. More serious adverse effects, usually associated with absorption of large amount of minoxidil through the skin, may include headache, nausea, vomiting, dizziness, change in heart rate or blood pressure, chest pain, swelling of hands or feet, or fatigue.

See also HAIR LOSS; HAIR REPLACEMENT SURGERY.

Moberg flap   See SKIN FLAP.

modified abdominoplasty   See ABDOMINOPLASTY.

modified radical mastectomy   See MASTECTOMY.

Mohs micrographic surgery   Technique to remove skin cancers using a microscope to identify malignant tissue so as to spare healthy tissue. This surgery, created by University of Wisconsin surgeon Frederick E. Mohs, is particularly valuable for plastic surgeons/dermatologists because it enables the surgeon to preserve the patient's appearance when removing skin cancers on the face.

Procedure

The surgeon outlines and removes the visible skin cancer, cutting into the skin on an angle to slice a thin section of tissue that includes a small border of apparently healthy tissue around the edges. Small sections of the edges of the excised tissue are microscopically examined for tumor cells. If tumor cells are discovered in the section from the edges, the surgeon again shaves away very thin slices of tissue and repeats the testing procedure. The remove-and-test procedure continues until the edges of the tissue are deemed free of malignant cells.

The surgeon closes the wound with fine sutures, or covers it with a skin flap lifted from an adjacent area and turned forward over the wound, or uses a SKIN GRAFT lifted from another part of the body. The closed wound is flushed clean with a saline solution and then covered with an antibiotic ointment and a pressure dressing to reduce swelling. For incisions closed with sutures or a SKIN FLAP, the dressing remains in place for 24 to 48 hours, then is removed and replaced once a day for several days. For incisions repaired with a skin graft, the pressure dressing remains in place for up to a week.

Risks and Complications

Bleeding, nerve damage, and infection are possible following this procedure. Using skin flaps or grafts may raise the risk of additional complications such as blood clots and/or failure of the transplant to survive.

Outlook and Lifestyle Modifications

Cosmetically, Mohs surgery is considered the standard procedure for completely removing a skin cancer with the least possible loss of healthy skin. In addition, its cure rate is higher than that for other surgical techniques. For example, the chance that a first-time basal cell cancer (the most common kind of skin cancer) will grow back within five years after Mohs surgery is 1 percent versus 10 percent for simple surgical excision, 8.7 percent for radiation therapy, and 7.5 percent for cryotherapy (freezing the tumor with liquid nitrogen).

mole   Nevus, beauty mark. Spot on the skin composed of pigmented cells (melanocytes); ranges in color from pink to tan to brown, black or blue. A small, dark facial mole is called a beauty mark. Sometimes an artificial beauty mark, such as a round piece of dark material or a dark mark is placed on the face to emphasize a light complexion.

Symptoms and Diagnostic Path

The signs and characteristics of moles varies according to the type of mole.

- A *congenital mole* is present from birth but may not be visible for several months.

- An *acquired mole* appears sometime in childhood; a common acquired mole (CAN, common nevus) usually begins as a dark spot but may lighten and rise above the skin later in life.

- A *hairy mole,* also known as a hairy nevus, is a benign mole that contains a hair follicle (the small pit in the skin from which a hair grows).

- An *atypical mole* (dysplastic nevi) may be flat or bumpy. Its appearance is described with the ABCD categories for pigmented lesions in which

    A = asymmetry rather than a smooth round or oval shape

    B = border, usually irregular with indentations and/or poor definition of the edges

    C = color variation, including white, tan, brown, red, black, and blue, alone or in combination

    D = diameter, larger than 6mm/0.2 inches, about the size of the eraser on top a pencil

- A *Hutchinson freckle,* or Hutchinson's patch, is a precancerous small brown spot, usually found on the face, named for British surgeon Jonathan Hutchinson (1828–1913).

- An *intradermal nevus* is a pigmented spot located under the surface of the skin, between the epidermis (top layer of skin cells) and the dermis (mid-layers of skin cells).

- A *stocking nevus* is a large birthmark on the part of the foot and leg normally covered by a sock or stocking.

Treatment Options and Outlook

Benign moles, such as hairy moles, are commonly removed for cosmetic reasons. (Note: A hairy mole must be completely removed by cutting out the hair follicle, otherwise the hair will grow back.)

Any mole that begins to bleed, darken, or grow larger is commonly examined by BIOPSY to rule out a malignancy. An incisional biopsy removes a small piece of the mole; a shave biopsy scrapes off the top of a raised mole, sanding down the surrounding tissue. Once the mole is removed, the scar may look lighter or darker than the surrounding skin. Eventually the color evens to match the surrounding skin; applying sunscreen for several weeks after biopsy or removal reduces darkening.

Risk Factors and Preventive Measures

Moles are present at birth; avoiding excessive exposure to sunlight may reduce darkening. Atypical moles, which sometimes run in families, may develop into MELANOMA, a potentially fatal form of skin cancer.

mucosal implant   See DENTAL IMPLANT.

muscle   Muscle, the specialized body tissue with the ability to contract and relax in response to electrical impulses from the nerves. Plastic surgeons use muscle tissue in plastic surgeries, either as one component of a SKIN FLAP or SKIN GRAFT, or as a single tissue muscle graft. These procedures are done to reconstruct tissue lost to injury or illness or to a surgery; for example, to remove a large tumor.

The three types of muscle tissue are skeletal muscle, the kind of muscle used in muscle flaps and muscle transfer; visceral (smooth) muscle; and cardiac muscle, the muscle tissue of the heart. Each of the three may also be described by its function (voluntary or involuntary) and its appearance (smooth or striated).

Types of Muscle

Skeletal muscle, the muscle tissue attached to the bones by strong fibrous cords called tendons, is voluntary muscle, meaning that a healthy person can move her skeletal muscles at will, for example to walk or lift or bend. Skeletal muscle is composed of long thin cells called muscle fibers containing smaller units called myofibrils with light (actin) and dark (myosin) protein strands.

The fibers in skeletal muscle are arranged in distinct patterns that make the light and dark protein strands look like stripes, so skeletal muscle is sometimes called striated (striped) muscle. Skeletal muscles act in pairs: flexor skeletal muscle bends a joint; extensor muscle straightens it.

Skeletal muscle is the tissue used by plastic surgeons for muscle flaps and muscle transfers. For example, a rectus abdominis flap is a piece of the muscle that stretches from the pubic bone to the abdomen or a piece of the muscle plus skin and fatty tissue from the same area. The muscle tissue alone may be used to repair a defect to the tongue or to the base of the skull. The muscle plus skin and fatty tissue may be used to build a new breast after mastectomy or to repair defects of the face or neck or lower leg.

Visceral (smooth) muscle is also made of muscle fibers, but in smooth muscles these fibers lie along side one another, so they look smooth, not striped. Visceral (smooth) muscle, found in the walls of a hollow organ such as the bladder, the blood vessels, the digestive tract, and the uterus, is called involuntary muscle because it is controlled by brain impulses not deliberate movement.

Cardiac muscle is found only in the heart. Like skeletal muscles, its fibers are arranged so that they look striped; like smooth muscle, its actions are involuntary. Cardiac muscle makes the heart beat by contracting and relaxing the four chambers of the heart, circulating blood throughout the body.

Muscle Tissue in Plastic Surgery

Plastic surgeons use muscle tissue alone for two types of PLASTIC SURGERY, the muscle flap and the muscle transfer.

The muscle flap is a piece of skeletal muscle tissue used in reconstructive surgery to repair a muscle defect or rebuild an area of the body. A simple muscle flap (muscle without skin or fatty tissue) is commonly used to replace infected muscle around a bone and provide new blood vessels to nourish the bone. A myocutaneous (musculocutaneous) or myodermal flap, which includes skin, fatty tissue, and muscle, is often used to rebuild a breast after mastectomy or to cover an area where the tissue layers have been destroyed by injury such as a burn or by infection such as a skin ulcer. A myofascial (fasciocutaneous) flap, which includes skin, muscle, and fascia (the tissue wrapped around muscles), is used to repair areas where a less bulky transplant is required, such as the lower leg or upper arm.

The term *muscle transfer* describes surgery to lift a piece of skeletal muscle from one place on the body and move it to another so as to enable function in the recipient site. For example, a surgeon may detach a muscle from the front of the knee (where it normally extends/straightens the knee) and move it around to the back of the knee, where it can be used to bend, rather than extend, the joint.

muscle flap   See MUSCLE.

muscle transfer   See MUSCLE.

Nager syndrome   See POLYDACTYLY.

nail   Fingernail, toenail; thin layer of specialized hardened epidermal cells covering the top of fingertip or end of the toes.

During any surgery requiring anesthesic, including plastic surgeries, the color of the nail bed—the pinkish skin visible through the nail—serves as a quick guide to the adequacy of blood circulation. To give the surgeon a clear view, the patient must remove any nail polish and/or fake nails. Note: Clear nail polish must be removed not because it masks color but because it may interfere with the accuracy of the pulse monitor, a small device that clips onto the finger to track heartbeat.

The visible section of the nail is called the body of the nail. The part of the nail back from the nail bed and moving under the cuticle and continuing under the skin of the finger is the germinal matrix/nail plate, where new nail cells are produced. Nails grow the same way hair does; as new nail cells are produced they push older ones out and onto the existing nail, making it thicker and stronger.

See also FINGERTIP REPAIR; VITAL SIGNS.

nasal reconstuction   See RHINOPLASTY.

nasolabial fold   See FACE-LIFT; FACIAL AGING; WRINKLES.

nasoplasty   See RHINOPLASTY.

natural skin lines   Naturally occurring creases or folds in the skin where plastic surgeons often make their incisions so that any scars will be less visible.

Relaxed skin tension lines (RSTL), also known as lines of expression or lines of minimal tension, are creases in the skin of the face and neck. Examples are the parentheseslike "smile lines" running down from the sides of the nose to the sides of the mouth, the frown lines caused by wrinkling the forehead, or the horizontal and vertical creases in the neck. Langer's lines, also known as tension lines or cleavage lines, occur at various points on the body such as under the breast, at the waist, or right above the pubic area, forming a pattern created by the alignment of the fibers in the connective tissue under the skin. Other prominent natural skin lines include those on the tips of the fingers and toes and on the palms and soles, forming patterns specific enough that they were once considered a conclusive tool in identifying an individual. (Today, DNA is considered the only completely accurate biological identifier.)

nd:yag laser   See LASER.

neck lift   Plastic surgery to tighten the skin and underlying muscles on the neck and under the lower jaw. One condition commonly treated by a neck lift is called witch's chin, an age-related sagging of fleshy soft tissue or a deep fold under the chin often coupled with a projecting lower jawbone.

Procedures

There are two basic types of neck lifts. A skin-only neck lift tightens only the skin on the neck and under the chin. A neck lift that tightens both the skin and the underlying muscle is called a plastysmaplasty after the platysma, the broad, flat muscle that extends down from the lower jaw to the breastbone on either side of the neck.

Skin-only neck lift The surgeon makes two incisions, one under or behind each ear, lifts the skin of the jaw and neck upward, trims away any excess tissue, and fixes the skin into its new position with suture or tissue glue.

Platysmaplasty The surgeon makes a transverse incision in the skin crease where the chin and neck meet just under the chin, lifts the skin, and removes excess fatty tissue underneath. She then tightens loose muscle tissue, pulls the skin and muscle toward the vertical midline, and sutures the edges of the incision in a straight line that will be partially hidden by the natural crease. This procedure is called a corset platysmaplasty because it wraps the tissue of the neck tightly to prevent glands in the neck from bulging under the skin. A hammock platysmaplasty is a procedure in which the surgeon adds sutures or surgical mesh to support the skin under the chin. In either case, the surgeon may also make an incision under or behind each ear and lift and tighten the skin around the lower jaw and chin.

Depending on the extent of the surgery required, the neck lift may be performed with general anesthesic, regional anesthesic, or LOCAL ANESTHETIC plus sedation. When the incision is closed, a pressure dressing is wrapped from the top of the head down to under the chin to reduce swelling.

To treat witch's chin, the folds under the chin may be corrected by pulling the sagging skin up closer to the chin bone via an incision inside the mouth and/or using an implant to fill in the extra skin. Reducing the projecting jawbone requires a separate surgery.

Risks and Complications

Bruising and swelling may occur following surgery. As with other facial surgery, the skin may be sensitive to sunlight for several weeks or months.

To reduce swelling, the patient may be advised to sleep with his/her head elevated. To avoid unnecessary tension on stitches in the neck, the patient may be advised to keep the head and neck as still as possible, turning the entire body rather than the neck when switching position.

Outlook and Lifestyle Modifications

The change in the skin on the neck is visible within a week after surgery, but swelling continues to diminish slowly over several months. As with any surgery to repair age-related stretching or sagging skin, how long the neck lift lasts varies from patient to patient. Due to the continued effects of natural aging, some patients may require a second procedure.

necrotizing fasciitis "Flesh-eating bacteria"; a potentially fatal bacterial infection of the fascia, the thin layer of connective tissue covering a muscle, commonly due to a streptoccoccus organism that destroys skin and the soft tissue underneath. If muscle is destroyed, the condition is called necrotizing myositis.

Once the initial infection is controlled and tissue damage stabilized, plastic surgeries, including SKIN GRAFTS, may be required to repair the damaged area. The extent of the plastic surgery required to repair the damage depends on the site and the extent of the original tissue loss.

Symptoms and Diagnostic Path

The symptoms of necrotizing fasciitis are common to any infection. Within 24 hours, there may be increasing pain either at the site of the injury or close by, upset stomach (nausea, diarrhea), and flulike symptoms such as dizziness or a general feeling of discomfort. Within four days, a patient may develop swelling and a rash in the area of the infection along with dark marks that turn into blisters, and dark or bluish white flakes due to death of tissue at the site of the injury. Within five days, the patient may experience critical symptoms, including a sudden severe drop in blood pressure and/or loss of consciousness due to organ failure caused by toxins released into the bloodstream by the bacteria.

The bacteria that cause necrotizing fasciitis release gas inside body tissue; imaging studies of the area (X-ray, CT-SCAN, MAGNETIC RESONANCE IMAGING [MRI]) will show the layers of tissue under the skin separated by air/gas. However, because other bacteria also release gas, imaging studies are suggestive not conclusive. To identify the bacteria causing the infection, the physician must take a tissue sample and culture (grow) the bacteria.

Treatment Options and Outlook

The first treatments for necrotizing fasciitis are intravenous antibiotics and debridement (surgical removal) of any infected tissue. The physician may prescribe medication to raise the patient's blood pressure, and/or hyperbaric oxygen therapy. For the latter, the patient may be put into a hyperbaric oxygen chamber, a sealed unit in which one breathes pure oxygen to increase oxygenation of body tissues and, coincidentally, destroy some of the bacteria causing the infection.

The outlook for a patient with necrotizing fasciitis may range from slight scarring where tissue has been lost to amputation of an infected limb to death from organ failure. The end result depends on the quickness of the diagnosis and the effectiveness of the treatment, which is determined to some extent by the virulence of the infecting organism.

Risk Factors and Preventive Measures

Staphyloccoccus organisms are common in the environment, carried by up to 30 percent of any given population. Infection may occur when the bacteria enter the skin through any injury from a tiny pinprick to a surgical incision. The best defense against infection is cleanliness: frequent hand washing and thorough cleansing of any wound.

Necrotizing fasciitis occurs most frequently among people older than 55 and is more common among women than among men. The risk of death is higher among women and among patients with a chronic disease such as diabetes or cancer, a widespread infection, or whose initial treatment was late.

neoscrotum construction   See PHALLOPLASTY.

neovaginoplasty   See VAGINOPLASTY.

nerve   See   NERVOUS   SYSTEM;   NEUROPLASTY; REPLANTATION.

nervous system   The brain, the spinal cord, and the nerves. NEUROPLASTY is PLASTIC SURGERY to repair the nervous system by transferring nerve tissue from one part of the body to another so as to ameliorate nerve damage due to an injury or medical condition.

Nerves are cordlike structures containing multiple fibers built of nerve cells (neurons). The fibers transmit motor impulses (messages that move the body) and sensory stimuli (messages for vision, hearing, taste, touch, smell, vision) back and forth between the brain and the body. A nerve block is a form of regional anesthesic that numbs sensation in one or more nerves in the same area. A nerve bundle or a mixed nerve is a nerve with more than one type of nerve fibers; a nerve tract is a bundle of nerve fibers in the brain. Nerve growth factors are naturally occurring chemicals that promote the growth of nerve tissue. A nerve plexus is a junction where fibers from different nerves are rearranged to form a single pathway from a specific part of the body. Most nerves contain both motor fibers and sensory fibers wrapped in a fatty sheath called myelin. If the myelin sheath is damaged, the nerve will no longer transmit impulses of stimuli.

In any surgery, including plastic surgery, surgeons strive to remove, repair, or reconstruct body tissue without damaging nerve tissue. Alternatively, plastic surgeons may be able to repair nerves damaged by an injury or illness by rejoining the ends of severed nerve fibers or by transplanting nerve tissue taken from the patient, a cadaver, or a living donor.

The brain and the spinal cord comprise the central nervous system. Nerves comprise two groups with specific functions: the somatic (voluntary) nervous system and the autonomic (involuntary) nervous system.

The central nervous system   Cranial nerves link the brain to the eyes, ears, nose, throat, head, neck, and some sections of the upper body. Spinal nerves come out into the body from the spaces between the vertebrae (bones in the spine) to carry messages to and from various parts of the body. Each spinal nerve has two roots emerging from the spine. The part of the nerve emerging from the front carries motor impulses from the brain to the body; the part of the nerve emerging from the back transmits sensory information to the brain. Cranial or spinal nerves that carry impulses from the central nervous system to the body are called efferent nerves (from the Latin *ad*, meaning "to," and *ferro*, meaning "carry"), while nerves that carry impulses from the body to the brain are called afferent nerves (from the Latin *ex*, meaning "from," and *ferro*, meaning "carry").

The somatic (voluntary) nervous system A group of 31 pairs of nerves originating in the spine and 12 pairs of nerves originating in the brain that transmit messages to and from the muscles to control the voluntary movements of the body; i.e., the movement of the muscles in the arms and legs. Somatic nerves also contain sensory fibers for sight, hearing, smell, taste, and touch.

The autonomic (involuntary) nervous system Two complementary sets of nerves, the sympathetic nervous system (SNS) and the parasympathetic nervous system (PNS), that transmit messages back and forth between the brain and organs such as the heart, lungs, and blood vessels, whose functions are usually considered beyond voluntary control. These messages travel via chemicals called neurotransmitters called catecholamines (acetylcholine, epinephrine, adrenaline, norepinephrine/noradrenaline) which are secreted by the outer covering (cortex) of the adrenal gland, a small structure sitting atop the kidney.

The nerves of the sympathetic nervous system send signals that step up protective body responses. This reaction to an emergency situation is commonly known as "fight or flight." The heart beats faster, pumping extra blood; the blood vessels constrict to reduce blood loss; breathing quickens and air passages expand to bring more oxygen into the lungs; the pupils of the eyes dilate to let in more light and improve vision; peristalsis slows; the production of diuretic hormones decreases; circular muscles such as those controlling the opening of the bladder and anus contract.

The parasympathetic nervous system is a calming agent that does exactly the opposite, sending messages that slow down the heartbeat, widen the blood vessels, slow the breathing, contract the pupils, step up the production of gastric juices and the contractions that move food through the intestinal tract, and relax sphincter muscles such as those at the opening to the bladder, anus, and uterine cervix.

See also BIOFEEDBACK.

neurofibromatosis NF; genetic disorder affecting the development of nerve cell tissue, leading to the growth of tumors on nerves, as well as changes in the skin and deformities of the bones. In many cases, PLASTIC SURGERY can remove NF tumors and/or alleviate the other signs of the disorder.

Symptoms and Diagnostic Path

There are two types of NF, neurofibromatosis type 1 (NF1/Von Recklinghausen's disease) and neurofibromatosis 2 (NF2/ bilateral acoustic neurofibromatosis). In both forms of NF, an important diagnostic clue is having a parent, sister, or brother with the disorder.

Neurofibromatosis type 1, the less severe form of the disorder, is identified by the following:

- appearance very early in life of flat light brown café-au-lait ("coffee with milk") spots on the skin
- bulging noncancerous tumors of the nerves called neurofibromas that may look like skin growths or cause bones to twist, sometimes causing curvature of the spine
- potentially lethal tumors in vital organs

Neurofibromatosis type 2, the less common form of NF, usually appears in young adulthood. Its symptoms are similar to those for NF1, but patients with NF2 also develop tumors of the brain (specifically the nerves that control hearing) and spinal cord that may cause deafness, loss of vision, chronic headache, and, in severe cases, paralysis or death.

Treatment Options and Outlook

The only treatment for NF1 is surgery to remove the nerve tumors and/or correct malformations of the bones; however, this does not prevent new tumors or new malformations.

For NF2, imaging techniques such as MAGNETIC RESONANCE IMAGING (MRI) make it possible to find very small tumors on the nerves that control hearing. Removing these tumors poses a risk of nerve damage leading to deafness; alternative treatments include simply watching slow-growing tumors or removing only part of the tumor or using radiation therapy to shrink the tumor.

Risk Factors and Preventive Measures

NF1 occurs in one in every 4,000 live births; NF2, in one in every 50,000 live births. Most people with NF inherit the disorder via a dominant gene on chromosome 17 (NF1) or chromosome 22 (NF2); each child born to a person with NF has up to a 50 percent chance of developing NF. As many as half of all cases of NF are due to a spontaneous mutation; once the gene has mutated, the person with NF can pass the disorder along to his/her children.

There are no preventive measures, but genetic testing can identify the gene in a person with a family history of NF.

neuroplasty Plastic surgery to repair severed or damaged nerves so as to restore or retain the ability to feel and move.

Procedures

The three basic methods of repairing damaged nerves are direct nerve repair, nerve graft repair (nerve tissue from the patient's own body), and nerve transplant repair (nerve tissue from a cadaver or a living donor). All three procedures are microsurgery performed with the surgeon using either an operating microscope or a loupe (a magnifying glass) and miniaturized instruments.

Direct nerve repair This procedure joins the ends of a nerve separated in a clean, sharply defined cut, with no frayed ends and minimal open space between the cut ends so that the joined nerve moves freely.

Nerve graft repair and nerve transplant repair These procedures are used to repair a nerve damaged by an injury that leaves frayed nerve ends far enough apart that joining the ends puts so much tension on the fibers that they are likely to separate after the surgery is complete.

All nerve repair begins with the surgeon's cleaning and trimming severed ends of the injured nerve.

Next, he positions the ends of the severed nerve or inserts and positions one or more grafts/transplants, being careful to match the sensory (touch) and motion fibers in the nerve endings. He sutures the nerve ends in place using as few sutures as possible so as to minimize scarring. Once the sutures are complete, the surgeon rechecks the stitching, especially if there are multiple grafts/transplants, moves the tissue to make sure that it moves freely, cleans the wound, and closes the skin.

Note: Nerve tissue taken from the patient usually comes from an area away from the original injury so that removing the tissue does not increase the loss of sensation or movement. Nerve tissue from a living donor is usually sensory tissue or duplicated nerve tissue; its loss does not create significant problems for the donor. A nerve graft is a reconstructive procedure to transfer nerve tissue from one part of the body to another or from one individual to a second to provide a base for the regeneration of axons, the part of the nerve cell that sends messages out from the cell. One type of nerve graft, a cable graft, is a strand made of several individual strands of nerve tissue twisted together like a wire cable. Cable grafts are used to repair damage due to the loss of a large piece of nerve tissue.

Risks and Complications

Failure of the rejoined or graft/transplant tissue to function is one risk. The complication specific to tissue transplanted from a cadaver or living donor is rejection transplant; the risk is less if the donor is a close relative. To reduce this risk, the patient must take antirejection drugs for a period of time (commonly up to two years) after the surgery until the body regenerates sufficient tissue to replace the graft/transplant.

Outlook and Lifestyle Modifications

The success of nerve repair depends on a variety of factors, including (but not limited to) the location and extent of the original injury, the timing of the repair surgery (the sooner, the better), the skill of the surgeon in positioning the nerve ends, and the patient's cooperation in using the affected body part safely soon after surgery so as to protect both nerve and muscle function.

nipple areola reconstruction PLASTIC SURGERY to construct a new nipple and surrounding tissue after breast surgery.

Procedure

The surgeon may lift a piece of tissue from the patient's healthy breast or from another area of the body and use the graft to build a small nipplelike projection on the breast. Once the graft has healed, the projection may be tattooed to resemble the dark skin of the nipple and areola. Note: In some cases, the surgeon may simply tattoo a nipplelike drawing onto the breast without actually building a nipple.

Risks and Complications

The most important risk is failure of the grafted skin to implant successfully at its new site.

Outlook and Lifestyle Modifications

Successful surgery results in a cosmetically acceptable breast.

See also BREAST REDUCTION.

nipple graft Transplant of nipple and areola tissue during BREAST REDUCTION surgery.

Procedure

If the original breast is very large, the surgeon may cut the nipple/areola from the breast to create a free graft. If the original breast is smaller, the surgeon may lift the nipple/areola partially from the breast, leaving it connected at one point to the breast as a pedicle flap. He removes excess tissue from the breast, manipulates the remaining tissue into shape as a new, smaller breast, sutures the tissue in place, and then sutures the free graft or pedicle flap onto the appropriate position.

Risks and Complications

Bleeding and swelling are common. Complications specific to the nipple/areola free graft include unnatural positioning of the tissue, fading color, loss of sensation in the nipple, and failure of the flap/graft to grow securely into place. These complications are much less likely to occur with a pedicle flap, which is transplanted with nerves and blood vessels attached and may retain milk ducts.

Outlook and Lifestyle Modifications

Successful surgery produces a natural-looking breast. Breast-feeding is impossible after a free graft because the graft does not include the milk ducts. A pedicle flap may include the milk ducts but cannot guarantee the ability to breast-feed.

noninvasive procedure Nonsurgical procedure; procedure that does not require inserting an instrument through the skin or into a body cavity. X-rays, CT-SCANS, MAGNETIC RESONANCE IMAGING (MRI), ultrasound, and nuclear medicine examinations are all noninvasive diagnostic techniques. Exfoliant chemicals are used to remove the rough top layer of skin cells during noninvasive facial rejuvenation. Medications such as MINOXIDIL (Rogaine®), FINASTE-RIDE (Propecia®), which may stimulate hair growth, are used for noninvasive hair replacement.

See also MINIMALLY INVASIVE SURGERY.

nonsurgical face-lift Also known as a "mini face-lift." Procedure designed to alter the contours of the face without surgery. One example of such a procedure is the use of low-voltage electrical current (GALVANIC CURRENT; the medical name for direct current or DC) in an attempt to reduce the visibility of fine lines by stimulating the facial muscles and increasing blood circulation through facial tissue. A second example is the use of radio frequency waves in an effort to tighten underlying connective tissue. The effects of these procedures are unproven.

See also FACE-LIFT; THERMAGE.

nose-lip-chin plane Imaginary line describing the ideal relationship of the tip of the nose, the lips, and the tip of the chin when viewed in profile; a schemata used by plastic surgeons in planning surgical reduction or enhancement of these features.

Ideally, a straight line drawn up from the front of the chin will cross slightly behind the edge of the lips and end at the middle of the nostril so that the tip of the nose is ahead of the chin. The upper lip is slightly in front of the lower lip, more so in women than in men. Obviously, the proportions of these features may vary with race and ethnicity; for example, the nose is commonly flatter among Asians than among Caucasians, and blacks commonly have fuller lips than do Asians or Caucasians.

See also CHIN LIFT; LIP AUGMENTATION; RHINOPLASTY.

nuclear medicine Imaging technique used to evaluate organ function, track blood flow through various parts of the body, and identify tumors, based on the detection of energy emitted from a radio-pharmaceutical (a medical substance containing radioactive material) given to the patient, either intravenously or by mouth.

Nuclear medicine is rarely used in PLASTIC SURGERY, two possible exceptions being to identify malignancy in the lymph nodes before breast surgery and to identify breast tumors after breast reconstruction when simple mammography may not produce a conclusive image.

Procedure

The patient is given a small amount of radioactive material either by intravenous injection or by mouth. The material collects in the organ or area to be examined, emitting energy (gamma rays) that will be recorded on a special camera. Note: Because some organs/areas pick up the material faster than others, the radioactive material may be administered right before the procedure, several hours before, and several days before.

During the procedure, which may last from a few minutes to an hour or more, the patient lies on a special table. The imaging camera hangs above the table, or the table may slide into a tube-shape machine with the camera inside, similar to the machine used for a CT-SCAN or a MAGNETIC RESONANCE IMAGING (MRI) examination. In either case, the camera records the gamma ray emissions, translating them into a picture on a television screen for the radiologist running the exam.

Risks and Complications

Minor discomfort from the injection or from having to lie still during the exam; allergic reactions to the radioactive material are rare.

The radiation exposure for this test is similar to that for a standard X-ray. After the exam, most of the radioactive material passes out of the body in urine or feces; the rest dissipates naturally through perspiration or breathing. There are no known long-term adverse effects.

This test is not recommended for pregnant women.

Outlook and Lifestyle Modifications

This test provides a clear diagnostic image without the trauma of surgery.

nutrients, nutritional deficiencies See DIETARY FAT; MINERALS; PROTEIN; VITAMINS.

nylon Durable elastic synthetic material created by E.I. du Pont de Nemours & Company chemist Wallace Hume Carothers. Nylon was first introduced in 1937 as single threads used as bristles for hairbrushes and as multiple threads woven into a silk substitute for stockings. Today, nylon is used as a suture in surgical procedures, including plastic surgeries. The suture may be a single thread or braided. Either way, the nylon is stronger than silk, less likely to cause an inflammation at the suture site, and is slowly encapsulated by connective tissue when used for internal suturing.

See also DACRON; SUTURE (SURGICAL).

obesity Excess body weight, so exceeding normal standards that it is considered unhealthy. In the United States, the National Health and Nutrition Examination Survey (NHANES) shows that approximately 119 million Americans, nearly 65 percent of all Americans age 20 to 74, are either overweight (body weight slightly above recommended weight levels) or obese (body weight extremely above recommended weight levels). The effect on health in general is an increased risk of chronic illnesses such as ARTHRITIS, diabetes, gallbladder disease, heart disease, high blood pressure, respiratory illness, stroke, and some forms of cancer. The effect on PLASTIC SURGERY appears to be a continuing increase in the number of cosmetic and reconstructive plastic surgeries (i.e., liposuction, abdominoplasty) designed specifically to reduce fat deposits and/or to eliminate excess skin remaining after massive weight loss.

Currently, the most reliable measurement of overweight and obesity for healthy adults—excluding women who are pregnant or nursing, athletes whose muscle mass may increase their weight, and all persons older than 65—is the BMI (Body Mass Index), an equation relating weight to height.

The original BMI equation, measured in kilograms/kg (weight) and meters/m (height), is $BMI = W/H^2$. In the United States, where weight is measured in pounds/lb. and height in inches/in.,

the equation is $BMI = W/H^2 \times 703$. Thus, a person who weighs 140 lbs. (63.6 kg) and stands 5.4 feet (64 in./1.64 m) tall measures his/her BMI as per the calculations illustrated above.

Health officials from different countries assign slightly different meanings to the BMI measurements. For example, the U.S. Institutes of Health and the World Health Organization consider a BMI lower than 18.5 underweight, BMI 18.5–24.9 acceptable, BMI 25–29.9 overweight, and BMI higher than 30 obese, while Health Canada labels a BMI less than 20 as underweight, BMI 20–24.9 acceptable, BMI 27 overweight, BMI higher than 30 obese. As for the effects of obesity on one's general health, according to Health Canada, both BMI lower than 18.5 and from 25.0–29.9 are labeled increased risk, BMI 30.0–34.9 high risk, BMI 35–39.9 very high risk, and BMI higher than 40 extremely high risk.

See also ABDOMINOPLASTY; ARM LIFT; BUTTOCK LIFT; LIPOSUCTION; THIGH LIFT.

2-octyl cyanoacrylate See WOUND ADHESIVE.

ocular implant surgery Plastic surgery to repair the bone socket surrounding the eye and/or insert an ocular prosthesis (artificial eye) following the loss of an eye due to injury or disease. The implant maintains the natural shape and structure of the area inside the socket and serves as a base on which to place the visible part of an artificial eye.

Procedure

The surgeon removes the damaged eye and inserts an orbital implant into the socket. The implant is

BMI in pounds/inches	BMI in kilograms/meters
$BMI = W/H^2 \times 705 =$	$BMI = W/H^2 =$
140/64 × 64) =	63.6/(1.625 × 1.625) =
140/4096 × 703 =	63.6/2.640 =
24.02 BMI*	24.09 BMI*

*The small difference between the final numbers is not significant; in common terms, both would be listed as BMI 24.

a small round structure made of porous polyethylene, aluminum oxide, or mineral derived from coral and treated to resemble hydroxyapatite, a mineral in human bone. The surgeon attaches the eye muscles to the implant and fixes the implant in place by covering it with the outer layers of the patient's natural eye. About a month after this surgery, the patient is fitted with an artificial eye, a thin porcelain, glass, or plastic shell colored to match the healthy eye and contoured to fit snugly under the eyelids.

Risks and Complications

Successful surgery to attach the eye muscles to the orbital implant enables the implant and artificial eye to move in tandem with the healthy eye. If the artificial eye does not move smoothly, the surgeon may be able to improve its function by inserting a titanium peg to anchor the false eye to the orbital implant.

Outlook and Lifestyle Modifications

Following successful reconstructive surgery, tissue from the patient's body grows into the implant, anchoring it more securely in place, and the eye looks completely normal. The artificial eye usually remains in place for up to several months at a time and is removed occasionally either to examine the implant and socket or simply to clean and polish the prosthesis.

oculoplastic surgery This is a general term for PLASTIC SURGERY on the eye. It includes surgery to rebuild the orbit (the circular cavity comprising parts of the forehead, nose, cheek, and upper jawbones that contains the eyeball and its associated muscles, nerves, and blood vessels). It may also include repair of broken bones after an injury, correction of a birth defect, or repair of the eyelids and/or the tear duct system.

See also EYE LIFT; OCULAR IMPLANT SURGERY.

OMENS OMENS classification; a system used by plastic surgeons to measure the severity of five specific defects affecting the facial features. The system is used when planning reconstructive surgeries or procedures to repair birth defects such as FACIAL CLEFT or HEMIFACIAL MICROSOMIA.

The defects evaluated with the OMENS system are

- *O*rbital asymmetry (unevenly placed eyes). For example, one eye socket may be higher or lower than the norm, or one eye socket may be farther toward the side of the skull, or both may be out of normal line. The more pronounced the deviation, the more severe the defect.
- *M*andibular hypoplasia (underdeveloped lower jaw). The smaller the jaw and the less aligned it is with the upper jaw, the more severe the defect.
- *E*ar deformity (ear missing CARTILAGE or a lobe, or an entirely missing ear). The more tissue missing from the patient's ear, the more severe the defect.
- *N*erve involvement (status of the nerves supplying the defective feature). The more damage to the nerves, the more severe the defect.
- *S*oft tissue deficiency (lack of supporting tissue under the facial skin; for example, the fat pad normally present under the cheek). The more tissue missing, the more severe the defect.

See also FACIAL CLEFT; HEMIFACIAL MICROSOMIA.

omentum Two-part layer of fatty tissue under the peritoneum, the membrane lining the inside surface of the abdomen. The larger part of the omentum (the greater omentum) hangs down from the bottom edge of the stomach to cover the intestines; the smaller part of the omentum (the lesser omentum) extends from the top edge of the stomach to the underside of the liver.

Plastic surgeons may harvest omentum tissue via laparoscopic surgery for use in replacing underlying fatty tissue lost from various parts of the body, most commonly the face and scalp. The omentum is also valuable for reconstructing the oral cavity because, like the tissue found normally in the oral cavity, gastro-omental tissue is a mucous membrane, secreting mucus that keeps the inside of the mouth moist.

See also FAT GRAFTING; SKIN GRAFT.

one-stage esthetic correction   A procedure in which several kinds of surgeries, including plastic surgeries, are performed at the same time by a team of surgeons whose specialties vary according to the requirements of the procedure. For example, the team assembled to reconstruct or repair an abnormally shaped nose and jaw might include an orthodontist/dental surgeon and a plastic surgeon specializing in maxillofacial (jaw and face) procedures, while surgery to reconstruct a hand might include a plastic surgeon and/or an orthopedic surgeon specializing in hand surgery.

See also HEMIFACIAL MICROSOMIA.

open   Surgical term used to describe a procedure performed with a standard, relatively long incision through the skin. For example, an open BROW LIFT is surgery on the forehead performed through an incision that stretches ear to ear along the hairline rather than via laparoscopic surgery through several small incisions. An open rhinoplasty is nasal surgery performed with an incision outside rather than inside the nose. An open miniabdominoplasty is contouring surgery performed with an incision stretching across the lower abdomen rather than through several small incisions.

When possible, modern PLASTIC SURGERY is more frequently performed with less invasive procedures so as to reduce the risk of complications such as infection and scarring.

See also ABDOMINOPLASTY; FOREHEAD LIFT; RHINOPLASTY.

orbitomeatal plane   Eye-ear plane; an imaginary anatomical reference line passing through the skull from the upper edge of the opening of the external ear canal on one side of the head, along the top of the bone under the eyes, and to the same point on the outside of the ear on the other side of the head. The orbitomeatal plane is used by plastic surgeons as a reference point in creating models and/or plans for proposed facial surgery, such as FACE-LIFTS or OCULOPLASTIC SURGERY. It is used by radiologists as a reference point in planning external radiation therapy for the head and neck.

See also EXTERNAL RADIATION THERAPY; RADIATION.

orchioplasty   Orchiopexy; PLASTIC SURGERY to release a testicle that has not descended from the abdominal cavity into the scrotum. The condition, which most frequently affects only one testicle, occurs in approximately 3 percent of newborn males, more commonly among premature infants. The surgery is usually done under general anesthesic, often on an outpatient basis.

Procedure

The surgeon makes an incision in the groin and frees the vas deferens (the tube through which sperm flow from the testicles to the urethra and out of the penis during ejaculation) and the associated blood vessels, nerves, and lymphatic vessels. Next, the surgeon carefully stretches out the vas deferens, makes a small incision in the scrotum, pulls the testicle down into the scrotum, stitches it in place, and closes the incisions.

Risks and Complications

Bleeding, infection, and reaction to the anesthetic are risks with this procedure. Adult patients are usually advised to rest for a few days and to avoid strenuous exercise for at least a month.

Outlook and Lifestyle Modifications

An undescended testicle increases the risk of infertility; once the testicle is moved into the scrotum, up to 90 percent of patients have normal hormone production and fertility. The risk of testicular cancer is up to 50 times higher for men born with an undescended testicle than for men born with normally descended testicles; as a result, men who have surgery to correct an undecided testicle should be examined regularly to detect any tumor.

otoplasty   See also EAR PINBACK; EAR RECONSTRUCTION.

overcorrection   In PLASTIC SURGERY, most commonly facial plastic surgery, a term used to describe the result of a surgeon's removing too much tissue, leading to complications such as an unnaturally tight facial appearance after a face-lift or the collapse of the nose after rhinoplasty. To remedy the problem, the patient may require a second surgery to replace lost bone and/or CARTILAGE.

Overcorrection may result from poor surgical planning or technique, or it may be the result of damage due to repeated surgeries that have damaged the bone or weakened the supporting tissues under the skin. It is sometimes done purposely to compensate for expected post-op changes, such as contraction of scar tissue or loss of flap volume due to resolution of edema.

The procedure to repair defects such as overcorrection due to complications from a previous surgery is commonly known as secondary surgery or sometimes touch-up surgery. Such surgery may be required, for example, to replace or reposition breast implants, to rebuild a nose from which much bone was taken, or to add more hair transplants after a hair replacement session. Another example is surgery to rebuild a sunken bridge of the nose caused by the surgeon's having removed too much supporting tissue during rhinoplasty.

Overcorrection may or may not constitute malpractice. Patients who believe their doctors are guilty of wrongdoing can seek legal recourse, although individual cases must be decided on their merits. It is possible for overcorrection to occur even when doctors plan and execute surgery appropriately.

See also FACE-LIFT; NECK LIFT; RHINOPLASTY.

pain Pain is a sensation triggered when body tissue is injured, either accidentally or during surgical procedures, including PLASTIC SURGERY.

Pain occurs when the damaged tissue releases histamines and cytokine, components of the IMMUNE SYSTEM that manage the inflammatory response. The histamines and cytokines latch onto the ends of nerve fibers, setting off the electrical impulses that travel along the nerve fibers to the spinal cord. In response, the spinal cord releases chemical signals that stimulate the nerve fibers that transmit a message to the brain, which identifies the message as pain of one sort or another. Analgesics and anesthetics alleviate pain by interrupting one or more of these reactions.

There are several types of pain reactions. These reactions are classified by the cause of the pain, the nerves or area of the body it affects, or how long it lasts.

Central pain is any pain sensation arising in the central nervous system (brain and spinal cord) such as that from a spinal cord injury or from an illness such as multiple sclerosis that attacks the central nervous system.

Neuropathic pain is pain that originates in a nerve and that arises from an injury or a nerve-related illness, sometimes resulting in a neuropathy, chronic pain that may last for weeks, months, or even years after the injury is healed or the illness cured. Some common causes of neuropathy are

- alcoholism
- amputation leading to phantom limb pain, the illusion of sensation in the missing limb
- diabetes
- exposure to toxins, including some chemotherapies

- nutritional deficiencies
- repetitive movement such as typing motions linked to CARPAL TUNNEL SYNDROME (pain in the wrist)
- shingles (herpes infection)

Note: Neuropathy is not a protective warning like other forms of pain but a sign of damage to the nervous system.

Nociceptive pain (from the Latin *nocere*, meaning "to injure") originates from an injury such as a burn, broken bone, bruise, cut, inflammation, or muscle stress. The sensation is limited to the area of the injury, and when the injury heals, the pain disappears. Peripheral pain (from the Greek *peri-*, meaning "around," and *phero*, meaning "carry") is nociceptive pain arising from an injury to muscles and/or tendons in the outer parts of the body, such as the arms and legs. Visceral pain is nociceptive pain originating in the viscera, the internal organs such as the stomach.

Persistent pain is a long-lasting sensation usually associated with damage to muscles and/or bones. It may alter the body's handling of pain signals, increasing the amount of chemicals released when a pain signal reaches a nerve ending or encouraging the growth of new nerves at the place on the spine where pain signals are received, so that persistent pain spreads out along nerve fibers, causing discomfort in parts of the body not directly related to the injury.

Phantom pain is discomfort at the site of an amputated limb; a burning, itching, tingling, or painful sensation creating an impression that the amputated limb is still in place. It can be treated as any other pain, with analgesics and/or mind/body therapies such as BIOFEEDBACK.

Referred pain is discomfort that arises due to an injury or illness in one part of the body but whose signals travel via nerve pathways to be felt somewhere else. For example, a person having a heart attack may experience pain in the left arm, while a person whose gallbladder is infected may feel pain in the right shoulder.

Pain Measurement Scale

To evaluate a person's perception of the severity of pain, doctors use a pain measurement scale. As a rule, adults are asked to rank their pain on a scale from 0 (no pain) to 10 (the worst possible pain). Children are asked to choose one of six pictures or drawings of faces whose expression ranges from smiling and happy to contorted as in severe pain. To assess pain levels in patients who cannot speak, pain experts observe vital signs (heart rate, respiration, pulse, and temperature) along with the patient's general level of calm versus restlessness or agitation, the latter being more common when people are in pain.

pain measurement scale   See PAIN.

palatoplasty   Plastic surgery to repair or reconstruct the palate, the tissues separating the mouth from the nasal passages. The hard palate is the arched top of the oral cavity over the tongue and teeth, a structure composed of bone covered with a mucous membrane. The soft palate, at the back of the mouth, is a fold of muscle covered with epithelial tissue that blocks the opening from the back of the nose during swallowing, thus preventing food and liquid from rising into the nose. The rounded tag hanging down from the soft palate at the back of the mouth is the uvula (from the Latin *uva*, meaning "grape"). The most common palatoplasty is surgery to repair a cleft palate; uraniscoplasty is surgery to form an artificial palate.

See also CLEFT LIP AND/OR PALATE.

parrot beak deformity   Nose with a tip that leans forward and down over the nostrils due either to a birth defect (underdeveloped bone structure of the nose) or to excessive removal of tissue during cosmetic or reconstructive surgery on the nose, leaving the tip without adequate support. The remedies for parrot beak deformity are similar to those for SADDLE NOSE, a related condition.

partial thickness   See BURNS AND BURN RECONSTRUCTION; SKIN GRAFT.

pathology   The study of the cause, development, and consequences of illness. During or after surgery, including PLASTIC SURGERY, a pathologist evaluates any tissue, such as a MOLE, removed from the body to determine whether it is benign or malignant.

The pathologist is a physician specializing in pathology; a board-certified pathologist is a person who has graduated from an accredited school of medicine, has a valid license to practice medicine, has completed a residency in pathology, and has passed the qualifying exams of the American Board of Pathology (ABP) in anatomical and/or clinical pathology. Persons accredited in these areas may also apply for certification in ABP subspecialties, including blood banking/transfusion medicine, chemical pathology, cytopathology, forensic pathology, hematology, medical microbiology, neuropathology, and pediatric pathology. ABP and the American Board of Dermatology offer a joint certification in dermatopathology; ABP and the American Board of Medical Genetics offer a joint certification in molecular genetic pathology.

pectoral augmentation   Surgery to insert material that will make the area around the pectoral muscle (from the Latin *pectoralis*, meaning "breast bone") more prominent.

Procedure

The surgeon makes an incision in the armpit and inserts a flexible silicone implant, maneuvering it into place behind the pectoral muscle. When one side is done, the surgeon closes the incision and repeats the process on the other side of the body.

Risks and Complications

Prior to this surgery, patients are usually advised to avoid working out for several weeks so as to reduce the risk of injury that might require postponing the procedure. After the surgery, the area will be sore for several days. Once the stitches are removed, patients are generally advised to wait two to six weeks before starting to exercise or take part in sports activities.

Possible complications include infection requiring removal of the implant; slippage of the implant requiring surgery to move it back into place; hematoma (blood clot); or temporary or permanent numbness in the upper arm due to nerve injury during surgery.

Outlook and Lifestyle Modifications

Successful surgery creates the appearance of a more powerful and more masculine chest but does not add muscle mass.

penile enlargement   Surgery that makes the penis look longer and/or wider without actually changing its size.

Procedures

The three most common cosmetic procedures for penis enlargement are penile ligament release, penalscrotal webbing release, and pubic liposuction.

Penile ligament release   During this procedure, also known as suspensatory ligament release, the surgeon makes an incision at the base of the penis (the underside of the point where the penis meets the groin) and cuts through the ligament anchoring the penis to the pubic bone. When the ligament is cut, a part of the penis that normally remains under the skin of the groin area slides forward, producing about one extra inch of external length. To maintain this extra length outside the body, the patient must wear weights on the penis for several months after the surgery, stretching the tissues so that the penis does not slide back under the skin.

Penoscrotal webbing release   During this procedure, also known as scrotum release, the surgeon detaches the underside of the penis from the skin of the scrotum (testes) so the penis moves forward

and looks longer; once again, there is no actual increase in penile length.

Pubic liposuction   The surgeon removes fat at the lower part of the abdomen, around the base of the penis. When the fat is removed, the penis appears longer and more prominent.

Risks and Complications

Bruising, swelling, scarring, and infection are risks for all forms of penile enlargement. Penile ligament release may keep the penis from standing upright when erect and/or may make it difficult or impossible to control movement of the penis during intercourse.

penile implant   A device designed to produce an erect penis in men unable to experience a natural erection. Generally used only after less invasive methods have failed, specifically in men whose erectile difficulties are due to physical problems such as blood vessel disease, diabetes, nerve damage caused by injury, or as a complication from pelvic surgery. Implants are not used as a treatment for erectile dysfunction due to psychological problems.

Three styles of penile implants are available: the semirigid malleable implant, the multipart inflatable implant, and the self-contained inflatable implant. None of the three either interfere with or guarantee ejaculation or orgasm; none affects libido (the desire for sex).

The semirigid malleable implant is a flexible rod-shaped silicone prosthetic. The device, which is surgically implanted into the penis, is normally bent down against the body and then straightened for intercourse. It is simple and relatively low-priced, but it does not increase the length or width of the penis, although it gives the impression of a permanent erection.

The multipart inflatable implant consists of two hollow cylinders that are surgically inserted into the penis; a pump in the scrotum; and a reservoir either inside the cylinders or as a separate part to be surgically inserted into the lower abdomen. To bring the penis erect, one squeezes the pump, sending fluid from the reservoir into the cylinders. The virtues of this device are that it is controlled by the owner, who is able to mimic the normal rise and fall of an erection with a natural-seeming increase in the length and width of the penis. The chief disadvantages are the device's high cost and the possibility of mechanical failure.

The self-contained inflatable implant consists of two parallel cylinders surgically inserted into the penis. To attain an erection, one squeezes the ends of the cylinders at the tip of the penis, releasing fluid to fill the cylinders, firming the penis in an apparently natural erection under the control of the user. This device does not lengthen or widen the penis, but it is easier to insert than the multipart inflatable implant, and it does not require any implants in the scrotum or abdomen. The chief disadvantage, as with the multipart device, is the possibility of mechanical failure. One type of self-contained inflatable implant is the Hydroflex penile implant.

Procedure

Surgery to insert a penile implant is performed under regional or general anesthesic. Once the patient is anesthetized, the surgeon inserts a thin flexible catheter into the urethra, the tube that carries urine from the urinary bladder out of the body. (In men, the urethra also carries sperm.) The catheter is left in place for about 24 hours after surgery to avoid any contamination of the surgical site.

Next, the implant is put in place through an incision in the penis; the multipart implant also requires an incision in the scrotum and lower abdomen to insert the pump and the reservoir. The patient usually stays in the hospital for a day or two. After leaving, men with a semirigid or self-contained implant generally should avoid tight underwear or trousers until the incision has completely healed. Men who have chosen a multipart implant may be advised to avoid tight clothing for up to six weeks so as not to displace the reservoir implanted in the abdomen.

Risks and Complications

The risk of infection after a penile implant is higher in men with a chronic condition such as diabetes, a spinal cord injury, or a history of urinary infections. To prevent infection, surgeons usually prescribe a course of antibiotics after implantation; if an infection occurs and is severe, the implant may have to be removed. Painful erection may also require removal of the implant. Other complications include the implant's being put in wrong or breaking through the skin of the penis or into the urethra. The most common complications with inflatable implants are leakage or mechanical failure.

Outlook and Lifestyle Modifications

Regardless of the type of implant chosen, a man can usually resume intercourse after about a month. During the waiting period, the inflatable implants should not be inflated.

The overall incidence of complications is low, between 1 and 4 percent, and the devices are all relatively durable; for example, even the multipart inflatable implant may last for 10 years or more.

penis implant See PENILE IMPLANT.

periareolar breast lift See BREAST REDUCTION.

periodontal disease Gum disease; infection caused by bacteria in plaque, a sticky colorless film that forms naturally on teeth. The bacteria excrete a toxin that inflames and may destroy gum tissue and, eventually, the bone supporting the teeth. This damage is commonly treated with surgical procedures designed to conserve and or replace bone.

Symptoms and Diagnostic Path

There are several forms of periodontal disease, each diagnosed by its symptoms. Gingivitis, the mildest form of periodontal disease, reddens the gums, which swell and bleed easily, symptoms that can be controlled with professional cleaning and rigorous home care. Chronic periodontitis, the most common form, is characterized by continuing gum inflammation, formation of "pockets" in the gum around each tooth along with continuing gum recession (shrinkage) bone loss. Aggressive periodontitis is characterized by sudden, rapid loss of gum and bone tissue in otherwise healthy people.

Necrotizing periodontal disease, characterized by the death (necrosis) of gum tissue, is most commonly associated with systemic conditions affecting the IMMUNE SYSTEM such as HIV/AIDS, malnutrition, or the use of immunosuppressant drugs after organ transplant.

Treatment Options and Outlook

The first step in treating periodontal disease is a maintenance plan: periodic professional cleaning (scaling) to remove plaque from the teeth and monitor the progress of the condition plus rigorous home care between dental visits. Progressive disease may require one of the following reconstructive dental surgeries:

- pocket reduction (surgery to cut away loose gum tissue, reducing spaces in which bacteria flourish)
- bone grafts (transplants of natural or synthetic material to strengthened damaged bone)
- soft tissue grafts (pieces of tissue lifted from the adjacent gum or the palate to cover areas where the original gum has been lost)

A patient who has already lost a tooth to periodontal disease may be interested in DENTAL IMPLANTS, a permanent tooth replacement option. Once bone loss leads to tooth loss, the patient may get dental implants, small devices inserted into the remaining jaw as anchors for replacement teeth. Note: Once a tooth is removed, the periodontal disease at that site ceases. It does not resume if a false tooth is inserted. However, is the patient fails to practice good oral hygiene, bone supporting the implant may be lost.

Risk Factors and Preventive Measures

Periodontal disease often runs in families; the most common risk factor is poor home care and lack of early treatment. A genetic susceptibility to the disease may affect as many as one in every three adults in the United States.

Several medical factors influence the progress and intensity of periodontal disease. Fluctuating levels of estrogen at puberty, menstruation, and during pregnancy can contribute to deterioration, because unlike testosterone, which builds new bone, estrogen plays a role in breaking down old bone. Emotional or physical stress can reduce the effectiveness of the immune system, making gums more susceptible to bacteria. Other factors include specific illnesses, such as diabetes, and certain drugs, including (but not limited to) oral contraceptives, antidepressants, and some medicines used to treat heart disease.

Other risk factors for periodontal disease include tobacco use and clenching the jaws or grinding the teeth, particularly while sleeping, which puts extra pressure on the teeth and may hasten bone loss.

Peyronie's disease This condition is characterized by the contraction of fibrous tissue under the skin of the penis, causing the organ to bend when erect. First identified by French surgeon François de la Peyronie (1678–1747), this problem may be relieved by reconstructive surgery to release the contracture.

phalloplasty Technically, any surgery on the penis; the term is most often used to describe surgery to build a penis during female-to-male gender reassignment surgery.

Procedures

Plastic surgeons commonly use one of two procedures to construct the new penis. The first is metoidoplasty, surgery to release the clitoris from its membrane tissue covering (hood) and the fibrous tissue underneath so that it can move forward in a multistage procedure that may also be used to replace a penis lost to trauma or disease. The second is penis construction with SKIN FLAPS.

Metoidoplasty The surgeon cuts the clitoris free of its membranes, moves the labia minora (small lips of the vagina) up to thicken and protect the freed clitoris, and may alter the tip of the clitoris to resemble the tip of a penis. The labia majora (large lips of the vagina) are moved downward, and implants are inserted to simulate a scrotum containing testicles. The surgeon may move the urethra (the tube leading from the bladder to the outside of the body) so that it opens at the tip of the newly created penis, enabling the patient to urinate while standing. After metoidoplasty, the patient may be given hormones to enlarge the clitoris so that it appears normal.

Penis construction with skin flaps First, the surgeon removes the female organs, including the uterus and ovaries. A year later, when the original surgery has healed, the surgeon will use a skin flap, commonly from the forearm, shoulder, or abdomen to construct a urethra and penis. When the new penis is attached to the body, the clitoral nerves are attached to nerves in the skin flap, and the newly constructed urethra is attached to the patient's original urethra. At the same time, the labia majora (the outer vaginal lips) are used to create a new scrotum. Several months later, when the patient has healed completely, the surgeon may insert testicular implants into the labia/scrotum, and a prosthesis into the penis to enable the patient to attain an erection.

Neoscrotum construction Part of both procedures described above is surgery to construct a natural-looking scrotum. The surgeon inserts tissue expanders to stretch the labia majora (large outer lips of the vagina) and periodically enlarges the expanders by filling them with a sterile saline solution. After several months, when the labial tissue has been sufficiently stretched, the surgeon removes the expanders and inserts silicon testicular implants, and then sutures the labia together so that they appear to be a normal scrotal sac.

Risks and Complications

Bleeding, swelling, infection. Complications specific to metoidoplasty include nerve damage to the erectile tissue in the clitoral members, and a risk of urinary leakage from the newly situated urinary opening. The latter problem may require a second, corrective surgery.

Complications specific to building a penis with skin flaps include scarring at the site from which the flaps were taken, failure of the skin flaps to thrive at the new site, and obstruction of the urinary tract, requiring corrective surgery.

Outlook and Lifestyle Modifications

The aim of this surgery is to produce a sexually functioning penis; success depends on the sur-

geon's skill and to a large extent on the patient's expectations.

See also GLANSPLASTY; PENILE ENLARGEMENT; SKIN FLAPS.

phlebectomy Surgery to remove a VARICOSE VEIN, a swollen, twisted vein, most commonly visible on the leg or ankle.

Procedures

There are two basic methods for removing a varicose vein: ambulatory phlebectomy (sometimes described as "stab avulsion" or "hook phlebectomy") and transilluminated powered phlebectomy.

Ambulatory phlebectomy The surgeon uses an indelible pen or surgical marks to outline the affected veins both while the patient is standing and lying down. Then, he numbs the area either with an injection of LOCAL ANESTHETIC directly into the vein or as a regional block (an injection that numbs a larger area around a specific nerve) or as an infusion or a large amount of anesthetic solution into the tissue around the vein. The latter technique makes the vein easy to reach, lengthens the effectiveness of the anesthesic, and compresses the area so as to reduce swelling after the surgery. When the anesthetic takes effect, the surgeon makes several small (1–3 mm/$^1/_{32}$–$^3/_{32}$ inch) incisions about 2–15 centimeters/1–6 inches apart along the vein. She next inserts a stripper, a hook-like instrument used to lift the vein free of the surrounding fatty and connective tissues, ties off the vein, and uses a small forceps to ambulate (push or pull) the vein from one incision to the next. The surgeon may remove part of the vein or the entire vein. Because the incisions are so small, no sutures are required.

Transilluminated powered phlebectomy The patient walks around for about 30 minutes to dilate the varicose veins, which are then marked with an indelible marker or surgical pen. If necessary, the surgeon may perform an ultrasound imaging study to ascertain the condition of the veins. Once the patient is given either local anesthesic, a spinal block, or general anesthesic, the surgeon makes small (3 mm/$^3/_{32}$ inch) incisions near the vein. She then inserts an irrigated illuminator, a lighted device with a channel through which the surgeon sends a large amount of an anesthetic solution into the area around the vein to lift the vein from the surrounding tissue. With the illuminator in place, the surgeon makes a second small incision and inserts a motorized resector, a bladed device attached to a suction pump. The resector draws in the vein, slices it up, and pulls the fragments out of the body. The surgeon repeats this sequence as needed to remove additional sections of the vein. The incisions are closed with a single stitch or an adhesive strip, and another anesthetic is injected to minimize bruising, pain, and blood clots.

The advantages of transilluminated powered phlebectomy appear to be fewer incisions (an average six versus 17 for ambulatory phlebectomy), a shorter operating time, more complete removal of the varicosities due to a better view of the field, and less pain several weeks after the procedure.

Risks and Complications

Swelling, bleeding, and superficial blood clots are common with phlebectomy. Other possible complications include scarring and reactions to the anesthetics or to dressings, commonly adhesives, and temporary numbness of the skin due to anesthesic or the surgical incisions. There may also be temporary discoloration of the skin and bumps caused by blood clots in the hollow left by the vein. These bumps usually disappear naturally within a few months.

The patient may see clusters of dilated blood vessels that represent areas still to be treated or may develop new clusters of varicosities due to an increase in venous pressure or the abnormal growth of new blood vessels as a response to tissue injury. If these clusters do not disappear spontaneously within a few months, very small vessels may be resolved with sclerotherapy or LASER therapy. Larger recurring varicosities may require further phlebectomy.

Outlook and Lifestyle Modifications

After either procedure, the postoperative dressing remains in place for two days. The patient commonly wears elastic support hose for two to six weeks and may also be asked to return to the doctor's office three times a week for two weeks for

ultrasound and other treatments to decrease pain and swelling.

The treated veins do not reappear, but new varicosities are possible.

See also SCLEROTHERAPY; VARICOSE VEINS.

Pierre Robin anomaly   See CHIN RECONSTRUCTION.

pigmentation mismatch   See CHEMICAL SKIN PEEL.

pig skin dressing   See SKIN GRAFTS.

plastic surgery   Any procedure to improve appearance or to improve the function of a body part. The evolution of plastic surgery as a medical discipline divides clearly into five distinct periods:

1. The creation of the written records in the ancient world.
2. The rebirth and consolidation of intellectual inquiry after the 900-year-long Dark Ages.
3. The expansion of medical knowledge and technique during the 18th and 19th centuries.
4. The establishment of a modern discipline between the two world wars.
5. The expansion of the discipline based on techniques developed on the battlefields of Europe, Korea, and Vietnam.

History of Plastic Surgery

The first written description of surgery to correct facial defects is the *Edwin Smith Papyrus* (ca. 3000 B.C.E.), named for the Connecticut Egyptologist who discovered it in Luxor in 1862. The manuscript, translated in 1930 by James H. Breasted, director of the University of Chicago Oriental Institute, contains 48 case histories, 27 of them head injuries such as deep scalp wounds and skull fractures.

Writing the early record   The *Samhita* (encyclopedia) by Sushruta is the classic text on Ayurveda, a system of healing arts based on creating harmony in one's body and life. The book, compiled during the first century C.E., was written in a period when amputation of the nose and genitalia was a common consequence of tribal warfare and an accepted punishment for criminal acts. As a result, the *Samhita,* which was eventually translated into Arabic, Latin, and German, is a source of reconstructive procedures such as rebuilding the earlobe with skin from the cheek and the nose with skin from the forehead (see CARPUE'S OPERATION).

The multivolume Roman *De Medicina* by Aulus Cornelius Celsus approaches the subject from both sides, presenting techniques for amputation as well as for repairing mutilated lips, ears, and noses. In Byzantium, the emperor Julian's personal physician Orabasius's 70-volume *Synagogue Medicae* (fourth century C.E.) had two chapters devoted entirely to the reconstruction of facial defects, including such advances as the advice to use SUTURES loose enough to allow a wound to heal without distorting the face, to clean exposed bone and removed damaged tissue so as to speed healing and prevent infection, to use SKIN FLAPS to replace lost skin and provide a normal facial appearance when repairing cheeks, ears, eyebrows, lips, and nose, and to retain the CARTILAGE support for ears and nose.

Despite the knowledge available in these classic texts, for 900 years, from the fall of the Roman Empire to the dawn of the Renaissance, intellectual commerce between Europe and the East came to a halt as did medical investigation. This left the Europeans to rely on dubious sources called "leech books," which were essentially collections of folk wisdom regarding illnesses, symptoms, and treatment. Occasionally, something new slipped through, such as the first description of a European attempt to repair a CLEFT LIP that appeared in *Bald's Leechbook* (ca. 920).

But as the Dark Ages receded, Western medical inquiry and conversation began anew. For example, it is clear European surgeons knew of the *Cerrahiyet-ul Haniyye* (imperial surgery) (ca. 15th century), the first illustrated Islamic surgical text, compiled by medical writer and inventor Serafeddin Sabuncuoglu. The book, or at least its contents, including a description of the first cosmetic BREAST REDUCTION, as well a various techniques for repairing damaged eyelids, was likely carried into southern Italy by invaders from the East. It was also the likely source for techniques described by Bolognese

philosopher-surgeon Leonardo Fioravanti in his *Il tesoro della vita humana (Thesis on Human Life),* ca. 1568.

Fioravanti's report included Indian nasal reconstruction refined by Sicilian physicians who used a skin flap from the arm rather than the forehead. This new "Italian method" lifted a piece of skin from the arm and attached it to the face but did not completely sever the skin from the arm until it (the flap) had become firmly affixed to the face. This new "Italian method" required the patient to assume an uncomfortable position—arm to face—as the wound healed, but it also assured a blood supply that kept the SKIN GRAFT alive on its new site.

Nonetheless, Indian RHINOPLASTY survived, thanks in large part to British surgeon Joseph Carpue of York Hospital in Chelsea, England, whose *Restoration of a Lost Nose* (1816) details his operations on two British officers, one who had lost his nose to arsenic poisoning, the other to a battle wound.

Approaching the modern age By and large, insofar as plastic surgery is concerned, the 1800s belong to the Germans such as Carl von Graefe, chief of surgery at the Berlin Charite, the first to link the word *plastic* with reconstructive surgery in the title of his *Rhinoplastik* (Rebuilding the nose) (1818). The book, a compilation of 55 previous reports of successful surgeries using both the Indian and Italian methods, also presents German innovations such as the use of a free graft (skin lifted entirely from the donor site) from the arm to rebuild the nose, as well as new approaches to eyelid surgery and CLEFT LIP AND/OR PALATE.

JOHANN FRIEDRICH DIEFFENBACH, von Graefe's successor at the Charite, was among the first to use anesthesic for rhinoplasty; his own text, *Die operative Chirurgie* (1845), is still considered a classic text of oral and facial surgery. Other German surgeons pioneered new grafting techniques such as the use of bone to rebuild damaged faces and experimented unsuccessfully with tissue from other species, such as ducks.

Equally important, these doctors introduced the concept of plastic surgery as a benefit to the psyche as well as the body, a radical departure in a society dominated by the Prussian belief that one accepted one's burdens, including physical deformity, in silence. The aesthetic approach was strongly endorsed by JACQUES JOSEPH, the Prussian-born, German-trained author of *Nasenplastik und Sonstige Gesichtsplastik* (Rhinoplasty and other facial plastic surgery, 1928), who is generally regarded as the father of modern reconstructive nasal surgery.

Charles C. Miller, an American "featural surgeon" (the sometimes derogatory term applied to those who believed in purely cosmetic procedures), wrote in the introduction to *The Correction of Featural Imperfections* (1908) that there is no longer any "doubt that featural surgery is destined to take its place as a recognized specialty." Miller, like the Germans, was strongly supported by St. Louis surgeon Vilray Papin Blair, whose innovative photographs of jaw reconstruction appeared in the *Journal of the American Medical Association* (1909) and whose *Surgery and Diseases of the Mouth and Jaw* (1912) remains a classic in its field.

Learning from battle From the beginning, the interest in facial reconstruction was driven by a desire to reduce the impact of injuries sustained in conflict of one kind or another. Not surprisingly, World War I, erupting on the heels of the 19th-century advances, became a seminal moment in the history of modern plastic surgery.

When the United States entered the war in 1917, reconstructive surgery took an immense step forward when the U.S. Surgeon General called on Vilray Papin Blair to set up military plastic surgery teams in specialized centers to repair and reconstruct damaged faces and bodies. The teams drew on the skills of surgeons from the Allied countries, many of whom left Germany for the United States after the war.

During the 1920s and 1930s, these men joined their American counterparts to secure professional recognition for plastic surgeons. They created the American Society of Plastic Surgeons, published a professional journal, and convinced the American Board of Surgery to conduct qualifying exams in plastic surgery and, in 1937, to establish an American Board of Plastic Surgery, thus ensuring a standard of excellence for its practitioners.

Entering the modern era Medical advances in the years after World War I made battlefield plastic surgery ever more valuable in World War II. The introduction of blood plasma and routine BLOOD TRANSFUSIONS kept wounded soldiers alive on the way to the surgeon; once there, safer anesthesic made surgery less risky. The invention of the dermatome, an instrument that enabled surgeons to shave off thin pieces of healthy skin with which to close an open wound, reduced the incidence of disfiguring contracted scars. The use of bone transplants made it possible to rebuild more normal facial structures. Finally, the introduction of antibiotics (sulfonamides and penicillin) saved countless lives by preventing infection after surgery.

As it had in World War I, the U.S. military once again set up specialized plastic surgery treatment and training centers, including centers specializing in the new field of hand repair. In 1945, when the war ended, there were more than 20 plastic surgery facilities in Europe to handle moderate injuries and nine in the United States to treat those whose complex wounds required multiple surgeries and longer rehabilitation.

In the 1950s, the Korean conflict produced its own contributions to plastic surgery such as internal wiring for facial fractures and yet more varieties of skin flaps to repair damaged skin, a trend that continued in Vietnam during the 1960s. Finally, there have been dramatic advances in microvascular reconstructive surgical techniques developed as a result of miniaturization and advances in optics "spun-off" from developments in the space race of the 1960s and 1970s.

Modern Plastic Surgery Procedures

Modern plastic surgery concentrates on cosmetic and reconstructive procedures to repair birth defects and reduce damage from injuries, while supporting research on new materials and the basic mechanisms by which the body builds and heals itself so as to improve healing and reduce scarring.

Cosmetic surgery This term describes any elective procedure to alter a normal body structure so as to enhance appearance, such as surgery to reduce the size of a large nose or a CHEMICAL SKIN PEEL to repair age-related damage such as roughness, WRINKLES, and/or unusual pigmentation. Also known as esthetic (or aesthetic) surgery, the primary aim of these medical procedures is to enhance appearance rather than to improve or restore body function. According to the American Society of Aesthetics Plastic Surgeons, in 2004 Americans spent more than $12 billion on nearly 2.2 million cosmetic plastic surgery procedures and 9.8 million nonsurgical cosmetics procedures, an increase of nearly 20 percent and 50 percent, respectively, over 2003. The five most popular cosmetic surgeries in the United States are LIPOSUCTION, BREAST AUGMENTATION, EYE LIFT, RHINOPLASTY (surgery to correct the shape of the nose), and FACE-LIFTS. The five most popular nonsurgical cosmetic procedures are BOTOX injection, LASER hair removal, CHEMICAL SKIN PEEL, MICRODERMABRASION to smooth the facial skin, and injections of FILLERS to round and smooth facial wrinkles. Women account for nine of every 10 cosmetic procedures. Nearly half of the patients seeking cosmetic plastic surgery are 35 to 50 years old; 31 percent are older; 24 percent are younger; 80 percent are white; 8.5 percent are Hispanic; 6.2 percent are African American; and 4.6 percent are Asians. The growing popularity of cosmetic surgery has generated the slang term *done* as in "She had her face done," referring to a tight, unnatural facial appearance resulting from multiple cosmetic surgeries.

Reconstructive surgery   This term describes any procedure to improve function by correcting an abnormality of a body structure due to a birth defect (such as cleft palate), an abnormality in development (such as LIMB-LENGTH DISCREPANCY), an injury (such as a burn), or to a disease (such as cancer). Reconstructive surgery may also have cosmetic benefits, creating a normal appearance while repairing a functional defect; for example, by reconstructing the face of a child born without a lower jaw or by tightening a drooping eyelid that is blocking vision. According to the American Society of Plastic Surgeons, in 2004 nearly 6 million reconstructive plastic surgery procedures were performed in the United States. The most common reconstructive surgeries were

- surgeries to remove a tumor (4,084,651)
- surgeries to repair a wound (314,844)
- breast reduction (105,592)
- jaw and face repair (84,469)
- breast reconstruction (62,930)

- birth defects (38,563)
- burn care and reconstruction (35,720)
- animal bite repair (44,801)
- breast implant removal (16,424)

Risks and complications of modern plastic surgery   As with any surgical procedure, plastic surgery may not be advisable for people with certain medical conditions, including (but not limited to) a recent heart attack or serious infection; a blood-clotting disorder; a chronic infectious disease such as hepatitis or HIV/AIDS; or some forms of cancer.

Some psychological conditions may also be disqualifying factors. Body dysmorphic disorder (BDD) is characterized by an obsession with an unrealistic body image (a person's perception of his/her own body) or an imagined or minimal flaw such as minor scarring or hair loss. For example, a thin person may see herself as overweight. BDD is a particularly important consideration in choosing candidates for plastic surgery because individuals with this condition may not only request unnecessary procedures but are also likely to be dissatisfied even with medically and aesthetically successful results.

Persons who undergo plastic surgery to repair a serious disfiguring condition such as a birth defect or injury due to a violent accident or crime may require follow-up psychological counseling.

Some risks associated with plastic surgery are similar to those linked to other forms of surgery: infection, reaction to an anesthetic, scarring, or nerve damage leading to loss of sensation, long-lasting pain, or discomfort. Others, such as the body's rejection of skin grafts or fat embolisms following liposuction, may be specific to plastic surgery procedures.

Qualifications of Modern Plastic Surgeons

In the United States, any licensed medical doctor, regardless of training, may legally perform plastic surgery and call oneself a plastic surgeon. In addition, surgeons certified by other medical boards may perform plastic surgery procedures related to their original specialties. For example, otolaryngologists (physicians who treat disorders of the ear, nose, and throat) may do surgery on the nose and face; ophthalmologists (eye specialists) may do surgery on the eyelids; and dermatologists may perform dermabrasion, chemical skin peels, laser surgery on the skin, and liposuction.

A "board-certified" plastic surgeon is a doctor who is certified as a plastic surgeon by the American Board of Plastic Surgery. To attain this status, the physician must

- graduate from an accredited medical school
- obtain a medical license
- complete at least five years of additional training as a surgeon with at least a three-year residency in an accredited general surgery program and at least a two-year residency in plastic surgery
- pass the American Board of Plastic Surgery's written and oral exams

In some states, the certification exam must be repeated from time to time; in others, physicians certified before a certain date are encouraged to seek recertification but are not required to do so. While board certification does not guarantee a perfect outcome, it does tell the patient that the doctor has taken the time and effort to pass a rigorous examination in his/her field.

A patient seeking to find out whether an individual plastic surgeon is certified by the American Board of Plastic Surgery may call the American Board of Medical Specialities at (800) 776–2378 or go online at http://www.abms.org/. The Web site requires a short registration procedure that gives the consumer access to the certification information about the physician.

The members of the American Board of Medical Specialities include

- American Board of Allergy and Immunology
- American Board of Anesthesiology
- American Board of Colon and Rectal Surgery
- American Board of Dermatology
- American Board of Emergency Medicine
- American Board of Family Medicine
- American Board of Internal Medicine
- American Board of Medical Genetics

- American Board of Neurological Surgery
- American Board of Nuclear Medicine
- American Board of Obstetrics and Gynecology
- American Board of Ophthalmology
- American Board of Orthopaedic Surgery
- American Board of Otolaryngology
- American Board of Pathology
- American Board of Pediatrics
- American Board of Physical Medicine and Rehabilitation
- American Board of Plastic Surgery
- American Board of Preventive Medicine

platelet Platelets (from the Greek *platys*, meaning "flat") are small, colorless, sticky, irregularly shaped disklike particles in blood essential for hemostasis (blood clotting). A sufficient amount of platelets in the blood prevents uncontrolled bleeding after an injury such as a surgical incision; one of the standard blood tests performed before any surgery, including PLASTIC SURGERY, assesses the patient's platelet count.

Platelets release and activate naturally occurring coagulation (clotting) compounds in the body while aggregating (clumping) together with calcium, vitamin K, fibrinogen (a protein in blood), and other platelets to form clots over injuries or to plug small holes in injured blood vessels.

Healthy adults have about 150,000–400,000 particles/mm^3 (millimeters cubed) blood. Lower platelet levels (thrombocytopenia) may occur with types of anemia and leukemia (cancer of the blood). The following medications, among others, can also lower one's platelet level:

- chloramphenicol (antibiotic)
- colchicine (antigout)
- H2 blocking agents (acid reflux)
- heparin (anticoagulant/blood thinner)
- hydralazine (high blood pressure)
- indomethacin (nonsteroidal anti-inflammatory)
- isoniazid/INH (tuberculosis)

- quinidine/Cardioquin
- Duraquin (heartbeat regulator)
- streptomycin (antibiotic)
- sulfonamide (antibiotic)
- thiazide diuretic/multiple brands ("water pills")
- tolbutamide/Orinase (antidiabetic)

Higher levels of platelets (thrombocytosis) may occur with leukemia, gastric bleeding (as from an ulcer), after removal of the spleen, or during and immediately after a heart attack or stroke.

platinum   See BREAST IMPLANT.

platysmaplasty   See NECK LIFT.

plumper filler   See LIP AUGMENTATION.

Poland syndrome   See FINGERS AND TOES, CONGENITAL STRUCTURAL DEFECTS.

polydactyly   A congenital defect involving the presence of more than five fingers on a hand or five toes on a foot; may occur alone as a dominant genetic trait. *Syndactyly* is fusion of fingers/toes. *Polysyndactyly* is a condition with extra fingers/toes, some of which are fused or joined with a tissue web. It is associated with Nager syndrome, a genetic disorder whose characteristic defects may include missing or webbed fingers or toes.

Symptoms and Diagnostic Path
The extra and/or fused digits are clearly visible, but the surgeon may use X-ray or other imaging techniques to show the exact nature of the bone or soft tissue defect.

Treatment Options and Outlook
The surgeon may remove fully formed extra fingers or toes or any webbing between them. Partially formed extra fingers or toes attached to the hand or foot by a stalk may be removed simply by tying

a surgical thread tightly around the stalk so that the finger or toe withers and falls off.

Risk Factors and Preventive Measures
Polydactyly occurs most often as a family trait among African Americans, or as a sign of a genetic disorder such as Trisomy 13 (one extra chromosome 13), in which case it may be associated with multiple defects, including mental retardation, seizures, deafness, small eyes, CLEFT LIP AND/OR PALATE, and congenital heart disease.

In January 2006, a report in the journal *Plastic and Reconstructive Surgery* suggested that a woman's smoking while pregnant might increase the risk of her delivering a child with finger and toe defects; the report remains to be confirmed.

port wine stain   *Nevus flameus*; a congenital malformation of capillaries (small blood vessels), most commonly on the face, neck, arms, or legs. Port wine stains appear first as flat pink marks, then darken and thicken, finally turning dark red or purple in adulthood. Plastic surgeons use LASERS to remove or reduce the color and/or size of the marks.

Port wine stains near the eyes or on the eyelids may be linked to glaucoma (increased pressure inside the eyeball) and/or seizures; infants born with a port wine mark in this area should have an ophthalmologic and neurological examination to rule out these complications.

Symptoms and Diagnostic Path
Port wine stains are clearly visible.

Treatment Options and Outlook
Cosmetics can be used to mask a port wine stain, but the most successful treatment is laser surgery with a yellow light laser such as a copper vapor laser, krypton laser, Nd-yag laser, or pumped dye laser, which obliterates capillaries without damaging the skin. The treatment, usually given every other month on an outpatient basis, may begin in infancy. The laser therapy may cause bleeding, crusting, or swelling, and it may darken or lighten the skin, but these effects are usually temporary. Permanent scarring is rare.

Up to 70 percent of those exposed to laser surgery will experience an improvement in the appearance of the port wine stain; 25 percent will experience complete clearing of the mark.

Risk Factors and Preventive Measures

In the United States, port wine stain occurs in three of every 1,000 infants. There is no known risk factor or preventive measure.

positron emission tomography (PET)   PET-scan; imaging technique that produces a picture of chemical changes in the living brain during activities such as thinking, watching, listening, or moving, by measuring the rate at which cells absorb and use glucose, the form of sugar found in blood once food is digested.

Before the procedure, the patient receives an injection of labeled glucose (glucose molecules attached to molecules of a radioactive element). The glucose circulates through the bloodstream to all parts of the body, including the brain. Then the patient lies with the head inserted into the opening of a machine lined with sensors that detect radiation emitted when positrons (charged particles produced by the radioactive material in the glucose) collide with electrons as the brain cells consume the glucose. The points of collision are fed into a computer that assembles them into a PET-scan, a cross section picture of the brain.

Unlike the images produced by CT-SCAN and MAGNETIC RESONANCE IMAGING (MRI), a PET-scan is in color, with different colors indicating the rate of glucose consumption by brain cells. The color for the highest brain activity is red, next is orange, then yellow, then green, and, last, blue. For example, when a person having a PET-scan is looking at something, the region of the brain that governs vision will show up red, while other areas, such as those that govern motion or speech, register in colors indicating less activity.

post-peel hypopigmentation   As the skin heals after a CHEMICAL SKIN PEEL, it may grow back lighter in color than it was before the peel. This permanent lightening of skin color may also occur after DERM-ABRASION or LASER SKIN RESURFACING on darker skin. In all three cases, the procedure may damage natural pigmented cells that give skin its color.

postsurgical depression   This phenomenon, commonly known as "third day blues," is a frequent reaction in the period immediately after cosmetic PLASTIC SURGERY, as the patient is recovering physically but the results of the surgery are not yet clear. Mild depression usually eases as swelling and bruising disappear. Some patients develop more serious depression, a reaction most likely to occur among those whose surgery has significantly altered their appearance or who entered surgery with unrealistic expectations of the procedure's ability to alter their lives. Those who have a presurgical history of depression or who have gone through surgery at a particularly stressful time in their lives are also at increased risk, as are patients going through several surgeries to repair a serious defect and who must wait until the final surgery for the complete results. In such cases, patients' reactions to the interval image and the patients appearance at one stage in a series, can influence their state of mind. If the depression persists, professional help may be required.

See also DEPRESSION (EMOTIONAL); PSYCHOLOGICAL EVALUATION.

premature aging   In general medicine, a synonym for progeria, a genetic condition in which the body ages at a dramatically quickened rate. In PLASTIC SURGERY, the term is used to describe changes in facial skin such as pigmented spots, WRINKLES, and loss of ELASTICITY, normally caused by aging but due instead to exposure to environmental factors such as sunlight or smoking. Patients often seek to correct these effects through plastic surgery, including such treatments as BOTOX injections, DERMABRASION, and FACE-LIFTS.

Preparation H™   Brand name for cream or ointment used to relieve itching or burning caused by hemorrhoids while shrinking the enlarged tissue. The original formula included live yeast cell derivative (LYCD), an ingredient reputed to reduce skin wrinkling. As a result some people used Preparation H on other parts of the body, such as the face and around the eyes, for cosmetic reasons. However, the Food and Drug Administration (FDA) found live yeast cell derivative ineffective in easing hemorrhoids, so it is no longer used in Preparation H manufactured in the United States.

protein Protein is an essential nutrient, used to build, maintain, and repair body tissue after injury, including surgical incisions such as those required for PLASTIC SURGERY and to synthesize new proteins such as

- enzymes (protein compounds that govern chemical reactions in the body)
- hormones (protein compounds that control growth and reproduction)
- nucleoproteins (compounds in chromosomes that carry an individual's genetic code)
- neurotransmitters (protein compounds that enable the transmission of messages between cells)

Proteins (from the Greek *protos,* meaning "first") are large molecules built of chemical compounds called amino acids, chemical compounds containing one or more amino groups (one nitrogen atom and two hydrogen atoms). Some amino acids are labeled "essential" because they cannot be made in the body and must be obtained from food. Others are called "nonessential" because they can be synthesized in the body from other nutrients, including other amino acids. The essential amino acids for human adults are isoleucine, leucine, lysine, methionine, phenylalanine, threonine, tryptophan, and valine; alanine and histidine are essential for children. The nonessential amino acids are alanine (for adults), asparagines, aspartic acid, citrulline, cysteine (cystine/two molecules of cysteine), gaba, glutamic acid, glycine, hydroxyglutamic acid, noleucine, proline, serine, and tyrosine. Glutamine, ornithine, and taurine fall somewhere in between essential and nonessential.

Simple proteins may contain as few as four different kinds of amino acids, while complex proteins usually contain more than 20. The quality of proteins in food is based on their similarity to human proteins. Proteins from foods of animal origin are considered "complete" or "high-quality" because they contain sufficient amounts of the amino acids essential for human beings. Proteins from plant foods are considered "incomplete" or "low-quality" because they have insufficient amounts of one or more of these amino acids.

The standard against which all dietary protein is measured is the egg, which is arbitrarily ranked as having a "biological value" of 100 percent, meaning that it is the most useful to the human body. Other foods may not be as valuable because proteins do not contain sufficient amounts of the amino acids required by the human body. For example, although dry beans have about twice as much protein per gram as do eggs, the protein in the beans lack essential amino acids and are thus not as valuable to human beings.

An average healthy adult man or woman requires approximately 0.8 grams of high-quality protein for every kilogram (2.2 pounds) of body weight, slightly less than 0.4 grams for every pound. For example, a 138-pound woman requires about 50 grams of protein a day; a 175-pound man, about 64 grams. Important dietary sources of protein include

- lean meat
- fish or poultry (21 grams per 3-ounce serving)
- eggs (6–8 grams each)
- prepacked fat-free cheese (5 grams each)
- bread (3 grams each)
- yogurt (10-gram/8-ounce serving)

Increasing the number of servings or adding other high protein foods raises the total.

Combining foods with limited proteins improves the nutritional quality of the dish in which they are used. For example, rice is low in the essential amino acid lysine, while beans are low in the essential amino acid methionine. Combining the two "complements" the proteins to provides complete proteins; many similar combinations such as dairy foods and grains or seeds (peanuts) are dietary staples in areas where animal proteins are scarce or very expensive.

psychological evaluation   Interview designed to evaluate a person's mental state and/or health. Psychological evaluation is sometimes used to identify appropriate candidates for PLASTIC SURGERY. Although the psychological evaluation is not a required part of presurgical planning, the American Society of Plastic Surgeons notes that "surgeons may recommend psychological counseling to ensure that the patient's desire for an appearance change isn't part of an emotional problem that no amount of surgery can fix."

The society describes the ideal candidate as a person with a strong self-image who simply wishes to correct what he or she perceives as a defect in physical appearance or a person whose self-esteem has been diminished by a congenital defect such as a CLEFT LIP AND/OR PALATE or a trauma-related defect such as a badly broken nose.

Inappropriate adult candidates include (but are not limited to)

- people in crisis, such as those experiencing the death of a spouse or close relative

- those with unrealistic expectations

- those who seek procedure after procedure in pursuit of an unattainable perfection

- those who fixate on a minor defect in the hope that repairing it will change their lives

- those who are mentally ill

pubic liposuction   See ABDOMINOPLASTY; PENILE ENLARGEMENT.

pulsed dye laser   See HEMANGIOMA; LASER; PORT WINE STAIN.

PUVA   This acronym stands for *p*soralen *u*ltraviolet *A* light, also known as psoralen phototherapy. The treatment is used to ameliorate the skin conditions psoriasis (patches of silvery scaling skin) and vitiligo (patches of white pigment-free skin). While this is more commonly performed by dermatologists, it may be used by plastic surgeons who also treat vitiligo with SKIN GRAFTS and tattooing.

Procedure

The patient may be given an oral medicine containing psoralens (substances that make the skin sensitive to sunlight), or creams/lotions containing psoralens are applied to the skin. The patient's skin is then exposed to ULTRAVIOLET LIGHT either from a sunlamp or from natural sunlight.

Risks and Complications

The possible risks include skin irritation, or, more seriously, an increased risk of MELANOMA, the most serious form of skin cancer.

Outlook and Lifestyle Modifications

The possible benefits include reduction of irritation and scaling in psoriasis and repigmentation of the skin in vitiligo. To prevent recurrence or spread, the patient is usually advised to use protective sunscreens and avoid excessive exposure to sunlight.

Q-switch   See LASER.

quadrantectomy   See MASTECTOMY.

quality of life   An evaluation of the patient's well-being and ability to perform the tasks of daily life from one's own point of view and that of a professional observer. The observer's view should be objective; the patient's may be colored by one's physical and emotional condition, pain, apprehension, restricted mobility, and diminished mental acuity.

Quality of life is an important criterion in evaluating the need for elective PLASTIC SURGERY, particularly cosmetic surgery. For example, plastic surgery to repair a deviated nasal septum so as to relieve breathing problems is generally considered a sensible way to improve a patient's physical quality of life, while the importance of cosmetic surgery to reduce a large nose may depend on the patient's self-image.

For example, one patient with an unusually large nose may be perfectly at ease with it, while another considers a large nose a detriment to quality of life. The first is unlikely to seek plastic surgery; the second may. The ultimate success of the surgery will depend in large part on having a realistic understanding of the limits of the physical and emotional changes plastic surgery can deliver. Because cosmetic surgery may trigger confusing emotional issues, reputable plastic surgeons often suggest a psychological consultation before surgery.

See also PSYCHOLOGICAL EVALUATION.

de Quervain's disease   Chronic discomfort and restricted movement of the thumb due to a thick-

ening of the tendons around the abductor pollicis longus and the extensor pollicis brevis, two muscles that run down from the forearm through the wrist to the thumb side of the hand. The thickening of the tendons prevents the muscles from moving smoothly and without pain. The condition, named for Swiss surgeon Fritz de Quervain (1868–1940), who first identified it 1895, may be relieved with PLASTIC SURGERY to release or reduce the tendons.

Symptoms and Diagnostic Path

The characteristic symptoms of this disease include inflammation, swelling, and tenderness at the wrist; hardened, thickened tissue on the wrist; sharp pain when moving the thumb or the thumb and wrist; and pain when bending the thumb across the palm in a diagnostic maneuver called the Finkelstein test, a procedure named for American surgeon Harry Finkelstein (1865–1939).

The lack of pain in the wrist joint differentiates this condition from ARTHRITIS, but if there is any question about the diagnosis, X-ray pictures may be useful in showing either the presence or absence of arthritic changes in the joint.

Treatment Options and Outlook

The treatment for de Quervain's disease may be medical or surgical.

Medical treatment   The simplest medical treatment for de Quervain's disease is splinting the thumb and wrist to relieve the discomfort. The benefit is relief from pain; the drawback is the inability to move the hand normally.

A second medical treatment is to inject cortisone into the wrist. As many as half of all patients get permanent relief from tissue thickening and/or discomfort from a single injection. Most patients get permanent relief after a second injection, given one month after the first. The risk is that the doctor may mistakenly inject the cortisone under the skin rather than into the "tunnel" through which the tendons travel, causing a loss of fatty tissue and shrinkage of the skin that may take up to six month to heal.

Surgical therapy Plastic surgery to release the thickened tendons and alleviate the discomfort of de Quervain's disease is an outpatient procedure, usually performed with local or regional anesthesic.

The surgeon begins with a short incision over the thickened part of the wrist, lifting the skin and exposing the tendons attached to the abductor pollicis longus and extensor pollicis brevis muscles. The surgeon loosens or cuts away part of the thickened tissues surrounding the tendons, closes the incision, and places a dry bandage around the wrists. The stitches are removed within 10 days. The area may be tender for several months, but patients are encouraged to use the hand as soon as it is comfortable to do so.

Successful surgery eliminates pain and restores mobility of the thumb and wrist. Risks and possible complications associated with this surgery include nerve damage and adhesions (abnormal healing of tissues under the skin that contract the wrist). Incomplete freeing of the tendons during surgery can lead to discomfort that may be relieved with cortisone injections or may require follow-up surgery.

Risk Factors and Preventive Measures
De Quervain's disease is more common in women than in men, occurring most frequently in the dominant hand, usually between age 35 and 55, often among new mothers who frequently lift the newborn. The most common cause, however, is a blow to the wrist. As with carpal tunnel syndrome, repetitive movement may be a precipitating factor.

See also CARPAL TUNNEL SYNDROME; HAND SURGERY.

question mark ear See EAR RECONSTRUCTION.

raccoon eyes   A slang term for bruising under and/or around the eyes. This type of bruising is a common complication of facial surgery, particularly surgery on the nose. The condition may be ameliorated with ice packs; it heals naturally within a week to 10 days.

See also RHINOPLASTY.

radial club hand   See CLUB HAND.

radial keratotomy   Surgery to correct nearsightedness by altering the shape of the cornea, the clear structure at the front of the eye. The cornea bends and focuses light to create an image on the retina at the back of the eye, a phenomenon called refraction. If the cornea and the eye are not perfectly shaped, the image they transmit is distorted. Because glasses or contact lenses can compensate for the imperfect shape, some consider this surgery to flatten the cornea a cosmetic procedure.

Procedure

Radial keratotomy requires a great deal of preparation. First, the surgeon numbs the patient's eye and marks (indents) the cornea with a "clear zone" over the center of the pupil. She then sets a pattern for the incisions, measures the thickness of the cornea to estimate the depth of the incisions, and sets the length of the surgical blade to correspond to this depth. She next rechecks the measurements and the blade and dries the eye to remove excess fluid on the surface. After this, she makes the correct incisions around the edge of the "clear zone" and flushes blood and debris from the eye.

Risks and Complications

Pain, occasionally severe, may occur for up to two days after surgery, and temporary sensitivity to light and swelling of the cornea are common. Less common complications include

- bacterial, viral, or fungal infection
- loss of close vision
- reduced ability to see in low light ("night vision")
- perforation (puncture) of the cornea leading to leakage of fluid from the eye
- a cut in the lens leading to cataract
- scarring and/or later tearing of the scars
- increased pressure inside the eye
- detached retina
- drooping eyelid due to nerve damage during surgery

To reduce the risk of complications, the surgeon may prescribe topical antibiotics for up to a week after surgery, as well as anti-inflammatory drops to reduce the risk of swelling, and artificial tears to alleviate the sensation of something in the eye.

Outlook and Lifestyle Modifications

The surgeon usually monitors the patient with follow-up visits the day after surgery, the week after, the month after, and three months later. Once the incisions have healed, the patient should have better distance vision.

See also LASIK.

Radiance®, Radiesse®   See FILLERS.

radiation Energy in the form of high-speed sub-microscopic particles and electromagnetic waves used to power technologies that produce images such as the X-rays that plastic surgeons use to diagnose and treat various defects as well as to plan complex surgical procedures.

Ionizing radiation, such as gamma rays, is radiation with enough energy to disrupt particles in an atom and cause tissue damage. A radiation absorbed dose (RAD) is a unit of energy absorbed from ionizing radiation. Nonionizing radiation such as microwaves and visible light may produce sufficient heat to damage tissue, but it does not disrupt atoms. Medical radiation is radiation such as X-rays used to diagnose a medical condition or as radiation therapy to treat a disease such as cancer. A radiation burn is an injury caused by overexposure to radiation. Any substance, such as plastic or paper that permits radiation to pass through, is radiolucent; any substance, such as lead that blocks the passage of radiation, is radiopaque. To make a radiolucent object such as a piece of plastic visible on an X-ray, the technician performing the X-ray will inject a dye into the patient's bloodstream to outline a radiolucent object, such as blood vessels inside a kidney, so that the object is visible on the X-ray picture.

See also BURNS AND BURN RECONSTRUCTION; CT-SCAN; EXTERNAL RADIATION THERAPY; IMAGING; X-RAY EXAMINATION.

radical mastectomy See MASTECTOMY.

rare earth elements See LASER.

recessive gene See GENETICS.

recipient site The place on the body to which tissue is transplanted; the opposite of the donor site. For example, a piece of skin taken from the forearm (donor site) may be used to repair a defect on the head (recipient site), or fatty tissue taken from the abdomen may be injected into the cheek or chin to round the contours of the face.

See also SKIN FLAP; SKIN GRAFT.

reconstructive ladder System that ranks surgical options in order of their increasing complexity. It is designed to enable plastic surgeons to choose the simplest, least invasive procedure that will restore function and preserve form when treating any particular medical situation. For example, applying moist dressings to burned skin so as to reduce the risk of infection and/or scarring is a simple solution at the bottom of the reconstructive ladder when treating burns. Performing a skin transplant to replace skin destroyed by the burn is a complex procedure at the top of the ladder. Similarly, cleaning a wound and allowing it to close naturally is at the bottom of the reconstructive ladder when treating an open injury. Suturing the skin is at the middle. Transplanting a graft of skin or a more extensive graft of skin plus underlying tissue and bone is at the top.

red light laser See LASER.

redundant skin Large folds of skin remaining after extreme weight loss, most commonly on the abdomen, upper arm, and upper leg. Stretch marks, also known as straiae gravidarum from the Latin word for pregnancy, is a term describing the redundant skin caused by the skin's failure to resume its former shape after a woman gives birth. Redundant skin is unattractive, and, depending on its location, it may also be heavy enough to impede movement or prevent clothes from fitting well. A plastic surgeon can remove the excess skin to smooth the body contour, most commonly at the upper arm, the abdomen, and/or the buttocks and top of the thighs with the appropriate surgical procedures such as ABDOMINOPLASTY, ARM LIFT, BUTTOCK LIFT, or THIGH LIFT.

Reiger flap See RHINOPLASTY; SKIN FLAP; SKIN GRAFT.

replantation Also called reimplantation; PLASTIC SURGERY to reattach an amputated body part or large piece of tissue such as an arm, ear, finger, nose, penis, or scalp. The procedure reestablishes blood circulation via microsurgery to reconnect severed blood vessels and restore function. Replantation may also be used to put a permanent tooth that has been knocked out back into its socket.

Procedure

At the site of the accident, the amputated/avulsed part should be wrapped in gauze, placed in a sealed plastic bag, and held in an ice bath at about 4°C/40°F for transport to the hospital. At the hospital, the surgeon cleans the amputated part, exposing and identifying the various blood vessels, and releases the connective tissue wrapped around muscle in the amputated part to allow for swelling after surgery. The surgeon then cleans and prepares the remaining stump of the finger or limb by cleaning and smoothing the bone and trimming tendons and muscles back to undamaged tissue. He identifies nerves and blood vessels, repairs blood vessels as needed, and again trims back to undamaged tissue. When this preparation is complete, the surgeon attaches the tissues in the amputated part to the tissues in the stump of the finger or limb. He then closes the skin over the injury, using SKIN GRAFTS if necessary, so that the closure is loose enough not to constrict the blood vessels or reconnected tissues underneath.

Risks and Complications

The primary complications following replantation surgery are infection and/or failure of the reattached blood vessels to maintain circulation to the reattached body part.

Antibiotics reduce the risk of infection. To reduce the risk of clots that can block circulation, the surgeon may elevate the reconnected body part, loosen the dressing/sutures, or prescribe anticoagulants such as heparin or medical leeches, whose saliva contains hirudin, a natural anticoagulant. Postsurgical tests to evaluate the condition of the blood vessels and track blood flow include

- arteriography (X-ray pictures of the blood vessels taken after a dye is injected into the bloodstream)
- Doppler ultrasound (use of sound waves to measure blood flow)

- intravenous fluorescein (injection of a dye that is visible on a fluorimeter that shows blood flowing through the vessels)
- pulse oximetry (use of a device that measures the amount of oxygen in the blood)

Outlook and Lifestyle Modifications

Even patients whose reattached finger/limbs heal properly may experience a loss of motion or sensation, continuing pain, and/or sensitivity to cold temperatures. The severity of these long-term complications depends to some extent on the conditions of the original injury. For example, patients with clean, sharply defined amputations are likely to have fewer problems than those whose stumps were crushed. As a rule, regardless of the initial injury, children recover faster and more completely than adults do.

residual scarring   Marks on the skin that remain visible after surgical incisions have healed and the primary scars have faded. Residual scarring may be made less obvious with resurfacing procedures such as DERMABRASION that remove the top layers of skin or with plastic surgery to relax or excise the scar.

See also RESURFACING; SCAR REVISION.

Restylane   See FILLERS; WRINKLES.

resurfacing   Resurfacing is a general term used to describe any plastic surgery procedure such as CHEMICAL FACE PEEL, DERMABRASION, or DERMAPLANING that smooths facial or body skin by removing the top layer of roughened, dead cells. The results are temporary. To maintain the smooth appearance, the procedure must be repeated at intervals that vary according to the patient's skin characteristics.

retinoic acid   Tretinoin; a vitamin A derivative used in lotions and creams that produces a superficial skin peel that lessens fine WRINKLES, reduces changes in skin color, and improves skin texture by sloughing off the top layer of skin cells and increasing the replacement of cells on the surface of the skin.

Products containing minimal amounts of retinoic acid are available in lotions and creams that look like cosmetics but are really over-the-counter (OTC) drugs. Products containing medically effective amounts of retinol are available only with a prescription. In the United States the prescription products containing retinoic acid are Renova™, Retin-A™, and Retin-A Micro™.

Both OTC and prescription products containing retinoic acid may cause burning and stinging, redness and irritation, severe dryness, sensitivity to sunlight, darkening of the treated area, and peeling skin. In some cases, these reactions may be severe enough to require medical attention. WARNING: Products containing retinoic acid are not recommended for women who are pregnant or nursing. Retinoic acid used by a pregnant woman has been linked to birth defects in the developing fetus.

rhinoplasty Nose job; PLASTIC SURGERY to improve the appearance and/or function of the nose, for example to reduce the size of a large nose or to straighten or widen the air passages inside the nose or to repair or reconstruct a nose damaged by a birth defect (such as a cleft) or an injury or a disease, such as cancer.

Depending on the extent of the surgery, rhinoplasty may be done either in an outpatient facility or in a hospital, under general or local anesthesic. The less complicated cosmetic rhinoplasty procedures such as tip plasty (surgery to alter the tip of the nose) commonly take about an hour; more complicated reconstructive procedures such as rebuilding an entire nose require more time. Rhinoplasty sometimes requires the use of an implant, such as a synthetic L-shaped implant used to reshape the cheek and/or to reconstruct the nose.

Procedures

In cosmetic rhinoplasty, the surgeon's aim is to create a straight nose with a smooth tip and narrow nostrils whose proportions fit the patient's other features. In reconstructive rhinoplasty, the surgeon aims to create a functioning nose with a normal appearance. In various types of nasal surgery, the surgeon may take a piece of CARTILAGE from the bridge of the nose and use it to strengthen the tip of the nose during nasal surgery. This is called a strut.

Cosmetic rhinoplasty Once the patient is anesthetized, the skin of the nose is separated from the underlying bone and cartilage. The surgeon then alters the shape of the nose, closes the various incisions, and replaces the skin over the newly shaped bone and cartilage. The surgery may be done with incisions inside the nose, called the endonasal approach, or with incisions inside the nose and outside, most commonly through the columella, the small piece of tissue between the nostrils, called the external approach. In general, cosmetic rhinoplasty aims to straighten the nose by removing any curve or bump in the bone or cartilage running down the length of the nose, and/or to reduce a bulbous (overly rounded) tip, and/or to narrow the nostrils. To straighten the nose, the surgeon cuts away excess bone and cartilage and/or makes controlled fractures to reshape segments of the nasal bones, carefully making certain to maintain the strength of the structure. If necessary, the surgeon will insert spreader grafts, pieces of cartilage that help hold the new shape. To reshape the tip of the nose, the surgeon removes excess cartilage via incisions inside the nostrils. To narrow the nostrils, she removes cartilage from the side of the nostrils and sutures the nostrils into a new, narrower position.

Reconstructive rhinoplasty The goal of this surgery is to reconstruct a damaged nose or to build an entirely new nose. The extent of the surgery depends on the extent of the defect. For example, the surgeon may simply use a SKIN FLAP to replace missing skin or she may use bone, cartilage, and skin lifted from the patient's own body to replace or create a missing structure. The most common source of skin grafts to repair defects of the nose is the patient's forehead or scalp. Skin taken from this area is generally the same color and texture of facial skin, and it has a plentiful supply of blood vessels to nourish the transplant as the skin grows into place at its new site. A piece of bone taken from the top of the skull and used to reconstruct a nose missing due to a birth defect or destroyed by an injury is called a cantilever bone graft. Another choice for skin grafts is skin lifted from the forearm. To repair structural deficits, the surgeon may take cartilage from the patient's septum (the wall separating the two chambers inside the nose) or the patient's ear; the cartilage is used to strengthen or build internal support for the reconstructed nose.

When the cosmetic or reconstructive surgery is complete, the surgeon may insert packing and/or soft plastic splints to stabilize the septum so as to maintain an open airway. Strips of surgical tape over the nose reduce the risk of swelling, secure bone segments, and provide padding for a cast. Packing is removed within a day; splints and/or a nasal cast may remain in place for up to a week to allow bones and cartilage time to knit.

Endonasal rhinoplasty This is a type of rhinoplasty performed via incisions placed inside the nose so as to enable the surgeon to feel changes being made inside the nose. It also reduces scarring and postsurgical swelling so that the nose assumes its new shape more quickly after surgery.

Indian rhinoplasty Repair or reconstruction of the nose with an Indian flap, a piece of skin separated from the forehead and turned downward to be used in reconstructing the nose. One of the oldest known techniques of plastic surgery, it was first documented in India around 600 B.C.E. The technique was brought to the West by British plastic surgeon Joseph Constantine Carpue, after which it was called CARPUE'S OPERATION.

Italian rhinoplasty This early technique for reconstructing the nose used a skin flap that lifted partially off the arm, but left attached to the donor site until it grew firmly anchored to the nose. It is also known as Tagliocotian rhinoplasty after its inventor, Italian surgeon Gasparo Tagliacotian (1546–99).

Tip plasty Surgery to reshape, repair, or reconstruct the tip of the nose by altering the fibrous greater and lesser alar (wing shape) cartilages in the tip of the nose and the nostrils. The greater alar cartilages form the tip of the nose, the separation between the front of the nostril and part of the outer side of the nostrils. The lesser alar cartilages run from the back of the greater alar cartilages on the top of the nostril to where the nostril meets the cheek. This surgery may produce a subtle change such as a slight narrowing of the tip or a more obvious change such as a reduction in a bulbous tip and/or a visible narrowing of the nostrils or, conversely, an augmentation of a too small tip.

Risks and Complications

Swelling and bruising, especially around the eyes, are common. Other possible complications include a reaction to the anesthesic, nosebleed several hours after surgery, or infection.

To reduce the risk of infection, patients with splints left in place may be advised to wash the nasal passages with saline (saltwater) solutions or to apply antibiotic ointment. To reduce the risk of bleeding and allow proper healing, patients may be advised to brush teeth gently, avoid strenuous chewing, and avoid blowing the nose for a week after surgery. It may also be necessary to avoid strenuous exercise (including sexual activity) for longer periods of time so as not to overheat the body and dilate blood vessels. Patients who use contact lenses can insert them soon after surgery; those who wear glasses may be advised to tape the glasses to the forehead until the nose is completely healed.

Surgery via internal incisions does not leave any visible scars. Narrowing the nostrils may leave barely visible scars. Depending on the procedure, reconstructive surgery may leave scarring. In either type of surgery, small red spots (broken blood vessels) may appear on the surface of the skin; in rare cases, these are permanent.

Both cosmetic and reconstructive nasal surgery may narrow the air passages inside the nose, leading some patients to experience breathing problems. If the surgeon removes too much cartilage in straightening the nose, the sides of the nose may be uneven or the nasal passages may be uncomfortably narrowed. It is also possible for the nose to collapse inward, necessitating a second surgery to repair the nose with cartilage grafts to strengthen the structure and skin grafts to cover the damage.

Outlook and Lifestyle Modifications

Applying cold compresses reduces swelling in the days immediately after surgery, but the final shape of the nose will not be clear until several months after surgery when all the swelling is gone.

See also SEPTOPLASTY.

rodeo thumb   An injury specific to rodeo riders. It occurs when there is a complete or partial amputation of a thumb caught between a rope and the horn of the saddle on which the victims were seated while performing in a rodeo. As with other accidental amputations, rodeo thumb may be repaired by PLASTIC SURGERY to reconnect the digit and reestablish a blood supply.

Roe, John Orlando (1848–1915)   Born in Rochester, New York, John Orlando Roe was an otolaryngologist who is believed to have performed the first intranasal rhinoplasty (in 1887), working inside the nose rather than outside on the surface of the face. That same year, he published "The deformity termed 'Pug-Nose' and its correction, by a simple operation," the first scientific paper documenting the repair of the deformity now commonly known as SADDLE NOSE. In 1891, he published the first article describing the use of a wire spring as an internal splint after surgery to alter or reconstruct the nose.

See also RHINOPLASTY.

Roentgen, Wilhelm Conrad (1845–1923)   German physicist, educated at the University of Zurich. He was a professor of physics and director of the Physical Science Institute at the University of Munich (1899–1920). Roentgen discovered X-rays in 1895, an achievement for which he was awarded the first Nobel Prize in physics (1901). The original name for X-rays was Roentgen (pronounced ren-ken) rays, but Roentgen preferred the term *X-rays* because it used the algebraic symbol (X) for an unknown quantity, an apt early description of radiation.

See also RADIATION; X-RAY EXAMINATION.

rosacea   Red nose syndrome; skin disease sometimes labeled adult acne due to its pimplelike outbreaks. Left untreated, rosacea, which causes small blood vessels just under the skin to dilate, may lead to rhinophyma, benign lumpy growths on the nose that can be removed only with PLAS-TIC SURGERY procedures. An enlarged, reddened nose with permanently dilated blood vessels due to rosacea (or sometimes the excessive consumption of alcohol) is called hammer nose. Facial redness, most commonly redness of the nose, is sometimes attributed erroneously to alcohol abuse rather than rosacea, such as in the slang terms *copper nose* and *rum nose*, for people who abuse alcohol.

Symptoms and Diagnostic Path

The temporary or persistent expansion of small blood vessels under the skin leads to redness (telangiectasia) and flushing; burning or sore skin and eyes; pimples and/or rash on the nose, cheeks, chin, and forehead. Rosacea is diagnosed primarily by the patient's appearance.

Treatment Options and Outlook

The cause of rosacea is unknown, but the condition may be linked to mites that live naturally on the skin or to the sensitivity of a patient's small blood vessels. Rosacea cannot be cured, but it may be controlled or lessened with antifungal lotion; topical or systemic antibiotics; and/or isotretinoin (Accutane) or tretinoin cream (Retin-A), the former for nonpregnant patients only. LASER therapy may reduce the redness associated with permanently expanded blood vessels. The success of these treatments varies from person to person.

The usual treatment options for advanced cases of rhinophyma are DERMABRASION, cryosurgery, or laser surgery, all of which remove existing swellings but do not prevent future ones.

Risk Factors and Preventive Measures

Rosacea is more common among people with fair skin, among those middle age (30 to 60 years old), and among women, although symptoms are often more severe among men.

A person with rosacea is likely to experience a flare-up when exposed to stimuli that cause blood vessels to expand, a list that includes but is not limited to: warm weather, ULTRAVIOLET LIGHT in sunlight or tanning lamps, exercise, spicy foods, and alcohol. Skin care products such as soaps, cleansers, or alcohol-based liquids that irritate the skin also expand the blood vessels, increasing the risk of flare-up. Applying makeup heavily may increase the risk of pimples in rosacea patients. Preventing flare-ups requires avoiding these triggers; using a nonalcohol-based sunscreen may help reduce the incidence of rosacea episodes linked to sun exposure.

See also VARICOSE VEINS.

Rubens flap   See BREAST RECONSTRUCTION; SKIN FLAPS.

ruby laser   See LASER.

Rule of Nines   See BURNS AND BURN RECONSTRUCTION.

S

S-plasty   See SCAR REVISION.

saddle nose   Pug nose, boxer's nose; sunken bridge of the nose creating a "pushed in," shortened nose with loss of support for the tip. The defect may be congenital, acquired due to an injury, or the result of an illness that attacks and destroys the supporting cartilage in the nose.

Symptoms and Diagnostic Path

The saddle nose is clearly visible. When viewed in profile, the deformity may be one of the following three degrees:

- mild, with only a slight variation from the normal relationship between the tip and the rest of the nose
- moderate, with a definite but not overwhelming loss of height in the middle of the nose
- major, with a true depression in the middle of the nose along with damage to the septum (the CARTILAGE separating the two interior chambers of the nose)

Treatment Options and Outlook

Medical treatment may be used to stabilize an illness and halt the destruction of nasal cartilage, but surgery is required to rebuild the nose. This is done either with material from the patient's own body (i.e., cartilage from the nose or the ear, or bone and cartilage from the ribs), or with tissue taken from a cadaver, or with synthetic implants.

Using tissue from the patient's own body results in a lower risk of infection and rejection, but natural tissues may eventually be absorbed by the body, requiring a second surgery. Synthetic materials are rarely rejected, but they have a higher rate of infection and inflammation, and in a period of time they may be extruded (pushed out through the skin).

Risk Factors and Preventive Measures

There are no known risk factors and therefore no preventive measures for congenital saddle nose. The two most common risk factors for saddle nose due to injury are nasal surgery and being a person continually exposed to the risk of facial injury (i.e., an athlete, specifically a boxer). To reduce the risk of the former, plastic surgeons generally remove as little tissue as possible during rhinoplasty; to reduce the risk of the latter, many athletes wear face masks.

Medical risk factors for saddle nose include recurring nasal infections, relapsing polychondritis (an autoimmune disease characterized by repeated inflammation and destruction of cartilage in ears, nose, larynx, trachea, and peripheral joints), Hansen's disease (leprosy), and advanced syphilis.

See also RHINOPLASTY.

salabrasion   See TATTOO REMOVAL.

saline   Saline is a sterile solution of salt and water. In PLASTIC SURGERY, saline is used in many different forms. A saline breast implant is a silicone sac filled with saline. A saline dressing is a gauze pad moistened with saline and used to keep the skin from drying. A saline-filled expander is a balloon-type device inserted under the skin, filled with an increasing amount of saline to expand the balloon and stimulate the growth of new skin over the expander, a technique used to create tissue for a SKIN GRAFT. Saline irrigation is a procedure to flush out a wound.

See also BREAST AUGMENTATION; TISSUE EXPANSION.

scalp lift   See HAIR REPLACEMENT SURGERY.

scar formation   Natural production of connective tissue to close a wound. Scar formation is a normal part of the healing process that ends when the tissue is strong enough to hold the skin together. If the body continues to produce connective tissue after a wound has closed, a thickened area called a hypertrophic scar forms. A hypertrophic scar that stretches beyond the area of the original injury is called a keloid. Scar tissue can be a problem when it affects one's appearance or limits mobility due to its tightness or thickness. In these cases, PLASTIC SURGERY may be required to remedy the problem.

See also HEALING PROCESS; KELOID; SCAR REVISION.

scar revision   PLASTIC SURGERY to reduce the size of a scar or to improve a patient's ability to move freely by releasing a contraction scar, an area where scarred skin has pulled the edges of the healthy skin tightly in toward the scar.

Procedure

To repair a small scar on the face, the surgeon may use a resurfacing technique such as dermabrasion or microdermabrasion to remove the top layers of skin, smooth the surface, and make the scar less visible. Alternatively, the surgeon may cut out a piece of tissue, including the scar, and close the incision with very small stitches to create a thinner, less noticeable mark. These are usually outpatient procedures, performed with LOCAL ANESTHETICS.

To repair a scar lying across the natural creases of the skin, the surgeon may use a Z-plasty, a Z-shaped incision, to reposition the scar so that it is parallel to the skin lines and thus less obvious. A curved form of Z-plasty, S-plasty, is used when straight-line incisions might be too visible, for example, on the face.

To repair a contraction scar (a scar due to the contraction of the tissue after an injury such as a burn), the surgeon uses a Z-plasty to release the scared tissue, or he may excise the scarred skin and replace it with a flap of healthy skin from an adjacent area or a graft of healthy skin taken from another area of the body. To obtain sufficient amounts of healthy skin for a large graft, the surgeon may insert a balloonlike device called a tissue expander under an area of undamaged skin, gradually adding saline solution to enlarge the expander as new skin grows over it, and then harvesting the skin for grafting. Scar revision requiring skin grafting is usually done in a hospital under general anesthesic.

Risks and Complications

Risks of scar revision include infection, bleeding, a reaction to the anesthesic, failure of grafted skin to thrive at the new site, or formation of a new unsightly scar. To reduce the risk of new scarring after excision of a scar and/or Z-plasty, the surgeon may inject steroids at the site of an incision during surgery and at regular intervals for up to two years afterward. If large areas of skin are grafted, the patient may have to wear elastic compression garments to prevent swelling and reduce the risk of new scars.

Outlook and Lifestyle Modifications

In most cases, the scar will be smaller and less visible, but the final results may not be apparent for some months.

See also DERMABRASION; MICRODERMABRASION; TISSUE EXPANSION; Z-PLASTY.

scarring alopecia   See HAIR LOSS.

sclerotherapy   Injection of a chemical solution such as saline (sterile salt water) into a varicose vein to sclerose (harden), block, and fade the blood vessel. This process is most commonly used to fade very small varicose veins (spider veins). The injected solution irritates the lining of the vein and clots the blood flowing through it, turning the treated vein to scar tissue that eventually fades. After sclerotherapy, the blood flow shifts from the treated veins to nearby healthy blood vessels; the treatment does not prevent the appearance of new spider veins in the future.

Procedure

Prior to sclerotherapy, the surgeon evaluates the area, observing the skin to check for swelling, sores, or changes in skin color that might indicate problems with larger blood vessels deep under the surface of the skin. He may also perform an ultrasound examination to rule out blockages in the deeper veins that must be corrected before sclerotherapy of the smaller surface blood vessels.

During the procedure, the patient feels the needle pricks and occasionally a burning sensation as the solution goes into the vein. The surgeon usually administers one injection for each inch of the vein being treated, then applies a compression bandage to each treated area. Once the injections are completed, the surgeon may prescribe a compression garment (support hose) to reduce swelling and the risk of blood clots.

Risks and Complications

Common aftereffects include bruising, inflammation, swelling, and allergic reaction to the sclerosing solution. Cosmetic side effects may include long-lasting brownish pigmentation in the skin around the treated area and new spider veins around the treated area. As with all surgery, blood clots are possible.

Outlook and Lifestyle Modifications

Each series of sclerosing injections makes the veins lighter, but more than one session may be needed to fade them sufficiently so that the skin looks clear. If more than one treatment is required, the surgeon usually spaces the sessions about one month apart.

See also COMPRESSION GARMENT; PHLEBECTOMY; VARICOSE VEINS.

scroll ear   See EAR RECONSTRUCTION.

scrotum release   See PENILE ENLARGEMENT.

septoplasty   PLASTIC SURGERY on the septum, the CARTILAGE membrane tissue dividing the two

chambers of the nose. It is most commonly done to straighten the septum or remove blockages so as to improve the flow of air, enabling the patient to breathe comfortably through the nose rather than being forced to breathe through the mouth.

Procedure

The surgeon makes an incision in the wall of the septum on one side of the nose, lifts the mucous membrane covering the cartilage, corrects a blockage or repositions the septum, recovers the cartilage with the membrane, and either stitches the septum and membrane into place or inserts packing into the nose to hold the septum in place as it heals; the packing is usually removed within a day after surgery.

Risks and Complications

Bleeding, swelling, and mild pain are possible following this procedure.

Outlook and Lifestyle Modifications

Successful septoplasty may cure or ameliorate headaches due to abnormal pressure inside the nose, recurrent nosebleeds due to a septal malformation, and sleep apnea (repeated interrupted breathing during sleep). It may also prevent repeated infection due to breathing through one's mouth, which dries the tissues and makes them more susceptible to invasion by microorganisms.

See also RHINOPLASTY.

short face syndrome   This congenital defect is a smaller-than-normal lower part of the face, a malformation of the upper or lower jaw that makes it difficult, if not impossible, for the jaws to meet properly. As a result, the patient is unable to chew normally.

Symptoms and Diagnostic Path

The deformity is diagnosed via physical examination. Physicians look for a lower jaw bone that ends too low at the back. Or they look for a prominent overbite due to a lower jaw that does not come far enough forward in front or the reverse. An upper jaw that does not come far enough forward in front or an upper jaw bone that does not come down low enough in the back are also signs of short face syndrome.

Treatment Options and Outlook

Plastic reconstructive surgery can lengthen and/or reposition the affected bone so that the teeth meet and the patient can chew naturally.

Risk Factors and Preventive Measures

There are no known risk factors or preventive measures for this birth defect.

short scar technique See BREAST REDUCTION (FEMALE).

silicone Silicone is a biocompatible, water-repellant solid, liquid, or gel material that holds its shape in different temperatures. Silicone liquid or gel may be used as a lubricant for surgical tools and devices. Solid silicone is used to build implants used in PLASTIC SURGERY procedures such as chin or breast augmentations. Once inserted into the body, the silicone device becomes encased in body tissue and can be easily removed, if necessary.

See also BREAST IMPLANT.

skin The largest organ in the body, and a major resource for plastic surgeons, providing tissue for grafts and flaps used to repair damage to injured skin or to reconstruct defects such as a missing earlobe. In addition, cosmetic procedures to smooth or lighten various areas of the skin or to repair the effects of normal aging such as drying, loss of ELASTICITY, pigmented spots, and WRINKLES, a condition called senile skin.

Skin is a multilayer covering known as the integumentary system. It regulates temperature; protects the body against heat, light, and microorganisms; stores water and fat; and sends sensory signals such as touch and pain to the brain.

Skin that shows characteristics such as drying, loss of elasticity, pigmented spots, and wrinkles associated with normal aging is called senile skin. This condition is a common motivation for cosmetic plastic surgery.

The three layers of the skin are the epidermis, the dermis, and the hypodermis (subcutaneous tissue).

Epidermis

The epidermis is the outer surface of the skin. It consists of the stratum corneum (horny layer), over the stratum granulosum (granular layer), over the stratum spinosum (prickle cell layer), over the stratum basale (basal cell layer). A fifth layer, the stratum lucidum (clear layer), is found between the stratum corneum and the stratum granulosum on the palms of the hand and the soles of the feet.

The top layers of the epidermis are composed of flat squamous cells. Beneath these are round basal cells, and under these are melanocytes, cells that produce melanin, the pigment that gives skin its color; people with fair skin have melanin only in the lower layers of the epidermis. People with dark skin have melanin in all layers of the epidermis.

Dermis

The dermis is a two-layer section of skin cells under the epidermis. It consists of the stratum papillare on top and the stratum reticulare underneath. The dermis contains blood and lymph vessels, hair follicles, and muscles that lift the hairs on the skin, sweat glands, and glands that secrete sebum, a waxy material that keeps skin supple.

Hypodermis

The hypodermis (subcutaneous tissue) is the lowest layer of skin. Like the dermis, the hypodermis holds sweat glands and blood vessels. It also stores fat that insulates and cushions the body.

See also FACIAL AGING; HEALING PROCESS; SCAR REVISION; SKIN BLEACHES/LIGHTENERS.

skin bleaches/lighteners Cosmetic creams and lotions designed to lighten relatively small areas of temporary or permanent hyperpigmentation (skin darkening) caused by a medicine or a medical condition such as chloasma (the "mask of pregnancy," a darkened area over the nose and cheeks triggered by excess hormone production during pregnancy).

The active ingredients in skin lightening products are melanin blockers, chemicals such as hydroquinone that keep the body from producing new melanin (pigment) in the treated area, thus lightening the skin. Hydroquinone is available either over the counter or in stronger prescription products, alone or in combinations with other melanin blockers such as arbusome, azelaic acid, glycomelanin, kojic acid, and licorice extract. High concentrations of hydroquinone are likely to irritate the skin. These chemicals may cause either permanent darkening or permanent loss of pigment in the treated areas, or black specks on naturally dark skin. Skin bleaches and lighteners have been banned in some European and Asian countries as suspected carcinogens.

Skin lighteners may be used alone or together with exfoliants (cosmetic products containing relatively mild acids that flake away the top layers of cells) or with skin resurfacing plastic surgery.

See also CHEMICAL SKIN PEEL; DERMABRASION; LASER; MICRODERMABRASION; SKIN COLOR.

skin color   Natural skin color is a genetic trait, determined primarily by the presence of melanin, a pigment produced by specialized structures called melanosomes in cells called melanocytes located in the epidermis (the upper layer of skin cells). All human beings have melanocytes and melanosomes, but these structures are larger and more numerous in people with dark skin. In addition, people with dark skin have larger amounts of eumelanin, a dark brown-to-black form of melanin, while those with light skin produce mostly pheomalanin (a red-to-yellow form of melanin). Skin color is also influenced by the presence of fat under the skin, the presence of the yellow pigment carotene, and (in light-skinned people) red blood cells flowing close to the skin's surface.

For the plastic surgeon, skin color is an important factor in determining a course of treatment for a particular patient. For example, an injury to the skin, including a surgical injury such as a CHEMICAL SKIN PEEL, may cause temporary or permanent hyperpigmentation (darkening of the skin). This side effect, called postinflammatory hyperpigmentation, is more common among people with naturally dark skin, as is the formation of heavy, sometimes pigmented scars, called keloids. Early treatment of the darkening and application of sun

blocks may prevent dark spots. Skin lighteners or, paradoxically, procedures such as superficial skin peels or DERMABRASION may also be used to fade postsurgical darkening by removing the top layer of darkened epithelial cells.

See also KELOID; SKIN BLEACHES/LIGHTENERS.

skin flap   Piece of skin (or mucous membrane, such as the lining of the mouth), with or without the underlying tissue (fat, blood vessels, muscle, bone), partially or completely lifted from one place on a patient's body (the donor site) and turned toward or transferred to another (the recipient site), to replace skin that has been damaged or entirely destroyed.

Skin flaps differ from skin grafts in that the flaps come with their own blood supply. The ideal flap also provides enough tissue to cover the wound and blends in with the color and texture of the site to which it is transferred. Once a flap is in place, the surgeon may prescribe anticoagulants (blood thinners) to reduce the risk of blood clots (the most likely complication after flap surgery) at the connection between the blood vessels in the flap and those in the recipient site.

Plastic surgeons characterize skin flaps in several ways: by the method of their transfer from one site on the body to another, by their blood supply, by their shape, by the site from which they are taken, or for the surgeon who created them.

Skin Flaps Classified by Method of Transfer

A local flap is skin lifted from an area close to the defect. A regional flap comes from an area somewhat more distant from the injury. An advancement flap (sometimes called a sliding flap) is skin lifted from the donor site and stretched forward to cover an adjacent donor site. A rotation flap is a triangular piece of skin turned forward on its base. A transposition flap is lifted and turned sideways.

A principal flap is a temporary covering used to encourage the growth of new tissue over a wound where bone is exposed, thus preparing the wound for a permanent graft. The surgeon lifts a piece of skin from a healthy site on the body, turns it to cover the wound, and leaves it in place for at least a week, allowing a thin layer of tissue to grow over the exposed bone so as to prepare the site for a permanent skin graft. The flap is then lifted off and returned to its original site; a day or two later, a permanent skin graft is placed over the wound.

A cross flap is skin or skin and muscle partially separated from one area of the body and grafted onto an adjoining area to grow there while still attached by a pedicle to the donor area. For example, a cross finger flap is a piece of skin partially separated from one finger and attached to the adjoining finger; it grows onto the second finger while still attached to the first finger. When the skin heals, the flap is cut, and the fingers separated. A lifeboat flap is an extra piece of skin to be used if the original skin cut for a flap fails.

Skin Flaps Classified by Their Blood Supply

A free flap is skin lifted entirely free of the donor site; its blood vessels are attached to blood vessels at the recipient site. A random pattern flap is skin and fatty tissue whose blood supply comes from the subdermal vascular plexus/deep dermal process, a group of blood vessels located at the juncture of the epidermis (top layer of skin cells) and the dermis (layers of skin cells under the epidermis). Because skin flaps must connect with or establish a new blood supply at the site to which they are transplanted, certain medical conditions, such as diabetes, which impede healing or interfere with blood circulation, may rule out the use of a random flap.

A pedicle flap is a piece of skin with a stalk containing blood vessels left attached to the donor site; when the flap grows into place at the recipient, the stalk is cut. There are several types of pedicle flaps. A bipedicle flap has two pedicles. A tubed flap (Gilles flap) has a pedicle rolled into a tube shape. An open flap/flat flap is a pedicle flap with the pedicle left unrolled. An interpolation flap is a pedicle flap lifted and turned forward to cover an injury on an adjacent area. A distant flap (Italian flap) is transplanted from an area relatively removed from the site of the injury; for example, from the abdomen to the arm, with a pedicle to the donor site for a short period of time (two to three weeks) to provide a continuing blood supply. Note: A pedicle flap is a delayed flap, skin lifted from the donor site in two or more stages so as to retain circulation in the flap and increase the chances of its surviving when moved to an adjacent site on the body.

Skin Flaps Classified by Their Shape

A bi-lobe flap has two rounded sections; the larger is used to repair a defect in an adjacent area, and the smaller, to repair the injury caused by lifting the first lobe. A caterpillar flap (waltzed flap) is a tube-shaped piece of skin moved end over end, one step at a time, from the donor site to the ultimate recipient site. An S-flap is an S-shape piece of skin and underlying fat used to rebuild the nipple during BREAST RECONSTRUCTION. A semi-lunar flap is a half-moon-shaped piece of gum tissue lifted and moved to cover the root of a tooth left bare by recession due to periodontal disease. A shutter flap, commonly used on the forehead, is two pieces of skin overlapping in the center like the shutter of a camera. A wraparound flap is a piece of skin, with the nail, taken from the big toe and used to repair a damaged or missing thumb. A VY flap (Y flap, Kutler flap, YV flap) is a piece of skin cut in the shape of a V with the broad end next to the area to be repaired. Once the skin is lifted, moved forward, and sutured in place over the injured area—usually a fingertip—the open edges of the site from which the flap was lifted are closed in a straight line to form a Y. An H-flap incision is made in the shape of a capital *H* under the eye to remove a large tumor from the lower eyelid.

Skin Flaps Classified by Their Tissue

A composite flap has more than one type of tissue. A sandwich flap has three layers of tissue, for example, skin on top and bottom with muscle in between. An axial pattern flap includes an artery. A fasciocutaneous flap contains skin and underlying fibrous (connective tissue); it is commonly used to replace missing skin on arms, legs, head, and neck. An innervated flap or a sensate flap includes skin, a nerve (motor or sensory), and muscle tissue. An island flap is skin plus the underlying connective/fatty tissue. A musculocutaneous flap—skin and muscle, or skin, muscle, and nerves—is used to repair defects in the hand or to restore movement to the face. An osteocutaneous flap is a free flap composed of skin and bone, often with an artery.

Skin Flaps Classified by the Sites from Which They Are Taken

Skin flaps lifted from various parts of the body are often named for the sites from which they come. (See chart below.)

Skin Flaps Named for Surgeons

An Abbe flap, also called the Abbe switch flap, is skin lifted from the side of an intact upper lip and part of the cheek to which it is attached and moved down to rebuild a lower lip or less frequently an upper lip. The technique is done so that the lip looks natural and moves naturally because it includes muscles from the lip and cheek. The flap is named for Robert Abbe (1851–1928), an attending surgeon at St. Luke's Hospital in New York City, a lecturer and fellow of the College of Physicians of Philadelphia, and vice president of the New York Academy of Medicine. Variations on the Abbe flap include the Abbe-Estlander flap, used at the corner of the mouth, and the Abbe-Sabbatini flap, used to reconstruct the center of the upper lip.

TYPES OF SKIN FLAPS TAKEN FROM THE PATIENT'S BODY			
Flap Name	Tissue*	Take From	Most Commonly Used to Repair/Reconstruct
Cervicofacial	Skin	face/neck	Nose/cheek
Cervicopectoral	Skin	neck/chest	Face/neck after cancer surgery
Deltopectoral	Skin, muscle	Under clavicle (shoulder bone) down to the fifth rib	Head, neck, oral cavity
Dorsonasal	Skin	Forehead, directly above nose	Nose
Epaulet	Skin	Shoulder	Neck
Forearm	Skin	Lower arm	Head/neck
Forearm, radial	Skin, underlying tissue, nerve	Lower arm	Head, neck
Glabellar	Skin	Forehead	Nose
Gluteal	Skin, underlying tissue	Buttock	Breast after mastectomy
Groin	Skin	Groin area	Hand, forearm
Lateral arm	Skin	Upper arm, outer side	Elbow
Lip-lip	Mucous membrane	Lip	Lip (upper to lower) membrane or one side to the other (same lip)
Moustache	Hair-bearing skin	Scalp	Male upper lip
Nasolabial	Skin	Side of nose/nostril	Area above lip
Omocervical	Skin	Shoulder, upper chest	Neck
Over-and-out cheek	Skin, underlying tissue	Cheek	Lip (with membrane side out)
Palatal	Mucous membrane	Roof of mouth	Gum
Parascapular	Skin	Shoulder	Various
Parieto-occipital	Skin, muscle	Scalp, over top (parietal)/ lower back (occipital) skull bones	Head, neck
Penile	Skin	Shaft of penis	Foreskin, penis, vagina (during gender reassignment surgery)
Platysma	Skin, muscle	Platysma (muscle down side of jaw to neck)	Floor of mouth
Scalping	Skin	Scalp	Scalp
Second-toe wraparound	Skin, underlying tissue	Toe	Finger
Septal	Mucous membrane	Septum (partition dividing chambers of the nose)	Nose (internal)

*Skin = epidermis plus dermis

A Cutler-Beard skin flap is a flap of skin or mucous membrane and the underlying tissue taken from the inside of the lower eyelid and used to repair a defect involving more than half the upper eyelid.

An Estlander flap, named for Finnish surgeon Jakob August Estlander (1831–1881), is tissue taken from one side of the patient's lip and used to repair an injury to the same place on the opposite side of the same (upper or lower) lip.

A Karapandzic flap is skin with blood vessels, nerves, and muscle lifted from one part of the upper or lower lip, turned and moved forward to cover a defect on another part of the lip. The flap was introduced in 1974 by Miodrag Karapandzic, onetime director of the Clinic for Burns, Plastic and Reconstructive Surgery of the Belgrade University Clinical Center. The flap remains attached to the original site to preserve the blood supply as the tissue grows into place in the new site. Approximately three weeks after the first surgery, a second surgery severs the connection to the original site.

A Moberg flap, named for Stanford University surgeon E. Moberg, is lifted from the palm of the hand and moved forward to cover or create a new thumb after amputation.

A Reiger flap is skin lifted from the forehead and rotated downward to cover a defect in the nose remaining after an injury or cancer treatment. The virtue of this flap lies in the fact that the skin from the forehead is similar in color, thickness, and texture to the skin covering the nose.

A Rubens flap is a piece of skin and underlying fatty tissue lifted from the hip area and moved up and forward to build a new breast after MASTECTOMY.

Tenzel's flap, named for ophthalmic plastic surgeon Richard B. Tenzel, is a semicircular piece of skin lifted from the outer edge of the upper eyelid and used to repair a defect on the same lid.

A Washio flap is hairless skin taken from the side of the skull in back of the ear to repair a defect of the nose. It is named for Hiroshi Washio, an American surgeon who introduced the technique in 1969.

A Zitelli flap is a bi-lobed (two-lobe/two section) flap made of two triangular pieces of lip and cheek skin, lifted, turned and brought together to repair defects of the skin on the nose. It was introduced in 1989 by dermatologist John A. Zitelli at Montefiore Hospital in Pittsburgh, Pennsylvania.

See also BONE REPLACEMENT; HAIR REPLACEMENT SURGERY; MUSCLE; SKIN GRAFT.

skin graft Piece of healthy skin lifted from one site on the body and moved to cover an area of the body where the skin is damaged or missing; for example, after a serious burn. Unlike a skin flap, a skin graft does not have its own blood supply; after the skin is transferred, the blood vessels in the grafted skin are joined to those in the recipient site so that the graft is vascularized (attached to local blood vessels). A graft is said to *take* (fix in place) when new blood vessels and scar tissue form in the injured area. All grafting, including grafts taken from the patient's own body, cause some scarring at both the donor and recipient sites.

Plastic surgeons characterize skin grafts by the source from which they are taken, the tissues they contain, the way they are constructed, or the way they function.

Skin Grafts Classified by Their Source

An autogenous graft (also called an autogenous transplant, autograft, autologen, or autologus graft) is tissue taken from one site on the patient's body and placed at another site on the body; for example, skin taken from the abdomen to replace burned skin on the neck. The surgery using material from the patient's own body is called autoplasty; the tissue used in the procedure is called autoplast.

An isogenic graft (isograft, isoplastic graft) is an exchange of tissue between individuals whose genetic makeup is sufficiently similar so as to avoid an immune response; e.g., a skin graft taken from one identical twin and given to another.

A homograft (syngraft) is tissue transferred from one member of a species to another member of the same species, for example from one human being to another. One important type of homograft is the cadaver skin graft, tissue lifted from a dead body and chemically treated to make it safe for use as a temporary skin graft, most commonly to replace skin lost to burns.

A heterograft (xenograft) is tissue transferred from a member of one species to a member of another. A zoograft is the transfer of tissue from an animal to a human being, for example, a porcine graft (pig skin) used as a temporary covering for areas of a human body where the skin has been destroyed by a burn.

Skin Grafts Classified by Their Structure

A full thickness graft is a piece of skin that includes both the epidermis (the top layers of skin cells) and the dermis (the two layers of skin cells under the epidermis). A split thickness graft (such as a pinch graft) is a piece of skin that includes the epidermis and the top part of the dermis. A dermal graft is a graft of tissue from the dermis, the second layer of skin cells. A mucosal graft is a piece of mucous membrane, such as the lining of the mouth, transferred from one site to another; for example, tissue from one side of the lip moved to the other side or a piece of tissue from the tongue used to rebuild or repair the urethra (the tube that carries urine from the bladder out of the body). A composite graft has two or more types of body tissue such as skin and fat or skin and connective tissue (CARTILAGE).

Skin Grafts Classified by Their Construction

An accordion graft (mesh graft) is a piece of skin, usually from the patient's own body, slit in many places and stretched to cover an area larger than the original graft; once the graft is in place, the patient's own cells begin to fill in the spaces in the graft, integrating the graft into the body. A postage stamp graft is a small piece of skin approximately 5 cm × 5 cm (2 inches × 2 inches), used either as a skin graft or as a base from which to grow larger pieces of the patient's own skin. A punch graft is a small, round piece of skin removed from one area of the body and transferred to another. Punch grafts, once commonly used in hair replacement, are now used to smooth small round ACNE scars or to transfer pigmented skin to nonpigmented areas for people suffering from vitiligo, a condition characterized by patches of skin where the pigment has disappeared. Skin tissue preserved by chilling and dehydration for use as a graft is called a freeze-dried graft.

A cultured skin graft is tissue grown in a laboratory, where a sample the size of a postage stamp can be sliced into a network and stretched to produce enough new skin to cover nearly an entire body. Cultured skin grafts are most commonly used in PLASTIC SURGERY to replace large areas of burn-damaged skin. A cultured epithelial autograft is skin grown from the patient's own epithelial cells. A cultured epithelial allograft is skin grown from cells taken from another human being.

Skin Grafts Classified by Their Function

An anastomosed graft is a skin graft with blood vessels in the graft joined end to end with those in the underlying area so to ensure the health and survival of the grafted tissue. A patch graft is a piece of natural or synthetic material inserted into the wall of a tubular structure such as the intestine or a blood vessel or a ureter (one of two tubes that carries urine from the kidney to the urinary bladder) so as to enlarge the interior of the tube.

See also BONE REPLACEMENT; HAIR REPLACEMENT SURGERY; SKIN FLAP.

skin substitutes See BURNS AND BURN RECONSTRUCTION.

smile lines See WRINKLES.

smoking Smoking is an important health risk factor for PLASTIC SURGERY patients. Before surgery, tobacco smoke dries the air around the face, thus drying the surface of the skin. Nicotine and other chemicals in the smoke constrict blood vessels, reducing the flow of nutrient-carrying blood to the skin. The lack of sufficient oxygen may reduce both the production of elastic fibers in the skin and the synthesis of supporting tissues (collagen) underneath it. Although the exact process by which smoking increases facial wrinkling is unknown, these effects, along with genetic factors, may contribute to it. During surgery, a smoker may have an increased risk of respiratory problems due to anesthesia. After surgery, a smoker's wounds usually heal more slowly due to constriction of the blood vessels supplying the skin, a smoking-related increase in blood clotting, and decreased collagen synthesis. In one review of 916 plastic surgeries involving SKIN FLAPS and SKIN GRAFTS, the risk of necrosis (tissue death at the site of the surgery) was three times higher for one-pack-a-day smokers than for nonsmokers, and six times higher for those who customarily smoke two packs a day.

Plastic surgeons are well aware of these findings. In fact, data from a University of Texas Southwestern Medical Center survey of 955 board-certified plastic surgeons published in the January 2002 issue of *Plastic and Reconstructive Surgery,* the official medical journal of the American Society of Plastic Surgeons (ASPS) and distributed by the American Society for Aesthetic Plastic Surgery, showed that about half of the surgeons surveyed limit the type of procedure they perform on smokers. Sixty percent "usually" or "always" perform a less invasive technique on smokers; a third "sometimes" change their technique. In treating smokers, nearly 90 percent of the surgeons surveyed perform procedures such as RHINOPLASTY, BREAST AUGMENTATION, or LIPOSUCTION that do not involve skin flaps or skin separation. Only 39 to 54 percent of the surgeons perform procedures such as BREAST REDUCTION, tummy tucks, or FACE-LIFTS that require significant incisions into and movement of the skin. Nearly half require patients to quit smoking for two weeks.

solar damage   Sun damage; tissue injuries related to exposure to ULTRAVIOLET LIGHT (UV) such as solar cheilitis (sun damage to the lips), solar dermatitis (sun damage to the skin), solar KERATOSIS (skin growth triggered by sunlight), and solar urticaria (an allergic reaction to ultraviolet light; hives).

Symptoms and Diagnostic Path
The first sign of solar damage is a suntan, an injury to the epidermis (top layer of skin cells) that occurs when exposure to UV signals the body to increase natural production of melanin, the dark pigment that gives skin its natural color in order to stop further UV damage. Further exposure to UV light leads to sunburn. Over time, continual tanning and/or burning damages deeper layers of the skin to cause premature thinning, wrinkling, roughening and spotting of the skin, a condition known as photoaging. Finally, if exposure to UV light is long enough and the damage goes deep enough, the result may be keratoses (dark, sun-roughened patches of skin) or, ultimately, injury to DNA in skin cells leading to skin cancer.

Most signs of UV injury are clearly visible: darkened SKIN COLOR such as the light brown color of a suntan; the reddened, swollen, painful, peeling and/or blistering of a sunburn; and the darkening, crusting, or bleeding spots on exposed areas of the body that may be early signs of solar-related skin cancers (the diagnosis must be confirmed by BIOPSY of the affected tissue).

Treatment Options and Outlook
Mild sunburn may be treated with cool or warm baths and mild pain relievers. Severe sunburn that damages several layers of skin is treated like any other burn (see BURNS AND BURN RECONSTRUCTION). Areas that show changes indicative of skin cancer must be biopsied; if malignant, they must be removed.

Risk Factors and Preventive Measures
People with lighter skin (as measured by the FITZPATRICK SKIN TYPE CLASSIFICATION) are at higher risk of UV injury in shorter periods of time than are those with darker skin. But if the exposure to UV light lasts long enough, every type of skin will show solar damage. To reduce the risk of solar damage, anyone who plans to spend time in the sun should

- use a protective sunscreen and reapply as directed on the package;
- avoid long periods of exposure to the sun when its UV rays are most intense, between the hours of 10 A.M. and 4 P.M.; and
- wear tightly woven clothing, including a hat to shield the face and neck.

somatic nervous system   See NERVOUS SYSTEM.

SPAIR technique   See BREAST REDUCTION (female).

spare parts surgery   Term used by plastic surgeons to describe a procedure used when reattaching an amputated body part, most commonly a finger. If the entire finger cannot be reattached at its original site, the surgeon may attach only a piece of the missing finger. If a patient has lost more than one finger and only one of the amputated fingers is complete enough to be replanted, the surgeon may cut the finger into two pieces, attaching each piece at the site of a missing finger, using the pieces of the salvageable finger as "spare parts" to restore a measure of function to the injured hand.

See also HAND SURGERY; REPLANTATION.

spot reduction, spot fat reduction   See LIPOSUCTION.

stem cell implants   Stem cells are the unspecialized cells from which all mammalian body cells develop. Embryonic stem cells come from the blastocyst, the hollow 200-to-250 cell sphere that develops within a week after a fertilized egg divides and then implants in the uterine wall. Adult stem cells are found in the umbilical cord ("cord blood"), or the placenta, or blood, bone marrow, skin, and other human tissue. For plastic surgeons, stem cell research, with either embryonic or adult stem cells, offers the possibility of creating natural implant material for reconstructive procedures. Such material could be used to replace a breast after mastectomy, fill in facial tissue after cancer surgery, replace tissue destroyed by an injury, or even simply to reduce facial wrinkling.

For example, in one series of studies financed by a grant from the National Institutes of Health's Institute of Biomedical Imaging and Bioengineering, researchers at the University of Illinois (Chicago) took stem cells via hypodermic needles from the bone marrow of healthy human volunteers. The cells, which have the potential to transform themselves into the cells that make CARTILAGE, BONE, and fat, were cultured (grown) in a nourishing bath, placed on an FDA-approved pliable mesh base similar to human tissue, and then implanted into the bodies of laboratory mice. When the implants were removed four weeks later, the cells had, indeed, developed into fatty tissue.

Results such as these suggest that FILLERS and implants created from stem cells are practical.

Clearly, further studies are required to test the reaction between the implants and living tissue. If animal studies continue to produce consistent positive results, and if eventual human studies do as well, the procedure may prove more practical and less intrusive than the two surgeries currently required to remove tissue from one part of a patient's body and then implant it at another; for example, lifting a large SKIN FLAP from the side and back to rebuild a breast after MASTECTOMY. In addition, the naturally created stem cell material may maintain its shape and volume better than synthetic implants do without a risk of rupture, leakage, or slippage.

See also BREAST RECONSTRUCTION.

stocking nevus   See MOLE.

stomach tightening   See ABDOMINOPLASTY.

Straatsma, Clarence Ralph (1896–1974)   Dutch-American plastic surgeon. Straatsma, a pioneering plastic surgeon in the United States, was a founder of the American Association of Plastic Surgeons, which he chaired in 1955 and the onetime chief of plastic surgery at Columbia University College of Physicians and Surgeons.

stretch marks   See ABDOMINOPLASTY; REDUNDANT SKIN.

strut   See RHINOPLASTY.

supratip   See PARROT BEAK DEFORMITY.

surgical staples   Stainless steel or titanium devices similar in design to ordinary office staples. Surgical staples are used during surgery, including plastic surgery, to close an incision on the scalp, arms, legs, abdomen, or back, or to connect the open ends of a large blood vessel or parts of the intestine after reconstructive surgery.

To insert the staples, the surgeon holds the edges of the incision together with his fingers or a forceps, holds the stapler against the skin, and squeezes a trigger to inject the staple into the skin to a depth controlled by his pressure on the stapler. Staples are usually removed with a special tool seven to 10 days after surgery.

Metal surgical staples can be put in more quickly than sutures and are less likely to cause infections, but they are more likely to leave noticeable scars if the edges of the wound or incision are not well aligned, and they cannot be used in areas such as the face or hand where the nerves are close to the surface of the skin. Note: A plastic staple that can be absorbed by the body within a few months, does not have to be mechanically removed, and does not leave a noticeable scar is currently awaiting approval by the U.S. Food and Drug Administration approval.

See also SUTURE (SURGICAL).

surgical support garment See COMPRESSION GARMENT.

surgical zipper A surgical zipper, also known as a medical zipper or an abdominal zipper, is an adhesive-backed plastic patch with a plastic zipper down the middle. It is used for wound closure and was approved by the U.S. Food and Drug Administration (FDA) in 2000 only for straight-line incisions such as one type of incision for ABDOMINOPLASTY.

Once the surgeon closes the internal layers of an incision with sutures, he removes a protective paper strip on the back of the zipper patch, places one edge of the adhesive-back patch on either side of the incision with the zipper open over the incision, and closes the zipper to pull the edges of the incision together. If necessary, the surgeon can open and close the zipper to follow the progress of the wound as it heals. When the wound heals, the patient peels off the zipper patch. The process of closing a wound with a surgical zipper is called zippering.

suspensatory ligament release See PENILE ENLARGEMENT.

suture (anatomical) Strip of connective tissue at the place where the edge of one bone plate in the skull meets another. For example, the coronal suture is the tissue between the two parietal bone plates at the top of the skull and the skull and the frontal bone, the plate that forms the forehead and the orbital (eye) and nasal cavities. At birth, the sutures are normally open. When bone plates in an infant skull fuse prematurely, it is called craniostosis (craniosynostosis). This condition makes the skull narrow, rather than round, and may restrict the normal growth of the brain. Plastic reconstructive surgery soon after birth can separate the plates, round the skull, and give the brain room to grow.

suture (surgical) Fine material (thread or wire) used to join tissues or close the edges of a surgical incision or a wound. Sutures are characterized according to the material from which they are made (natural or synthetic), the way they are constructed (monofilament or multifilament), their interaction with the body (absorbable or nonabsorbable), their size, and the method used to place them in the body tissue.

Sutures Classified by Their Material

The most familiar natural material used in sutures is sterilized *gut*, a twisted threadlike absorbable wound closure, originally derived from catgut; it is now made from beef (bovine gut suture) or sheep (ovine gut suture) intestinal connective tissue. It is derived from the fibers in the intestinal submucosa, which is the layer of tissue underneath the mucous membrane lining of the intestines. Other natural materials used for suturing are raw silk, cotton fibers, and surgical steel wire composed of an iron-chromium-nickel-molybdenum alloy. Synthetic materials used in making surgical sutures include polymers (substances composed of long chains of molecules) such as plastics and woven fabrics such as NYLON and DACRON™.

Sutures Classified by Their Construction

Sutures may be monofilament (consisting of a single strand) or multifilament (consisting of several strands braided or twisted together). Monofilament sutures are easier to tie, pass more easily through tissue, and are less likely to collect bacteria once in place. Multifilament sutures are more flexible, less likely to break or crimp, and stronger once in place.

Both natural and synthetic monofilament and multifilament sutures may be coated with substances that make them easier to handle, improve their ability to pass smoothly through body tissue so as to avoid excess injury, to reduce the risk of reaction with body tissues, and to maintain the suture's strength by slowing absorption or dissolution. Some sutures are colored with dye to make them more visible to the surgeon.

Sutures Classified by Their Interaction with the Body

Sutures may be absorbable or nonabsorbable. Over time, absorbable sutures will be dissolved by body fluids; nonabsorbable sutures must be removed by a surgeon.

Absorbable sutures may be made of natural material, such as gut, or synthetic materials. Plain gut sutures lose their original strength (ability to hold an incision closed) and are absorbed within a week to 10 days; they are completely absorbed within two months. These sutures often react with body tissue, leading to inflammation at the site of the suture. Chromic gut sutures are treated with chromium compounds to slow absorption and reduce any reaction with body tissue. They hold their original strength for as long as 21 days; they are completely absorbed within three months. Fast-absorbing gut sutures (plain gut treated with heat to increase the speed with which they are absorbed) hold their original strength for about one week; they are completely absorbed within two to four weeks. The first absorbable synthetic suture material, polyglycylic acid (Dexon™), was introduced in 1970; modern synthetic absorbable suture materials include

- polyglactin 910 (Ethicon ™, Vicryl™)
- polydioxanone (Ethicon ™, PDS™)
- polycaprone glycolide (Monocryl™)

Gut sutures are degraded by enzymes in the body within two months. Synthetic absorbable sutures are dissolved by water in the body over a period ranging from six weeks to four months, depending on the material.

Nonabsorbable sutures such as surgical cotton and various synthetic plastic fibers are most frequently used to close incisions in the skin. They may also be used inside the body; i.e., stainless steel wire sutures used to join pieces of bone. Nonabsorbable sutures in the skin are removed as soon as the incision has healed sufficiently to remain closed on its own, usually within a week after surgery. Internal nonabsorbable sutures are eventually covered and encased by connective tissue. Note: Although surgical silk is commonly classified as a nonabsorbable suture material, it may be degraded by enzymes over a two-year period.

Sutures Classified by the Size of the Thread

The United States Pharmacopoeia (an official list of drugs published each year by the United States Pharmacopoeial Convention) has established standard sizes for sutures as measured by the diameter of the suture. Currently, standard sutures range in size from 3 to 4 (the largest) down to 12/0 (the finest). For comparison, a 0 suture made of any material other than catgut is 0.350–399 mm in diameter; a 6/0 suture made of any material other than catgut is 0.070–0.099 mm in diameter. Sutures smaller than 7/0 can only be seen through a microscope. Plastic surgeons use the thinnest possible sutures for incisions in the skin during cosmetic surgery, so as to create the least visible scarring. They may use a variety of suture materials for reconstructive plastic surgery that involves internal incisions and the construction of a body part, such as a rebuilt ear or nose.

Sutures Classified by Their Insertion

Surgeons use one of four basic techniques to suture an incision. Simple interrupted sutures are individual stitches, equally spaced along the incision. A continuous or running suture is a single thread pushed in and out of the skin at equally spaced intervals along the surface of the incision. A continuous subcutaneous suture is a single thread pushed back and forth across the incision below the surface of the skin. A mattress suture is an individual stitch that closes the incision with the edges of the incision pushed together and up.

See also SURGICAL STAPLES; SURGICAL ZIPPER; SUTURELESS CLOSURE; WOUND ADHESIVE.

sutureless closure Method of closing internal incisions, including those made during major PLASTIC SURGERY procedures such as ABDOMINO-PLASTY. Sutureless closure is also used to attach cut ends of large blood vessels. To produce the closure, a surgical adhesive such as BioGlue™, a compound made of a PROTEIN found in cow's blood that forms links to body tissue, is applied to close the incision. In the United States, the Food and Drug Administration (FDA) has approved the use of several surgical adhesives as an adjunct to classical closures such as sutures and staples and to reinforce soft tissue.

See also LASER; SURGICAL ZIPPER; WOUND ADHESIVE.

tarsoplasty See EYE LIFT.

tattoo (medical) Also called intradermal micropigmentation, cosmetic tattoo, permanent makeup; a design drawn by injecting droplets of ink under the surface of the skin. Plastic surgeons use tattooing in reconstructive or cosmetic surgery to alter the appearance of tissue so as to make it appear more natural. For example, the surgeon may tattoo the skin to simulate the pigmented tissue of a nipple and areola on a reconstructed breast. Tattooing is also used to draw on eyebrows lost to alopecia or to an injury such as a burn, to darken depigmented spots on the skin as may occur with a skin condition such as vitiligo, or to lighten scarred skin. Finally, tattoos may be used to improve appearance by defining the edge of a lip where the color of the vermilion border has faded due to aging, to provide an indelible eyeliner, or to emphasize the eyelashes for patients who have difficulty applying regular makeup.

Procedure

The first step in applying a tattoo is usually a patch test. The surgeon applies a small amount of ink to the patient's skin, covers the area, and leaves the covering in place for several days or a week or more to see if an allergic reaction occurs. If no allergic reaction takes place, the surgeon may go ahead with the procedure.

To create the tattoo, the surgeon begins by applying a topical anesthetic to numb the skin. Once the skin is numb, the surgeon uses hollow, vibrating needles to inject the sterile surgical ink solution, repeating the process until the tattoo is complete. Immediately after the tattooing is finished, the surgeon may apply cold compresses to reduce inflammation and swelling and antibiotic ointment to reduce the risk of infection.

Risks and Complications

Slight stinging during the tattooing process and redness and swelling afterward are common. Allergic reactions to the ink are less common but may develop up to several years after the original tattooing process. Other possible complications include granulomas, small bumps that form when the body reacts to a foreign substance, such as the tattoo ink. In rare cases, scarring may occur at the site of the tattoo.

Infection after tattooing is most commonly associated with a procedure done in a nonmedical setting with nonsterile equipment; it rarely occurs following medical tattoos. Using nonsterile equipment may also transmit skin infections and blood-borne bacterial and viral diseases such as hepatitis and HIV/AIDS.

Outlook and Lifestyle Modifications

Immediately after the procedure, the tattoo colors are darker than expected; they fade to final color within approximately three weeks.

In rare cases, people with tattoos have developed swelling or a burning sensation at the site of the tattoo during or after magnetic resonance imaging (MRI). No reason for this reaction has been conclusively identified. One theory is that it occurs due to the presence of minuscule metal particles in the tattoo inks. To be safe, a patient with a tattoo should alert the radiologist before undergoing MRI.

See also BREAST RECONSTRUCTION; EYEBROW REPLACEMENT; EYELASH TRANSPLANT; HAIR LOSS; MAGNETIC RESONANCE IMAGING (MRI); NIPPLE AREOLA RECONSTRUCTION.

tattoo removal   Plastic surgery procedures to fade, erase, or remove a tattoo. It is most commonly used to erase a decorative tattoo.

Procedures

The three basic methods for fading, erasing, or removing a tattoo are excision, abrasion, and laser surgery.

Excision   The surgeon numbs the area of the tattoo with local anesthetic and then excises (cuts away) several layers of ink-impregnated skin cells, producing a shallow wound. When the entire tattooed area has been excised, the surgeon applies an antibiotic cream and a bandage to reduce the risk of infection.

Abrasion   The surgeon numbs the area of the tattoo and then abrades (rubs the surface of the skin) with a roughened instrument to remove the top layers of ink-impregnated cells. The abrasive techniques used to erase/remove tattoos are salabrasion (abrading the skin with gauze pads saturated in a salt solution) and dermabrasion (abrading the skin with a high-speed rotating surgical brush or a sandpaper-covered device). When the tattoo is removed, the surgeon applies an antibiotic cream and covers the shallow wound with a protective bandage to reduce the risk of infection. Salabrasion uses fine grain salt or a salt and water solution to rub away the top layer of pigmented skin cells.

Laser surgery   The surgeon fits the patient with protective eye-shields and then tests various lasers to see which is most effective in fading the tattoo ink. For example, black tattoo ink absorbs and is degraded by all types of lasers; other color inks respond only to specific types of lasers with specific energy levels.

Depending on the site of the tattoo, the surgeon may numb the area with a LOCAL ANESTHETIC before placing the laser device against the skin and activating it in a series of pulses designed to break up the ink pigment with a beam of high-intensity light. The larger the tattoo, the more pulses are required to obliterate it. After the laser treatment, the surgeon usually applies an ice pack to reduce swelling and an antibiotic cream to reduce the risk of infection.

Immediately after laser surgery, the tattoo may darken temporarily and then becomes lighter. A series of laser treatments may be needed to fade the tattoo completely, but the tattoo will become lighter after each session.

Risks and Complications

Redness and swelling are common after tattoo removal. Infection and scarring are less common. The risk of infection is highest with excision. Scarring is most likely to occur with excision or salabrasion.

Both dermabrasion and laser surgery may cause permanent darkening or lightening of the skin around the treated area. To reduce the risk of sun-related darkening, the patient is usually advised to apply protective sunblock.

Outlook and Lifestyle Modifications

The U.S. Food and Drug Administration (FDA) considers the inks used for tattoos cosmetics, but does not regulate them as tightly as other cosmetic products. As a result, the composition and density of the inks may vary widely. In addition, during tattooing, the ink may be deposited at different levels under the skin. As a result, although laser surgery often gives the best results, complete fading, erasure, or removal of any tattoo is a difficult task and by no means guaranteed.

See also DERMABRASION; LASER.

T cell   See IMMUNE SYSTEM.

tea   *Camellia sinensis*; tea leaves contain tannins, naturally occurring astringent chemical compounds also found in coffee beans, the bark of oak, chestnut and mangrove trees, and various other plants. Tannins, originally used to process animals skins into leather, form complexes with PROTEINS, including proteins in the skin. Cool wet tea bags or gauze pads soaked in strong tea may be used today as a home remedy: the tannins do produce a slight, temporary reduction in puffiness under the eyes, and they may also soothe a small area of a minor burn or sunburn.

See BURNS AND BURN RECONSTRUCTION; EYE LIFT.

Tessier classifications   System for classifying craniofacial clefts of bone and soft tissue introduced by

French surgeon Paul Tessier in 1973. Tessier's system identifies 15 distinct facial bone and soft tissue defects, each defined by the position of the defect in relation to the sagittal midline, an imaginary line that divides the body into two symmetrical halves, in this case, two halves of the face/skull.

Tessier clefts are numbered beginning with cleft #0 (the center of the nose), moving out toward cleft #7 at the ear and then coming back across the forehead to cleft #14, a cleft in the center of the skull. The numbers 0 through 7 identify facial clefts; the numbers 8 through 14 identify the clefts' extension to the skull. For example, Tessier cleft #1 runs from the top of the inner edge of the eye down through the nostril and perhaps into the upper jaw. Its extension, Tessier cleft #13, runs up from the top of the inner edge of the eye up the skull. The entire cleft is described as "Tessier cleft #1–13."

The virtue of the Tessier system is that it enables plastic surgeons to treat a defect involving the eye, nose, mouth, and skull as a single defect to be corrected in a limited number of surgeries with several specialists working as a team rather than in a series of surgeries performed by one specialist, one procedure at a time. This sequence is less stressful for the patient.

See also CLEFT LIP AND/OR PALATE; FACIAL CLEFT.

testicle expander A silicone sac implanted into the scrotum after removal of a cancerous testicle. It is implanted with a valve opening at the skin that permits the surgeon to periodically expand the sac with increasing amounts of saline (sterile salt water). When the sac is fully expanded, it may be left in place or removed to allow the surgeon to insert a prosthesis that creates a natural-looking scrotum.

See also TISSUE EXPANSION.

Thermage™ Form of nonsurgical FACE-LIFT; a noninvasive treatment employing a special device, called a Thermacool™, to transmit radiofrequency (RF) energy into the skin, heating the connective tissue underneath so that it contracts to make the face look smoother. Thermage was approved by the U.S. Food and Drug Administration (FDA) in 2001.

Procedure

The doctor fits a grid over the patient's face to guide the Thermage device and, as during an ULTRASOUND SCAN, applies a fluid to the skin to ensure successful contact. The device also releases a cooling spray to reduce the risk of burning the skin. When the device touches the skin, the patient may feel no difference, or warmth, or in rare cases pain. The treatment may last up to two hours, depending on the number of areas to be treated.

Risks and Complications

Redness, swelling, a tingling sensation, or soreness are common. Serious complications include burns, blisters, scarring, or (rarely) pits in the skin due to overheating that causes shrinkage of the fat under the skin or excessive tightening of the connective tissue.

Note: Unlike LASER SKIN RESURFACING, another heat-related procedure, Thermage does not cause permanent changes in pigmentation; it can be used on all SKIN COLORS.

Outlook and Lifestyle Modifications

Thermage is not a substitute for a surgical facelift, but it may reduce fine WRINKLES around the nose and mouth or tighten skin that has loosened slightly with age. Because this is a new technique, there are no reliable reports as to how long these improvements may last.

thigh lift Thighplasty, thigh reduction; PLASTIC SURGERY to remove excess skin and/or fat from the thighs. The various nonmedical names for this excess dimpled skin caused by fatty deposits include cellulite, cottage cheese skin, Chesterfield sofa skin. (Cellulitis, a condition that can affect this part of the body, is an infection in connective tissue under the skin.)

Procedure

A thigh lift, which is done with general anesthesic, may be a single surgery to tighten the entire thigh, or one surgery to tighten either the inner part of thigh or the outer part of the thigh. The thigh lift may also consist of two separate surgeries, several weeks or months apart, one for the inner thigh and one for the outer thigh.

The site and length of the incisions depend on which procedure is performed. For example, if the entire thigh is to be lifted, the surgeon makes a relatively long incision around the top of the thigh in the natural crease between the thigh and the trunk (pelvis). If only the inner or outer thigh is to be tightened, the surgeon will make a shorter incision on the appropriate surface.

Whichever incision is chosen, the surgeon lifts the skin and underlying tissue, pulls it up toward the trunk, cuts away excess skin, removes excess fatty tissue, and sutures the newly tightened skin in place and fits the patient with a compression garment to reduce swelling and speed the healing process.

Risks and Complications

Common complications include bruising, swelling, bleeding, and recurrence. The degree of pain varies according to the extent of the surgery.

Outlook and Lifestyle Modifications

As the swelling recedes, the alteration in the shape of the thigh becomes visible within four to six weeks after surgery. The final shape is usually attained within six months.

See also BUTTOCK LIFT; COMPRESSION GARMENT; TOTAL LOWER BODY LIFT.

third day blues See POSTSURGICAL DEPRESSION.

thread lift This minimally invasive surgical technique for lifting and tightening facial skin at eyebrows, forehead, and midface is commonly used for patients with minimal age-related sagging.

Procedure

The surgeon numbs the forehead with LOCAL ANESTHETIC, then passes absorbable surgical sutures under the skin at the hairline. She pulls the sutures tight, secures them to tiny hooks that anchor the skin and hold it smooth, and then cleans the fore-head and applies a dressing. Afterward, the patient avoids wrinkling the forehead or sleeping on her face so as to reduce tension on the threads until the skin heals.

Risks and Complications

Bruising, swelling, and a pulling sensation as the skin heals around the SUTURES are common.

Outlook and Lifestyle Modifications

The thread lift is not permanent. It is less traumatic than a standard FACE-LIFT, but the results may not last as long. As the patient ages, the skin will once again stretch and sag, often within three to four years, compared to five to 10 years for the more complex face-lift.

See also FOREHEAD LIFT.

thrombophlebitis Blood clot in a vein in the leg. Deep vein thrombophlebitis (a clot in a blood vessel deep inside the leg) is a possible complication following surgery or being confined to bed for a prolonged period of time. Superficial thrombophlebitis (a clot in a blood vessel near the surface of the skin) may occur as a complication of varicose veins.

Symptoms and Diagnostic Path

The clot generally causes pain, sometimes severe enough to make it difficult for the patient to walk more than a short distance at a time. Blood clots in the veins in the leg are diagnosed via an ULTRA-SOUND SCAN or with an X-ray taken after a contrast agent (dye) is injected into a large vein in the foot or ankle to outline the clot. A blood test showing an elevated amount of D dimmer, a naturally occurring blood thinner, may be used as a diagnostic tool, but it is less conclusive than either the ultrasound or the X-ray.

Treatment Options and Outlook

The three treatment option for thrombophlebitis are medication, support stockings, and surgery.

Medication Anticoagulants ("blood thinners") are used to dissolve an existing clot and keep particles in blood called platelets from sticking together to form new clots. For most patients, the medication is a temporary rather than a long-term option.

Support stockings Before surgery, support stocking may offer some relief from discomfort due to varicose veins; after surgery, they are used to maintain pressure that keeps veins from swelling and prevents blood from pooling at around valves in the veins. People with recurrent swollen veins may require stronger prescription stockings to control swelling.

Surgery If there is a chance that a clot in a vein in the leg may break loose, the surgeon may insert a small umbrella type device called a filter into the vena cava, the large vein in the abdomen through which the clot might flow upward into the lungs, a potentially fatal development. Other possible surgical treatments include removing the clot, or bypass surgery (removing the blocked vein and creating a new circulatory pathway), or inserting a small mesh tube called a stent that expands inside the vein to hold the vessel open so that blood flows freely though it.

Risk Factors and Preventive Measures

Using oral contraceptives increases the risk of blood clots. Varicose veins are also a risk factor, as is any major surgery. Using another form of contraception reduces the risk. Patients with varicose veins may be advised to wear stronger prescription support stockings and/or take anticoagulant drugs.

To prevent clots after surgery, the patient is fitted with compression stockings to maintain the flow of blood up through the veins and/or given anticoagulants.

See also COMPRESSION GARMENTS; VARICOSE VEINS.

tip plasty See RHINOPLASTY.

tissue expansion Plastic surgery procedure to grow extra skin for use in PLASTIC SURGERY to repair an area where skin is missing due to an injury, a disease, or a birth defect.

Procedure

The patient is given either local or general anesthesic. The surgeon makes a small incision adjacent to the area to be repaired, creates a small pocket, and inserts a balloonlike silicone device called a tissue expander under the skin. The expander has a small tube with a self-sealing valve at the surface of the skin into which the surgeon injects a small amount of sterile saline solution to inflate the expander.

Over the next several months, the patient returns periodically to the surgeon who injects larger amounts of sterile saline solution into the expander, enlarging the expander to stretch and grow new skin above it. When enough new skin has grown, the surgeon performs a second surgery to remove the expander and fix the new skin in place.

Risks and Complications

As additional saline is added to the expander, the patient may feel mild discomfort. Occasionally, the expander may break or leak, releasing saline solution into the body. The solution is harmless, but the expander must be removed and replaced. Infection at the site of the expander also requires that the device be removed; it may be replaced once the infection has cleared.

Outlook and Lifestyle Modifications

Tissue expansion is valuable because it yields skin that matches the color and texture of the skin to be replaced, is connected to blood vessels and nerves in the immediate area, and is compatible with the patient's own body. These factors greatly increase the chance of successful plastic surgery.

toe transfer Plastic surgery to amputate a toe, usually the big toe, and use the toe to replace a missing finger, usually the thumb.

Procedure

Once the patient is anesthetized, the surgeon amputates the toe and then closes the wound. She transfers the toe to the site of the missing thumb, attaches blood vessels and nerves as required, and closes the wound.

Risks and Complications

Bleeding, swelling, and infection at either the site of the amputation or the transplant is possible.

Failure of the grafted digit to grow into place at the new site is a more serious complication.

Outlook and Lifestyle Modifications

Because the structure of the large toe is similar to that of the thumb, if the graft takes and the nerves grow together, the transplanted toe can function as well as a thumb.

If only a small amount of tissue is removed, the surgeon will simply close the incision, in some cases repairing the defect with a small SKIN GRAFT.

tongue reconstruction   Surgery to repair the tongue after removal of a tumor.

Procedure

If part of the tongue is removed, the surgeon may rebuild the tongue either by moving tissue from the healthy part of the tongue into a new position or by lifting tissue from another part of the body, commonly the forearm, and grafting it onto the remaining tongue tissue.

If the entire tongue is removed, the surgeon may reconstruct a tongue, using one or more pieces of tissue lifted from another part of the body. The most common donor sites are the thigh, the latissimus dorsi (the broad flat muscle on the side of the back behind the arm), and the rectus abdominus (the broad muscle on the back wall of the abdomen), each offering bulky, muscled tissue.

If bone has been removed along with part or all of the tongue, the tissue for repairing the tongue must include bone into which teeth can be implanted. The most common donor sites for the bone are the fibula (the slim bone attached to the side of the tibia, the broader bone in the lower leg) and the iliac crest (the flat bone at the top of the hip bone).

Regardless of the procedure and the site from which the tissue is taken, the surgeon must attach blood vessels and nerves in the graft to those in the tongue or tongue area so as to assure the survival of the new tissue and retain or restore the patient's ability to move the tongue effectively.

Risks and Complications

Bleeding and swelling; infection; pooling of liquid at the surgical wound; infection; leakage of saliva from the mouth; or failure of the transplanted tissue to attach successfully in its new site.

Infection is treated with antibiotics to prevent it from spreading. Small pools of liquid may be aspirated (suctioned) to prevent infection; large pools of liquid may require a second surgery to drain the liquid. Leakage of saliva due to poorly aligned incisions may require a second surgery to correct the misalignment.

Failure of the tissue to grow into place most commonly results from a poor blood supply. To prevent this (or catch it early), the surgeon may monitor the shape and elasticity of the newly implanted tissue or use ultrasound to evaluate the flow of blood through the newly attached blood vessels. If the new tissue does not assume a normal shape or seems rigid or if blood is not flowing normally, a second surgery may be required to correct the blood flow.

tongue splitting   Forked tongue; an elective cosmetic surgery to divide the tongue in two, while maintaining sensation and motion in both halves.

Procedure

Once the patient is given either local or general anesthesic, the surgeon uses a scalpel, cautery, or LASER to cut the tongue about 1–2 inches down the middle, separating it into two sections. Then the surgeon stitches the exposed edges of the tongue closed to prevent their growing back together.

Risks and Complications

Bleeding, swelling, pain, and difficulty in eating and speaking are common for the first few days until the patient learns to manipulate the newly forked tongue. As with all surgery, infection is a possibility. Keeping the mouth clean reduces the risk, as does the use of antibiotics.

Outlook and Lifestyle Modifications

Some people experience a permanently altered sense of taste, loss of sensation due to nerve damage, and lingering speech problems (such as a lisp) after tongue splitting.

When the tongue is split, no tissue is removed, so this surgery can be reversed with a second operation to remove the healed tissue on the inner edges of the split tongue and stitch the two halves together.

See also BODY PIERCING.

tooth bonding   See DENTAL BONDING.

tooth caps   See DENTAL CROWN.

tooth veneer   See DENTAL VENEER.

tooth whitening   Cosmetic DENTISTRY to remove stains on the surface of the tooth or inside the tooth. Surface stains may be due to tobacco, coffee, or tea. Stains inside the tooth may be due to

- influences on the embryo such as exposure to tetracycline antibiotics
- excessive consumption of fluoride during tooth formation
- death of the interior of the tooth (the pulp)
- heredity (a natural tendency to darker teeth or cavities or a natural heightened response to staining agents)
- systemic medical conditions such as jaundice

Procedures

The two basic techniques for lightening the color of teeth are bleaching and microbrasion. Before beginning any lightening process, the dentist applies protective gel to the patient's gums and inserts a rubber device to protect the interior of the mouth. Before bleaching, he may also use pumice to remove superficial stains or debris from the tooth surface.

Bleaching   To bleach vital teeth (teeth with a healthy pulp and nerve), the dentist isolates the teeth to be whitened, protects the gum tissue, and applies a bleaching paste every 15 to 20 minutes. This application is followed by exposure to a specific lamp, which helps activate the bleach and hasten the procedure.

Alternatively, the dentist may apply a lightening paste or gel to the surface of the teeth and then use two LASERS to activate the gel. The first laser, an Argon laser, emits a blue light that activates the gel; the second laser, a CO_2 laser, emits infrared light that bleaches deeper layers of the surface of the tooth.

Kits for bleaching the teeth at home provide a bleaching compound and "bleaching trays" that the patient can wear over the teeth for up to four hours. These kits are less expensive than bleaching in the dentist's office, but they require repeated application over a longer period. Also they are usually less effective because the bleaching solution is weaker than the one used by the dentist and because the patient may not comply completely with all instructions.

To bleach nonvital teeth (teeth from which the nerve has been removed) the dentist drills a small opening in the back of the tooth, inserts a bleaching paste, and covers the hole with a temporary seal that can be removed to change the bleach paste once a week, as required, until the tooth is the desired color. This procedure, a walking bleach, lightens the tooth from the inside out; several visits to the dentist may be required to renew the bleach solution in order to lighten the tooth properly.

Microbrasion   First, the dentist uses a fine abrasive such as pumice to remove stains on the outer surface of the tooth. Then, he applies an acid or acid/abrasive paste to the surface of the tooth. The acid oxidizes and removes stains, dissolves white calcium deposits, and smooths the enamel surface of the tooth so that the tooth reflects light more cleanly.

Risks and Complications

The strong bleaches used by dentists rarely injure the gums due to the protective covering or damage the surface of a healthy tooth.

Excessive use of the peroxide bleaches in home bleaching kits may alter the bacterial content of the mouth, increasing the risk of infection. Repeated use of the bleaching trays in these kits may alter the bite and/or trigger temporomandibular disorder (TMJ), a pain in the side of the face. Etching or microbrasion may make teeth more sensitive to heat and cold.

Outlook and Lifestyle Modifications

Bleaching a vital tooth does not produce a permanent change. Repeated touch-up procedures usually maintain results, but after a few years, the tooth may gradually darken again, requiring a second procedure. Teeth with multiple restorations (fillings, veneers, caps) or insufficient or cracked enamel may not respond well to bleaching.

Microbrasion does not lighten teeth; it simply removes stains so that the surface of the tooth resumes its natural color.

See also DENTAL BONDING; DENTAL VENEER.

Toronto facial grading system (TFGS) A scale for evaluating facial nerve damage based on visible characteristics. This scale may be used to determine how to proceed with FACIAL REANIMATION, PLASTIC SURGERY to restore nerve activity to facial muscles.

The indicators on the scale include symmetry of the face when resting and symmetry of the face during voluntary movement such as smiling or frowning. Another consideration is how well the muscles on both sides of the face move together; for example, whether the muscles on the right and left side of the mouth lift the lips equally when the patient smiles.

total autogenous latissimus (tal) breast reconstruction See BREAST RECONSTRUCTION.

total body surface area Also called TBSA, body surface area, BSA; the complete outer surface of the body. This measurement used along with body weight and the patient's age when calculating various medical measurements, including (but not limited to) drug dosages, surgical anesthesic, and the amount of intravenous (IV) fluids to be given during and after surgery, including PLASTIC SURGERY. TBSA is also used in evaluating kidney and heart function and as one of the guides by which to estimate the total amount of skin and underlying tissue lost by burn patients.

There are various ways to determine TBSA, but the one most frequently used in Western medicine was published by biochemist Raymond D. Mosteller in *The New England Journal of Medicine* in 1987. Mosteller's "simplified" equation measures body surface area in square meters:

$$\text{Body surface area} = \text{the square root of } \frac{(\text{weight/in kilograms}) (\text{height/in centimeters})}{3,600}$$

As a general rule, 1.7 square meters (18.3 square feet) is considered a normal TBSA for an adult, but the true figure may vary according to age and gender. For example, the realistic average TBSA for an adult man is 1.9 square meters (20.45 square feet); for an adult woman, 1.6 square meters (17.22 square feet); for a child, 1.03 square meters (10.76 square feet) to 1.33 square meters (14.32 square feet), depending on the age of the child.

See also BURNS AND BURN RECONSTRUCTION.

total lower body lift Multiple cosmetic and/or reconstructive PLASTIC SURGERIES performed simultaneously to remove excess skin from the waist, abdomen, buttocks, thighs, and legs following extreme weight loss. A total body lift adds a breast and/or upper arm lift to the list of surgeries. Total lower body lifts and total body lifts are extraordinarily complex procedures with a long recovery period and the risk of multiple complications. These surgeries are most commonly seen on television shows about plastic surgery. In actual plastic surgery practice, the operations are likely to be done separately, several months apart so as to allow sufficient time for recovery.

See also ABDOMINOPLASTY; ARM LIFT; BREAST LIFT; BUTTOCK LIFT; THIGH LIFT.

transconjunctival blepharoplasty See EYELID RECONSTRUCTION (COSMETIC, LOWER LID).

transcyte See under BURNS AND BURN RECONSTRUCTION.

transosseous osteosynthesis See under LIMB-LENGTH DISCREPANCY.

tummy tuck   See ABDOMINOPLASTY.

Tweed's facial triangle   The pattern formed by teeth and jaws; most important, the degree of protrusion or recession of the teeth in relation to the upper and lower jaw bones. This diagnostic tool was created by American orthodontist Charles H. Tweed for use in planning orthodontic treatment. It may also be used in planning PLASTIC SURGERY or cosmetic dental surgery to create a more pleasing appearance.

See also JAW.

ultrasonic liposculpting   See LIPOSUCTION.

ultrasonic liposuction   See LIPOSUCTION.

ultrasound assisted lipectomy (ual)   See LIPOSUCTION.

ultrasound scan   Sonogram; noninvasive, radiation-free imaging technique employing the Doppler effect, an alteration in the perception of sound or light due to the movement of the source of the sound or light and/or the person observing it, a phenomenon identified by Austrian mathematician Christian Andreas Doppler (1803–53). For example, the sound of an automobile siren will remain the same so long as both the automobile and the person who hears the siren stay in the same position. If the car moves closer (or farther away) or the person moves forward (or back), the sound of the siren will get louder (or softer).

Doppler mapping is the use of an ultrasound device called a *transducer* or *Doppler scanner* to create a visual image of sound waves (ultrasound) to produce a picture of the internal organs. Ultrasound is most commonly used to create a picture of blood flowing through blood vessels during echocardiography, a diagnostic technique that shows a picture of a beating heart; fetal monitoring, a picture of the fetal heartbeat; and the evaluation of tumors, tracking the blood vessels into and out of the tumor. Plastic surgeons may use ultrasound to visualize internal organs before reconstructive surgery.

Procedure

For six to eight hours prior to a scan of internal organs, the patient generally avoids eating and drinking foods and beverages other than water; for some ultrasound examinations, the patient may be told to drink up to six glasses of water to make the organs more visible.

The technician smooths a gel on the patient's skin and presses the transducer against the gelled-site. The transducer converts electricity into high-frequency sound waves (ultrasound) that are directed through the skin into the patient's body, creating vibrations (echoes) that are converted back into electric signals that produce a picture of the sound on a television monitor visible to the technician running the test. The picture is then recorded on film or videotape.

Risks and Complications

There are no known adverse effects associated with ultrasound scans.

Outlook and Lifestyle Modifications

The scan produces a clear picture for diagnosis.

ultrasound surgery   Surgery employing an ultrasound (high-frequency sound waves). An ultrasonic scalpel concentrates ultrasound energy (high-intensity focused ultrasound [HIFU]) at a specific point in the body, producing heat sufficient to destroy tissue. Plastic surgeons often use ultrasound during liposuction to turn solid fatty tissue to liquid tissue so it can be easily suctioned away with less injury to muscle, nerves, and blood vessels.

Ultrasound energy can also be used to eradicate a varicose vein, clot blood inside a blood vessel, or stop bleeding from a severed one. It can also produce vibrations sufficient to shatter solid material. For example, lithotripty is a procedure employing ultrasound to break kidney stones into small particles that can be eliminated painlessly from the body in urine.

See also LIPOSUCTION; VARICOSE VEINS.

ultraviolet light Radiation in sunlight or from a tanning bed or sunlamp that triggers the release of melanin, a pigment in skin cells that ordinarily protects the body from absorbing excess ultraviolet (UV) radiation. This causes premature aging of the skin that may be reversible with some PLASTIC SURGERY techniques such as CHEMICAL SKIN PEEL or DERMABRASION.

There are two types of ultraviolet radiation, ultraviolet A (UVA) and ultraviolet B (UVB). Ultraviolet A (UVA) radiation, which is most common at higher elevations and equally available during most daylight hours, penetrates deeper into the body than does UVB. Exposure to UVA ages skin rapidly, triggers the release of existing melanin from pigment-producing skin cells called melanocytes, and is a primary cause of MELANOMA, a potentially fatal skin cancer. UVA rays are not blocked by most sunscreens. Ultraviolet B (UVB) radiation, which is most common at lower elevations and during midday, signals the body to produce new melanin and stimulates the production of vitamin D in the layer of fatty tissue just under the skin. On the down side, UVB exposure causes most sunburn, ages skin (but more slowly than UVA), leads to the emergence of skin MOLES and some types of skin cancer other than melanoma, and damages DNA. UVB is blocked by most sunscreens and some protective clothing. Note: Both UVA and UVB radiation may affect the melanin-producing cells in the eye, resulting in melanoma.

See also FACIAL AGING; FITZPATRICK SKIN TYPE CLASSIFICATION; GLOGAU PHOTOAGING CLASSIFICATION.

umbilicoplasty Surgery to reshape the umbilicus ("belly button") scar tissue left when the umbilical cord joining a fetus to its mother's placenta is cut at birth and the layers of the abdominal wall (skin, fat, muscle) fuse. Ordinarily, the scar tissue turns inward; occasionally the mass of scar tissue protrudes. The former scar is commonly known as an "innie"; the latter, an "outie."

Procedure
After administering LOCAL ANESTHETIC, or local anesthetic plus sedatives, the surgeon trims extra skin from the naval, often via an endoscopic incision with absorbable SUTURES. The incision is hidden in the navel, leaving no visible scar.

Risks and Complications
In rare cases, the patient may experience minor swelling, bruising, or discomfort.

Outlook and Lifestyle Modifications
Unless the patient gains or loses a large amount of weight, including weight gain during pregnancy, the reshaping is permanent.

Unna, Paul Gerson (1850–1929) German dermatologist who was the first scientist to identify a link between exposure to sunlight and the development of skin cancer (1894). He was also the first to document the effective use of salicylic acid, resorcinol, phenol, and trichloroacetic acid (TCA) as a CHEMICAL SKIN PEEL to smooth, lighten, and repair the skin.

uvulopalatoplasty PLASTIC SURGERY to relieve sleep-related breathing disorders such as loud snoring and sleep apnea (interrupted breathing during sleep) due to an unusually large uvula, the rounded piece of tissue that hangs down from the roof of the back of the mouth. The large uvula may vibrate, producing noisy snoring, or it may temporarily block the airway, causing sleep apnea.

Procedure
The surgeon uses a scalpel or a LASER (laser-assisted uvulopalatoplasty [LAUP]) to trim the uvula. The surgery is commonly performed with a LOCAL ANESTHETIC, and the patient goes home the same day.

Risks and Complications
Bleeding and or temporary swelling of the tissue may occur.

Outlook and Lifestyle Modifications

Uvulopalatoplasty relieves snoring, but the snoring may return within two years after the surgery, requiring a second surgery. According to the American Academy of Sleep Medicine, LAUP is not a reliably effective treatment for sleep apnea. About one-third of those treated with LAUP improve, while about one-third stay the same. About one-third of those treated get worse.

vaginal agenesis A congenital defect, which results in an abnormally short or completely absent vaginal canal, commonly corrected by PLASTIC SURGERY.

Symptoms and Diagnostic Path

The external genital area is normal, so the first sign of vaginal agenesis is commonly a failure to menstruate at puberty. The lack of a vagina is diagnosed via a physical gynecological examination, usually followed by imaging tests such as an ULTRASOUND SCAN of the pelvic area to ascertain the presence and condition of the uterus and ovaries and/or a MAGNETIC RESONANCE IMAGING (MRI) to show details of the reproductive tract.

Treatment Options and Outlook

The treatment depends on the severity of the defect. The most common treatments of choice are

- vaginal dilation for a patient with an existing, but shorted vagina
- vaginal reconstruction with bowel tissue for a patient with an extremely short vagina or a remnant of the vaginal canal
- vaginal reconstruction with SKIN GRAFTS for a patient who has no vaginal canal

Neither form of vaginal reconstruction leaves external scars.

Vaginal dilation The patient may be able to widen and lengthen the vaginal canal by pressing a tube-shaped device called a vaginal dilator firmly against the skin for up to 20 minutes, once a day, usually after bathing, when the skin is softened.

Vaginal reconstruction with bowel tissue The surgeon makes an incision in the patient's abdomen and removes a short portion of the colon, sets it aside, and closes the opening between the remaining parts of the colon. Then, she closes one end of the excised section and sutures the colon section onto the vaginal remnant, inserting a vaginal mold that remains in place for at least three days to shape the colon section. If the vagina begins to tighten later, the surgeon will numb the area and dilate the tissue.

The bowel tissue used to create the new vagina secretes some lubricants, but the patient may require additional lubrication for comfortable sexual intercourse.

Vaginal reconstruction with a skin graft First, the surgeon lifts a thin piece of skin from the patient's buttock and drapes it over a mold in the shape of a vaginal canal. Then the surgeon makes an incision at the normal site for the vagina and inserts the graft-covered mold. A week or later, when the grafted skin has attached itself, the surgeon removes the mold. To maintain the shape of the newly constructed vagina, the patient wears a vaginal dilator 24 hours a day for a period of up to three months, removing the dilator when she urinates, defecates, bathes, or has sexual intercourse. Then she uses the dilator only at night for another six months. After that, if the vaginal tissue begins to tighten, the patient may use the dilator periodically to maintain the vaginal canal.

Unlike normal vaginal tissue, the skin grafts used to create the new vagina do not secrete lubricating substances; the patient must use lubricants during sexual intercourse.

Risk Factors and Preventive Measures

Vaginal agenesis occurs once in every 5,000 live female births. Slightly less than one-third of girls born without a vaginal canal also have a defective or missing kidney. One in eight may have skeletal defects. There are no known risk factors or preventive measures for vaginal agenesis.

vaginal rejuvenation   See LABIAPLASTY.

vaginoplasty   PLASTIC SURGERY on the vagina; a term commonly used to describe construction of a vagina during male-to-female gender reassignment surgery, or to construct a vagina for a female child born with VAGINAL AGENESIS (the absence of a vagina), or to reconstruct a vagina destroyed by disease such as vaginal cancer.

Procedures

During gender reassignment, the surgeon removes the penis and testicles, redirects the urethra (the tube that carries urine from the bladder out of the body), and employs one of three procedures to build a vaginal canal:

- vaginal construction with SKIN GRAFTS
- vaginal construction with bowel tissue
- penile inversion

Once the vagina is created, the surgeon may use the glans (tip of the penis) to create a clitoris and the scrotal skin to create labia (the lips of the natural vagina).

Vaginal construction with skin grafts   The surgeon lifts a thin piece of skin from the penis or the patient's buttock and drapes it over a mold in the shape of a vaginal canal. Then the surgeon makes an incision at the normal site for the vagina and inserts the graft-covered mold. A week or later, when the grafted skin has attached itself, the surgeon removes the mold. To maintain the shape of the newly constructed vagina, the patient wears a vaginal dilator, a cylindrical device ranging in size from about 1.1–1.5 in./28–38 mm in diameter and 4–6 in./102–152 mm in length, 24 hours a day for a period of up to three months. The patient removes the dilator when urinating, defecating, bathing, or having sexual intercourse. Next, the patient uses the dilator only at night for another six months.

After that, if the vaginal tissue begins to tighten, the patient may use the dilator periodically to maintain the vaginal canal.

Unlike natural vaginal tissue, the skin grafts used to create the new vagina do not secrete lubricating substances; the patient must use lubricants during sexual intercourse.

Vaginal construction with bowel tissue   The medical name for this procedure is intestinal substitution vaginoplasty. The surgeon makes an incision in the patient's abdomen and removes a short portion of the colon, sets it aside, and closes the opening between the remaining parts of the colon. Then, he closes one end of the excised section and sutures the colon section into place at the site of the natural vagina, inserting a vaginal mold that remains in place for at least three days to shape the colon section. If the vagina begins to tighten later, the surgeon will numb the area and dilate the tissue.

The bowel tissue used to create the new vagina secretes some lubricants, but the patient may require additional lubrication for comfortable sexual intercourse.

Penile inversion   The surgeon removes the skin covering the penis, turns it inside out, and uses it to create a vaginal canal. Although the patient will still need lubrication for comfortable sexual intercourse, the inner surface of the penile skin provides some sensation. The use of the skin from the penis also reduces the risk of adverse effects that may be associated with lifting skin from another site for a SKIN FLAP or removing part of the colon.

Risks and Complications

Risks include infection, bleeding, damage to the bladder or prostate, and vaginal-rectal fistula (an abnormal opening that permits feces to leave the body through the vagina rather than the rectum/anus, requiring a second, corrective surgery). After construction with skin grafts, the skin may fail to survive at its new site; a vagina constructed with a section of bowel may be odorous, produce excess mucus, and bleed during intercourse.

Outlook and Lifestyle Modifications

Successful vaginoplasty creates an esthetically pleasing vagina that allows comfortable sexual intercourse.

varicose veins Enlarged veins; commonly large twisted veins visible on the surface of the legs and ankles. Other types of varicosities include

- hemorrhoids (varicose veins around the anus)
- reticular veins (flat blue-ish veins, usually in the back of the knee)
- spider veins (small reddish/purple/blue veins [capillaries] in a web- or tree-shape pattern on the surface of the skin)
- telangiectasias (reddish clusters of fine blood vessels, usually on face or upper body)
- venous lakes (pool of blood in a vein, usually on the face or neck)

Note: THROMBOPHLEBITIS is the enlargement of a vein due to a blood clot. Superficial thrombophlebitis is due to a blood clot and inflammation in a small vein near the skin. Deep vein thrombophlebitis is due to a blood clot in a vein deep inside the leg that may cause redness, swelling, and pain. The condition, which is potentially fatal because the clot may break free and travel to the lung, requires immediate medical attention.

Symptoms and Diagnostic Path
Varicose veins may cause inflammation or changes in skin color or open sores or bleeding after even a minor injury at the site of the vein. Aching, burning, throbbing, muscle cramps, and swelling are common, especially after prolonged standing or sitting in one position.

Varicose veins on the surface of the skin are identified by simple observation; an ULTRASOUND SCAN may be used to check for a blood clot in veins under the surface of the skin.

Treatment Options and Outlook
The common treatments for varicose veins include PHLEBECTOMY ("vein stripping"), SCLEROTHERAPY (injections of an irritating solution to scar and close the vein), or LASER surgery or ULTRASOUND SURGERY (directing heat into the vein to seal the vessel).

Risk Factors and Preventive Measures
A varicose vein develops when a valve controlling the flow of blood through the vein malfunctions, causing the blood to pool in and stretch the vein. Valve function may be affected by age, gender, body weight, an increase in blood volume and/or a shift in hormones production. As a result, varicose veins are more common among older people, women, the obese, pregnant women, and prior to a menstrual period or during menopause. Genetics also play a role; varicose veins may run in families.

There are no known ways to prevent varicose veins, but exercising to improve circulation, controlling one's weight, avoiding tight clothing, and changing position frequently while sitting or standing may relieve discomfort.

vascular birthmark See HEMANGIOMA; MACULAR STAIN; PORT WINE STAIN.

vermillionectomy Surgery to remove cancerous or precancerous tissue from the vermillion border (also known as the vermillion margin or carmine margin), the pink-pigmented outer surface of the lips and then to reconstruct the lip(s).

Procedure
The surgeon numbs the lip(s) and uses a scalpel or a chemical peeling agent or a CO_2 LASER to remove the damaged tissue. Depending on the amount of tissue removed, the area of the surgery may be left to heal on its own or may be rebuilt with a myomucosal flap, a piece of the lining of the lip and the underlying muscle lifted and turned forward, up or down, to cover the surgical defect.

Risks and Complications
Bleeding and swelling may occur. The most serious complications is the failure of the flap to grow firmly into place at its new site.

Outlook and Lifestyle Modifications
Medically, this surgery removes the malignant tissue. From a cosmetic point of view, even after successful surgery, the lip may appear unnaturally flattened.

vital signs Blood pressure, pulse rate (heartbeats per minute), respiration (breaths per minute), and

NORMAL RANGE OF VITAL SIGNS IN HEALTHY ADULTS

Blood pressure	100/60–140/90 mm Hg*
Pulse rate	50–90 beats/minute (at rest)
Respiration	12–16 breaths/minute
Temperature	97.8°–99.1°F

*In 2003, the Heart, Lung and Blood Institute of the National Institutes of Health set the following standards for blood pressure measurement categories: 140/90 mm HG = hypertension (high blood pressure); 120–139/80–89 mm HG systolic pressure = prehypertension; > 120/80 = normal blood pressure.
Sources: Oregon Health and Sciences University, "Cardiovascular Diseases: Vital signs." Available online. URL: http://www.ohsuhealth.com/htaz/cardiac/vital_signs.cfm. Accessed July 28, 2006. University of California, San Diego, "A Practical Guide to Clinical Medicine," August 23, 2005. Available online. URL: http://www.medicine.ucsd.edu/clinicalmed/vital.htm. Accessed July 28, 2006. "Vital Signs," MedLinePlus. Available online. URL: http://www.nlm.nih.gov/medlineplus/ency/article/002341.htm. Accessed July 28, 2006.

temperature; physical signs of life. Vital signs are used to measure health and/or physical function, particularly after illness or surgery, including PLASTIC SURGERY.

Modern diagnosticians often add pain as a fifth vital sign, because being in physical distress may affect the original four indicators. For the same reason, some mental health experts suggest including emotional distress as a sixth vital sign.

The "normal" ranges for the vital signs may vary with age, gender, weight, and physical condition.

See also PAIN.

vitamins   Vitamins are organic chemicals, substances that contain carbon, hydrogen, and oxygen. As opposed to dietary minerals, which are elements that contain only one type of atom, vitamins are complex molecules that contain many types of atoms.

In addition to regulating various body functions, vitamins are essential for the synthesis of proteins and other substances required for the new tissue that the body builds to heal a wound, including the wounds of PLASTIC SURGERY.

Human beings require at least 11 specific vitamins: the fat-soluble vitamins A, D, E, and K; the water-soluble vitamins C; and the B complex (thiamin/vitamin B1, riboflavin/B2, niacin, B6, folate, and B12). Two more B vitamins, biotin

and pantothenic acid, are also believed to be valuable.

Vitamin A reduces early inflammation around the wound and enhances the production of new skin cells to repair tissues and reduce scarring. Vitamin K produces specialized proteins in blood plasma (the clear fluid in blood), including prothrombin, the protein that clots blood and helps form a scab over an injury. Even surgical patients who are not deficient in vitamin A may heal quicker if they take vitamin A supplements of if vitamin A is applied topically to the wound.

Vitamin C develops and maintains connective tissue and increases the production of new cells after a wound. A patient who is deficient in vitamin C may experience slow healing of wounds, including the wounds of plastic surgery. Vitamin C supplements may reduce the risk of bedsores (pressure sores, decubitus ulcers), but there is no evidence that giving vitamin C supplements to patients who are not deficient in vitamin C will speed healing after surgery.

The B vitamin niacin increases the flow of oxygen into body tissues to hasten healing. Folate, another B vitamin, participates in the synthesis of amino acids used to build new body cells. Biotin is used to make fatty acids and amino acids, and pantothenic acid protects hemoglobin, the protein in red blood cells that carries oxygen throughout the body.

Vitamin E is a special case. On the one hand, it is an anti-inflammatory; applied to the skin, it reduces redness and swelling at the site of the wound. On the other hand, if applied to a wound, it may interfere with the production of connective tissue, slowing the healing process and causing the scar to spread out. While some experts recommend the use of topical vitamin E products to reduce scarring, the product is applied only after the wound (scar) is completely healed.

Note: Each of the effects specific vitamins exert on wound healing occurs when the vitamins are taken as part of a normal healthy diet. With the single exception of onetime large doses of vitamin A, there is no evidence to show that taking supplements after an injury or after surgery speeds healing.

See also DIETARY FAT; MINERALS; PROTEIN.

RECOMMENDED DIETARY ALLOWANCES FOR HEALTHY ADULTS (2006)

Age (Years)	Vitamin A (RE/IU)	Vitamin D (mcg/IU)	Vitamin E (alpha-TE)	Vitamin K (mcg)	Vitamin C (mg)
Males					
19–24	900/2970	5/200	15	120	90
25–50	900/2970	5/200	15	120	90
51–70	900/2970	10/400	15	120	90
71+	900/2970	15/600	15	120	90
Females					
19–24	700/2310	5/200	15	90	75
25–50	700/2310	5/200	15	90	75
51–70	700/2310	10/400	15	90	75
71+	700/2310	15/600	15	90	75

Age (Years)	Thiamin (Vitamin B1)(mg)	Riboflavin (Vitamin B2)(mg)	Niacin (mcg/NE)	Vitamin B6 (mg)	Folate (mcg)
Males					
19–24	1.2	1.3	16	1.3	400
25–50	1.2	1.3	16	1.3	400
51–70	1.2	1.3	16	1.7	400
71+	1.2	1.1	16	1.7	400
Females					
19–24	1.1	1.1	14	1.3	400
25–50	1.1	1.1	14	1.3	400
51–70	1.1	1.1	14	1.5	400
71+	1.1	1.1	14	1.5	400

Age (Years)	Pantothenic acid (mg)	Biotin (mcg)
Males		
19–24	5	30
25–50	5	30
51–70	5	30
71+	5	30
Females		
19–24	5	30
25–50	5	30
51–70	5	30
71+	5	30

W abdominoplasty   See ABDOMINOPLASTY; W PLASTY.

Wallace Rule of Nines   See BURNS AND BURN RECONSTRUCTION.

wart removal   Medical or surgical treatment to remove a wart on the skin, a benign growth caused by a human papilloma virus (HPV), one of a family of more than 100 different viruses.

HPV organisms are classified as either "low risk" or "high risk," depending on their potential to cause malignant growths. The HPVs that cause common skin warts and some forms of genital warts are low risk; the HPVs linked to cervical cancer and perhaps to some cancers of the neck (tonsils) are high risk.

Procedures

Warts may be removed with conventional surgery (an incision), laser surgery (heat), caustic chemicals, cryotherapy (cold), and/or drugs that stimulate an immune response.

Conventional surgery   Warts on the skin or in the genital area may be removed by loop electrosurgical excision procedure (LEEP), during which the surgeon passes a sharp loop-shaped instrument under the wart to lift it off the skin or mucous membrane.

Laser surgery   A pulsed dye laser may be used to "burn off" warts on the skin. A CO_2 laser may be used to remove large warts in the genital area. The anesthesic choice, whether local or general, depends on the size of the area and the number of warts to be treated.

Caustic chemicals   To remove warts on the skin, the surgeon applies a caustic substance such as salicylic acid (the active ingredient in Compound W®) or cantharidin, a chemical derived from a species of beetles. To remove genital warts, the doctor may apply once a week a solution of podophyllin, an extract from the root of the American mandrake that kills warts by interrupting the natural growth processes of skin cells. Podofilox (Condylox®), a form of podophyllin available as a cream, may be applied to the warts at home twice a day for three days, skipping four days, then repeating the cycle until the warts are gone.

Cryotherapy   The surgeon applies liquid nitrogen to freeze the wart, allows it to dry (it will turn white), then scrapes off the residue, including the wart. The process may have to be repeated two to four times to destroy the wart completely.

Immune system stimulants   The surgeon injects an antigen or combination of antigens at the site of the wart to stimulate the patient's immune system to attack and destroy the virus causing the wart. In cases of stubborn infection, interferon may be injected into the wart twice a week for up to two months to boost the body's immune response to the wart virus.

Risks and Complications

All treatments to remove warts may leave the skin irritated, painful, and/or swollen. Conventional surgery and caustic chemicals leave a scar; laser surgery and immune system stimulants do not. After cryotherapy, the treated area may be lighter in color than the skin around it.

Outlook and Lifestyle Modifications

Some warts disappear spontaneously. Others require medical treatment. No medical treatment is guaranteed to destroy warts permanently.

See also CRYOSURGERY; IMMUNE SYSTEM; LASER.

Wassel classification   System created by American surgeon H. D. Wassel to describe the various kinds of duplicated thumb, for example, extra bones in the thumb or a split down the middle of the thumb that creates two thumbs. Duplicated thumb is a birth defect that occurs most frequently among African Americans (1/300 live births vs. 1/3000 live births among Caucasians and Asian Americans). PLASTIC SURGERY may repair the defect.

waxing   Cosmetic technique to remove excess hair on various parts of the body, most commonly the face, arms, legs, pubic area ("bikini wax"), and anal area.

Procedure

The technician applies warm wax to the skin, allows it to cool and harden, and then peels it away, taking with it hairs and their roots.

Risks and Complications

The possible adverse effects of waxing are skin irritation or in rare cases burns caused by very hot wax.

Outlook and Lifestyle Modifications

Waxing produces a temporary but longer-lasting result than shaving; the result may last up to six weeks, depending on how fast an individual's hair grows. Continued waxing lengthens the time between treatments and reduces the amount of hair that grows back.

webbing   See FINGERS AND TOES, CONGENITAL STRUCTURAL DEFECTS; FINGERTIP REPAIR.

wen   Pilar cyst; a bump on the skin filled with sebum (fatty material) secreted by a block pilosebaceous gland, a gland with a hair growing out of it.

wet-to-dry dressing   Multilayer, absorptive, non-adhesive bandage; typically, a layer of gauze soaked in saline solution (salt water), covered with a layer of petroleum jelly coated gauze, covered with a dry layer of gauze. It is used to promote the growth of new tissue on a moist wound such as a bedsore. The dressing does not injure the skin when it is removed so long as it is not allowed to dry out. However, it must be replaced frequently to prevent its drying and sticking to the wound, and when removed, it may leave residue behind.

W incision   See W PLASTY.

windblown hand   See FINGERS AND TOES, CONGENITAL STRUCTURAL DEFECTS.

witch's chin   See CHIN LIFT; NECK LIFT.

wound adhesive   Natural or synthetic glue used to close a wound or surgical incision, primarily straight incisions or incisions in areas such as the upper eyelid, the face, and the scalp where the skin is not under tension. Wound adhesives are not suitable for areas such as the hands, feet, joints, or inside of the mouth where the surface is subject to repeated movement that can stress the glue and cause it to peel off the wound. For a short time after surgery, the adhesive closure is weaker than sutures; as time passes, its strength equals that of stitches.

Synthetic wound adhesives have an added benefit: they form a waterproof dressing that lowers the risk of infection. The synthetic most commonly used as a wound adhesive is 2-octyl cyanoacrylate, a member of the family of chemical adhesives created by Kodak Laboratories researcher Harry Coover in 1942. Unlike the original cyanoacrylate compounds, including methyl-2-cyanoacrylate (Crazy Glue®), 2-octyl cyanoacrylate does not irritate the skin. In 1998, the U.S. Food and Drug Administration (FDA) approved this glue as a substitute for sutures in closing the skin over the wounds and surgical incisions (sutures are still required for closing layers of tissue under the skin). In 2001, the FDA approved the use of cyanoacrylate dressings (Dermabond™, Traumaseal™) as a barrier against common disease-causing bacteria such as staphylococci, pseudomonads, and E. coli. In 2004, the FDA approved the use of a second surgical glue, butyl-2-cyanoacrylate. Cyanoacrylate glues are also used in orthopedic surgery, dental, and oral surgery (Soothe-n-seal™), and simple bandages (Band Aid® Liquid Bandage). Note: Cyanoacrylates approved for medical use contain plasticizers that enable the closure to bend with the skin, thus remaining in place until healing is complete. Ordinary household cyanoacrylate glues do not contain the requisite plasticizers; in addition, they are strong irritants not meant for medical uses.

The virtue of wound adhesives is that unlike sutures (stitches) they are a needle-free technique that lowers the risk of infection from blood-borne viruses such as HIV. Wound adhesives may be used to close the surface of deep wounds after the subcutaneous (under-the-skin) edges of the wound are stitched together. But they cannot be used inside any wound; even a glue made of natural materials is a foreign body that may trigger an immune reaction, or raise the risk of infection, or cause inflammation and tissue damage that interferes with healing.

See also IMMUNE SYSTEM; SUTURES.

wound dressing See ABSORBENT FOAM; FOAM WOUND DRESSING; HYDROCOLLOID DRESSING.

W plasty Surgical incision in the shape of a *W*, created by outlining two triangles on either side of a straight line, with the tip of one triangle placed in the center of the base of the other; used in surgery such as abdominoplasty or to relax the skin and reduce tension in a straight-line scar. In abdominoplasty, this technique enables the surgeon to make both sides of the abdomen equal, without leaving skin folds or a visible straight-line vertical scar (the horizontal W scar is hidden in the pubic hair). In addition, the W incision creates longer-lasting results because it stretches the abdominal skin farther and tighter than do other incisions.

See also ABDOMINOPLASTY.

wrinkles Lines in the face most commonly associated with normal aging of the skin and/or exposure to environmental factors such as air pollution and ULTRAVIOLET LIGHT (sunlight).

As a person ages, cells in the epidermis (the top layer of skin cells) and the dermis (layers of cells underneath the epidermis) thin and reproduce more slowly. The sebaceous glands grow larger but produce less sebum, the natural oil that keeps skin supple. The amount of elastin (protein fibers that give skin its ELASTICITY) declines, and the collagen (connective tissue) network that supports the skin sags. As a result of these changes, natural ridges on the skin surface flatten, and cells in the layer of fat under the skin shrink. At the same time, exposure to air pollution and/or ultraviolet light (sunlight) thins and dries the epidermis while encouraging the production of enzymes that damage collagen and accelerate the wrinkling process.

Symptoms and Diagnostic Path
There are two types of facial wrinkles, dynamic wrinkles and fine wrinkles (crepe-paper wrinkles), both diagnosed by simple observation.

Dynamic wrinkles These wrinkles are associated with normal aging. They appear along wrinkle lines, also called relaxed skin tension lines (RSTL), the natural lines of tension associated with the muscles used to create facial expressions. Repeated use of these muscles to smile, frown, purse the lips, or squint causes mild wrinkles that deepen and become permanent with age, most commonly around the lips, between the eyebrows, and at the side of the eye. An example of dynamic wrinkles are glabellar furrows, age-related, deep vertical wrinkles in the glabella, the skin above the nose between the eyes. Smile lines, fine lines around the corners of the mouth created by repeated movement of the facials muscles used to create a smile, are another common example.

Fine wrinkles (crepe-paper wrinkles) These wrinkles, usually found on the cheeks, are commonly linked to environmental factors such as sunlight, smoking, or the age-related loss of the underlying facial fat pads.

Treatment Options and Outlook
Mild dynamic wrinkles such as crow's feet, scowl lines, forehead creases, and lip wrinkles may be reduced with BOTOX injections. To reduce deep

dynamic wrinkles such as skin folds around the mouth, the surgeon may inject filler such as collagen, fat, or hyaluronic acid (Restylane), or perform a face-lift to remove excess skin and tighten sagging skin. Fine wrinkles (crepe-paper wrinkles) may be smoothed with a chemical skin peel or dermabrasion, techniques that remove the top layer of skin cells.

See also CHEMICAL SKIN PEEL; DERMABRASION; FACE-LIFT; FACIAL AGING; FAT INJECTION.

xanthelasma Benign, soft, yellowish plaque (raised spot), composed of xanthoma cells, foamy cells packed with fat, primarily cholesterol. The spots commonly occur on the eyelid, most frequently on the upper lid. The plaques tend to enlarge; if there are two or more, they may join together to form one plaque. If the spots are annoying or cosmetically unattractive, they may be removed with PLASTIC SURGERY.

Symptoms and Diagnostic Path
Xanthelasmas are diagnosed by observation. If there is any question about the nature of the spot, a BIOPSY may be performed. Because about half of all patients with xanthelasma have lipid (fat) disorders, the doctor may also order a cholesterol blood test to determine cholesterol levels.

Treatment Options and Outlook
Surgical treatment for xanthelasmas include excising (cutting away) small lesions. Both large and small lesions may be treated by one of the following methods:

- chemical cauterization (agents such as trichloroacetic acid that coagulate proteins and dissolve fats)
- cryotherapy (freezing the lesion)
- electrodesicccation
- laser surgery

Each treatment has risks and benefits. For example, surgical excision is rarely used for larger lesions because removing a relatively large amount of tissue risks ectropion (an eyelid that folds out and up or down) or may require EYELID RECONSTRUCTION. Chemical cauterization is unlikely to cause scar-

ring. Cryotherapy, which often requires more than one treatment, may cause scarring and loss of skin color. Electrodessication may also require repeated treatments. Laser surgery can cause scarring and changes in SKIN COLOR, but it is quick and requires no SUTURES.

Finally, recurrence of xanthelasma after removal is common. Some studies suggest that the recurrence rate after surgical excision may be as high as 40 percent.

Risk Factors and Preventive Measures
Xanthelasmas occur more often among women than among men. They are most likely to appear between age 30 and 50 and are most common in people with high cholesterol levels, and/or high levels of low-density lipoproteins (LDLs, the "bad" cholesterol), or low levels of high-density lipoproteins (HDLs, the "good" cholesterol). Uncontrolled diabetes, which is often accompanied by high cholesterol levels, is also a risk factor for xanthelasmas.

Xenon (Xe) One of the noble gases, a group of relatively nonreactive elements listed in Column VIIIA/Group 0 of the periodic table of the elements that also include argon (Ar), helium (He), neon (Ne), krypton (Kr), radon (Rn), and ununoctium (Uuo).

Xenon is a source of energy in LASERS used by plastic surgeons and high-intensity xenon lamps used by cosmetic dentists. The xenon lamps emit high-intensity light (ultraviolet, near-infrared) produced by electrical discharge in a mixture of the element xenon and antimony vapor or xenon and mercury vapor under high pressure. The xenon/antimony lamp produces a higher level of ULTRAVIOLET

LIGHT than the xenon/mercury combination. The light from a xenon lamp is used to "cure" (harden) materials used in cosmetic dentistry for veneers and other cosmetic tooth coverings and dental restorations.

See also DENTAL BONDING.

xerography Xeroradiography; a noninvasive imaging technique that may be used to produce an image of an area to be treated with PLASTIC SURGERY. Xerography creates a visible record by projecting an image onto an electrically charged, photoconductive (light-absorbing) plate, developing the plate with dry ink powder, and transferring the image to plain paper that is heated to produce a print. Xerography was invented in 1937 by American physicist Chester F. Carlson (1906–68); developed by the Haloid Company, which named the process xerography, created the name *XeroX* (with two capital X's), sold the first Haloid Xerox Copier in 1950, and changed its corporate name to Xerox in 1961. In 1981, Carlson was posthumously inducted into the National Inventors Hall of Fame. The image produced by xerography is a xerogram.

xerostomia Failure of the salivary glands to produce sufficient saliva leading to excessive dryness ("cottonmouth") that can make speech and swallowing difficult, increase the risk of cavities because the teeth are no longer continuously bathed in mineral-rich saliva, and raise the risk of oral infection. It may also increase the likelihood of halitosis (bad breath) and cause damage to the tissues inside the mouth, requiring PLASTIC SURGERY/cosmetic dentistry.

Symptoms and Diagnostic Path

The symptoms, dry tissues due to lack of sufficient moisture in the mouth, are clearly visible on physical examination.

Treatment Options and Outlook

If the underlying cause of the dryness cannot be eliminated, treatment is designed to reduce the incidence of cavities and infection by avoiding anticholinergic medications, keeping the mouth moist by drinking sufficient quantities of sugar-free liquids, using a commercial saliva substitute mouthwash, and keeping the mouth as clean as possible.

Risk Factors and Preventive Measures

Xerostomia may be associated with an illness such as diabetes or Sjögren's syndrome (dryness of the membranes in eyes, nose, and mouth), or to the side effects of anticholinergic medicines (products such as decongestants that decrease the secretions of the mucous membranes). It may also be related to an injury to the salivary glands or to radiation therapy in the area of the salivary glands.

X-linked condition See GENETICS.

X-ray examination Imaging technique; this noninvasive diagnostic tool utilizes a form of radiation that passes through solid material such as flesh or metal to show details of the internal structure such as bones inside the body or flaws in metal objects. It is sometimes used by surgeons as a guide in planning a PLASTIC SURGERY procedure. For example, a panoramic radiograph is an image produced by a camera that moves around the head, creating one long film that shows an image of all the teeth in both the upper and lower jaws, along with portions of the jaw. Commonly used in DENTISTRY, this type of X-ray is also valuable to surgeons planning a procedure to alter the shape or size of the jaw.

Procedure

The patient is positioned in front of, under, or over a special camera that releases radiation that passes through the patient's body to create an image captured on photographic paper as a negative in which solids appear white and spaces appear dark gray or black. The picture is also called an X-ray.

Risks and Complications

X-rays are ionizing radiation, the form of radiation that breaks apart molecules. Ionizing radiation can damage body tissues. Depending on the part of the body exposed, excess exposure to X-rays may cause

- anemia
- cataracts
- skin irritation (X-ray dermatitis)
- burns
- cancer
- abnormal sperm production
- testicular atrophy
- male and female infertility
- fetal damage, including birth defects, mental retardation, and childhood leukemia

Outlook and Lifestyle Modifications

A clear picture of solid structures, i.e. bones, inside the body may improve the chance for successful surgery.

X-ray therapy Any treatment (usually for cancer) involving X-rays. External radiation therapy (XRT) is radiation delivered from outside the body. Internal radiation therapy is radiation delivered via radioactive seeds implanted in the body, such as the treatment sometimes employed for a localized tumor such as a prostate cancer that has not moved outside the prostate gland. X-ray therapy may be used in preparation for PLASTIC SURGERY; for example, to treat persistent skin ulcers in advance of SKIN GRAFTS to repair the ulcerated area.

Y

YAG laser   See LASER.

yellow cartilage   See ELASTICITY.

yellow light laser   See HEMANGIOMA; LASER; VARI-COSE VEINS.

yttrium   See LASER.

yttrium-aluminum-garnet   See LASER.

Y-plasty   A surgical incision in the shape of a *Y*. Like Z-plasty, a surgical incision in the zigzag Z shape, Y-plasty is most commonly employed as a technique to relax and smooth tissue and thus increase mobility in a scarred area of skin, particularly after a severe burn injury.

See also BURNS AND BURN RECONSTRUCTION; Z-PLASTY.

yttrium-aluminum-garnet Nd laser   See LASER.

Z

ZF suture Place where the *zygomatic* bone (cheekbone) meets the *frontal* bone (the flat bone on the forehead and side of the face).

Human infants are commonly born with the various sutures on the skull slightly separated rather than fused, as in the adult skull. As the child grows, the sutures come together to close the skull. Premature closure of the sutures during pregnancy produces an abnormally shaped skull that may compress the brain. In some cases, plastic surgeons may separate and reposition the bones, altering the shape of the skull so as to give the brain room to develop normally.

zippering See SURGICAL ZIPPER.

Zitelli flap See SKIN FLAP.

Z mammaplasty See BREAST REDUCTION; Z-PLASTY.

Z-plasty Zigzag plasty. This surgical incision in the shape of a *Z* is created with three incisions: one down the length of the existing scar; the second, down to the left at a 60-degree angle from the top of the existing scar; and the third, up to the right at a 60-degree angle from the bottom of the existing scar. The three incisions allow the surgeon to create two triangular SKIN FLAPS that are turned and moved forward, the top to the right and the bottom to the left. When the flaps heal, if the original scar was vertical, the new one is horizontal (and vice versa).

Z-plasty is used to relax the tension on a straight-line scar, releasing the surrounding tissue so as to make the scar less visible and permit freer movement. The Z-plasty is also used to remove an abnormal connection such as webbing between fingers or toes, or to repair a natural skin defect or to repair the scar caused by a surgical injury such as the opening cut into the throat to insert a breathing tube. Very long scars may require more than one Z-plasty.

See also INTUBATION; POLYDACTYLY.

Zyderm™ See FILLERS.

zygoma The cheekbone. In describing the face and/or PLASTIC SURGERY to repair facial defects

- the zygomatic arch is the point where the cheekbone joins the flat temporal bone that comes down the side of the face next to the eye
- the term *zygomaticofacial* refers to the cheekbone and the face
- the term *zygomaticofrontal* refers to the cheekbone and the frontal bone (the bone over the eye)
- the term *zygomaticomaxillary* refers to the cheekbone and the maxilla (upper jaw bone)
- the *zygomaticoorbital* region is the area that includes the cheekbone and the orbit, the boney socket around the eye
- the term *zygomaticotemporal* refers to the cheekbone and the temporal bone

Zyplast™ See FILLERS.

APPENDIX
WEB SITES

Searching for medical information on the Internet can be risky. Given the open nature of the Internet, which encourages the exchange of anecdotal (and sometimes misleading) evidence, it may be difficult to vouch for the quality and reliability of the information on a specific site. Not so with the Web sites listed here.

At first glance, some of these sites may seem distant from the subject at hand, plastic surgery. But look closer: each site deals with medical conditions that may require plastic surgery or with an aspect of surgery in general or with the history and lore of medicine and surgery. Furthermore, each is run by a thoroughly professional organization or individual posting only up-to-date and accurate information. And each makes clear that the best source for personal medical advice is one's own physician.

Plastic Surgery

American Society for Aesthetic Plastic Surgery*
http://www.surgery.org

ASAPS is the professional organization of board-certified plastic surgeons specializing in cosmetic plastic surgery such as adominoplasty ("tummy tuck"), breast augmentation, eyelid surgery, face-lift, liposuction (lipoplasty) and rhinoplasty, as well as nonsurgical cosmetic procedures such as hair removal, skin resurfacing, and Botox injections.

Click the Public Site in the bar at the top of the home page to bring up consumer-related features such as finding a surgeon, a gallery of

Note: * indicates that the site offers some information in Spanish and/or other languages.

pictures showing the results of cosmetic surgery, information on patient safety, and a description of injection techniques such as injections of collagen filler.

For patients who have not yet selected a doctor, the site provides an online Find a Surgeon form, a toll-free 800-number surgeon referral service, a free brochure on cosmetic surgery (by mail or download), and an interactive form that allows patients (or prospective patients) to ask an ASAPS surgeon a question about cosmetic surgery.

American Society of Plastic Surgeons*
http://www.plasticsurgery.org

ASPS, founded in 1948, is the largest and oldest professional association for board-certified plastic surgeons who perform both cosmetic and reconstructive surgery. The society's site is the most complete one designed specifically for plastic surgery patients.

Begin on the home page by clicking Procedures to open the superb list of articles about cosmetic and reconstructive procedures, each written in clear, patient-friendly language, and each available in both a brief version and a longer, more technical one.

The site also has a before-and-after photo gallery showing the results of plastic surgery procedures, a guide to choosing a plastic surgeon, a Find a Plastic Surgeon button at the top of the home page that brings up an interactive form allowing the reader to choose a surgeon by name/locale/procedure, a toll-free surgeon referral phone number, and an Ask the Plastic Surgeon e-mail form.

Finally, for patients interested in plastic surgery statistics, typing "statistics" into the search bar yields a wealth of yearly totals on the number and success of various procedures.

Related Medical Disciplines

American Academy of Cosmetic Dentistry
http://www.aacd.com

AACD, founded in 1984, is the largest international association of cosmetic and reconstructive dentists, dental laboratory technicians, educators, researchers, students, and hygienists. The academy's site explains modern cosmetic dentistry techniques and offers several interactive services.

On the home page, click Public to bring up several quick links. The two most valuable are How to Choose Your Dentist and Ask an AACD Member Dentist Your Dental Question.

The first link sets out the obvious standards for professional care: make sure the dentist belongs to AACD, ask for before-and-after pictures of the dentist's patients, get references from other dentists (and other patients), check to see that your dentist participates in continuing education courses to keep his knowledge and techniques up to date. The second link goes to a form you can use to e-mail or print and fax your question to the AACD. There is also an 800-number for patients who prefer live talk.

American Academy of Dermatology*
http://www.aad.org

AAD, established in 1869, counts among its membership most of the practicing American dermatologists. The academy's consumer-friendly site provides information regarding skin conditions that are often treated with plastic surgery.

To access the information, go to the Public Center box on the home page and click on Derm A–Z. When the page comes up, you may either type in a subject at the top in the box that searches the site or go to Dermatology Health Topics Quick Access on the right side of the page and select the section of the alphabet under which your topic appears.

Searching the site brings up professional and consumer articles; using the alphabetical listing produces a variety of material.

For example, type "aging skin" into the search bar, and you get 1,090 articles related to aging, skin, or aging skin. Alternatively, choose Topics A–E on the left side of the home page, scroll to "aging

skin," and the offerings include a pamphlet on Mature Skin, available free by mail or download; the standard FAQs; access to AgeingSkinNet, a second AAD site; and a plethora of clearly written articles such as "What's Ahead for Aging Skin," "Ways to Counter Aging," and "How Old Can Skin Get?" and such plastic surgery-specific topics as "Need a Lift? New Non-Invasive Radiofrequency Treatment Is an Alternative to the Traditional Facelift."

American Academy of Orthopedic Surgeons*
http://www.aaos.org

AAOS, founded in 1933, provides continuing education for orthopedic surgeons; a subsidiary division, the American Association of Orthopaedic Surgeons, founded in 1997, advocates healthy policy and patient care.

The AAOS site is valuable for people whose plastic surgery involves replacing or reconstructing bones or boney structures. Scroll to the left of the home page and click on Patient Information to bring up a page offering general information about orthopedics, plus special sites for children, preventing injuries, replacing joints, osteoporosis, patient care, patient stories, sports and exercise, bone tumors, women's health. To view everything at once, click View All Articles.

Click on Ask a Question to get an e-mail form to send your query directly to an orthopedic surgeon. You can also scroll through other patients' questions (and the answers); no names, of course.

American Cancer Society*
http://www.cancer.org

The ACS's 13 divisions and more than 3,400 local offices deliver cancer prevention, early detection, and patient services programs. Clearly, the site is devoted primarily to basic information about cancer: prevention, warning signs, symptoms, diagnosis, treatment, and patient care.

Typing "plastic surgery" into the search box on the home page produces more than 100 articles that are also useful for plastic surgery patients. These include (but are not limited to) information on reconstructive surgery, including skin grafting, the use of permanent or temporary prostheses, and general advice about feeling well during or after surgery/treatment (i.e., "Beauty Shown More Than Skin Deep: Survivors With Attitude").

American Pain Foundation*

http://www.painfoundation.org

Effective pain management is a relatively new medical specialty. The American Pain Foundation, created in 1997 to promote research and advocate for increased access to effective pain management, has designed its site to raise public awareness of the deleterious effects of pain and the benefits of pain treatment.

The resources available on this site include, but are not limited to, news about developments in pain management, basic questions and answers for people in pain, a comprehensive online pain information library, and a guide to clinical trials for specific pain conditions, including pain before and after surgery.

American Psychiatric Association*

http://www.psych.org

The American Psychiatric Association represents physicians who specialize in the treatment of mental disorders, including mental retardation and substance-related disorders.

While this has no listing for plastic surgery, it provides reliable information about mental health conditions such as depression that may affect a patient's view of his/her body. The site also offers brochures, tips, and articles on psychological issues that affect physical and emotional well-being, and "referral tools," the link that makes it possible to find a psychiatrist either through an online e-mail form or a toll-free 800-number.

American Psychological Association*

http://www.apa.org

The American Psychological Association represents professionals with a doctoral degree in psychology (the study of mind and behavior) from an accredited university or professional school.

While this has no listing for plastic surgery, it provides reliable information about mental health conditions such as depression that may affect a patient's view of his/her body. The site also offers brochures, tips, and articles on psychological issues that affect physical and emotional well-being, and "referral tools," the link that makes it possible to find a psychologist either through an online e-mail form or a toll-free 800-number.

New Zealand Dermatological Society

http://dermnetnz.org

This excellent and accessible site, launched in 1996, provides authoritative information about dermatological conditions, many associated with plastic surgery. The list includes, but is not limited to, aging skin, birthmarks, camouflage makeup, pigmentation problems, skin grafting, and the like.

The articles may be opened from the home page either by typing a subject into the search bar or by clicking on the appropriate letter in the alphabetical listing. Either way, the writing is clear and thorough. Another feature, a list of medical abbreviations, is a useful tool for any nonprofessional working his/her way through medical sources.

General Medical Information

American Academy of Family Physicians*

http://www.familydoctor.org

The AAFP (formerly the American Academy of General Practice) publishes the medical journal *American Family Physician* and maintains this site specifically for patients.

The home page is studded with click-on buttons. Conditions A to Z, in a green-tinted box on the home page, makes it possible to choose information about a disease or medical condition by clicking on a letter of the alphabet. Choose "D," for example, and you get a list that begins with "Dandruff" and ends with "Dysthmic disorder" (depression).

When the list does not have what you are looking for—there is no entry for "plastic surgery" under "P"—typing the subject (plastic surgery) into a search box at top right brings up a list of pertinent articles, each starred to show how closely the article matches the search. The more stars, the closer the match.

The site also facilitates searches through the usual health topics such as healthy living, women, men, over-the-counter guide, smart patient guide (with tips on how to choose a doctor), parents and kids, seniors, and health tools (dictionary, find a doctor, BMI [body mass index] calculator, drug info, search by symptom). In sum, just the sort of thing a patient wants his/her doctor to talk about.

Answers.com
http://www.answers.com

An excellent site for general information on multiple topics, including medicine, delivering multiple entries from a wide range of sources for each search.

For example, typing "plastic surgery" into the Tell Me About search bar on the home page brings up three dictionary definitions (*American Heritage Dictionary of the English Language, Stedman's Medical Dictionary,* and *New Dictionary of Cultural Literacy*), three encyclopedia articles (*Britannica Concise Encyclopedia, Columbia Electronic Encyclopedia,* and *Gale Encyclopedia of Surgery*), and two Web site entries (WordNet, Wikipedia). Every entry is sourced; every source is reliable.

eMedicine
http://www.emedicine.com

This online medical library is one of three sites maintained by WebMD (see below). eMedicine's distinguishing feature is its willingness to accept questions posed in slang terms as well as medical language. For example, entering the words "nose job" into the search box on the home page produces the same 40 articles returned when one enters in the medical term "rhinoplasty." The articles, drawn from a variety of professional journals, are sophisticated but still accessible to the informed reader.

Note: To use this site, the reader must register; registration is free.

Health A-to-Z
http://www.healthatoz.com

A reliable site with clear, nontechnical information. While its entry on plastic surgery is limited to cosmetic procedures, the articles on specific procedures are well organized and useful. For example, the entry for rhinoplasty defines the procedure, explains the rationale for the surgery, lists precautions ("Rhinoplasty should not be performed until the growth spurt is complete")

describes the surgery itself (and aftercare), presents directions on how to prepare for surgery, and lists the possible risks. To accommodate the general public, each entry defines relevant medical terms such as *cartilage*. To please the curious, each concludes with a list of books, periodicals, and organizations for follow-up.

MedicineNet.com
http://www.medicinenet.com

This online health care/medical publishing company, run by board-certified physicians, is one of three sites maintained by WebMD (see below).

The site provides access to an extraordinary range of articles on health subjects from medical journals, medical institutions such as the Cleveland Clinic, government agencies, and MedicineNet's own roster of experts. For example, typing the words "plastic surgery" into the search bar brings up 43 articles on disease and conditions, one on medications, 29 on procedures and tests, 35 on health news, five on doctor's views of the subject, 32 from medical dictionaries, 75 on health facts and other categories, and 42 on related information.

The only problematic feature on the site is Sponsored Links, a list of paid advertisements such as (in the case of plastic surgery) individual surgeons, plastic surgery clinics, and purveyors of over-the-counter products ("eye serum").

WebMD
http://www.webmd.com

WebMD, the company that also owns and operates eMedicine.com and MedicineNet.com, produces and publishes original articles on medical subjects written by experts in the relevant field. As with articles in print medical journals, WebMD's pieces are vetted by independent reviewers. In addition, this site offers access to articles from standard medical journals and other sources, including reliable medical Web sites.

The amount of material offered on WebMD is so vast it may occasionally seem overwhelming. For example, typing "plastic surgery" into the search bar brings up more than 700 articles, videos, and links to other Web sites, including interactive sites on subjects ranging from the mundane ("Is Plastic

Surgery a Teen Thing?") to the esoteric ("Latest Plastic Surgery Trends and Stats").

As with eMedicine, the only problematic category is Sponsored Links, which for plastic surgery means ads for individual surgeons, plastic surgery clinics, and purveyors of over-the-counter products.

Technical/Medical Information

American Association for Clinical Chemistry*
http://www.labtestsonline.org

This site explains lab tests and test results in terms accessible to laypersons.

One way to begin is to click on Understanding Your Tests on the left side of the home page. Opening this section brings up a list of articles on basic subjects related to medical tests: "Reference Ranges and What They Mean," "Evidence-Based Approach to Medicine Improves Patient Care" (the role of laboratory testing in its application), "How Reliable Is Laboratory Testing?," "The Universe of Genetic Testing," "How Clinical Laboratory Tests Get to Market," "Home Testing," "Coping with Test Pain, Discomfort, and Anxiety," "Staying Healthy in an Era of Patient Responsibility," and "Test Preparation: Your Role."

A second way into the site is to scroll to the right side of the home page that offers indexes for tests, conditions, and screening. A click on the box marked Tests brings up a list of common laboratory procedures. Choosing one produces a clear and complete description that includes alternative names for the test, who gets the test, when the test is used, what sample is required, the actual test procedure, common questions about the test, and best of all, a form that allows you to ask a question about the test and get a confidential reply by e-mail.

There are similar indexes of medical conditions and screening procedures for specific demographic groups such as infants or people older than 50.

The Doctor's Doctor
http://www.thedoctorsdoctor.com

This site is run by pathologists, physicians who specialize in medical diagnosis and are sometimes described (in the site's title) as doctor's doctors.

The special feature of this site is its translation of pathology reports into terms any patient can understand. Begin by clicking on the circle marked "Home," then "Translating a Report." When that page appears, scroll down to the last three entries: "A Typical Surgical Pathology Report," "Examples of a Translated Report," and "Order a Translated Report."

The first entry explains how a pathology report is organized. The second entry explains each section of a sample report, using a two-column page with the traditional diagnosis ("Fibroadenoma with Lobular carcinoma in situ") in column A and the translation ("1. Fibroadenoma. This is a benign nodule composed of a mixture of breast lining cells and the fibrous tissue that supports it. 2. Lobular Carcinoma in Situ: This is a proliferation of cells that have a malignant appearance but have not invaded into the surrounding breast fibrous tissue. These cells are present within the fibroadenoma") in column B.

The third entry is a form to fill out and mail or fax along with a copy of a pathology report to the Doctor's Doctor for a translation. The only drawback is the cost, as of this writing, a hefty $200 per translation.

Online Metrics Conversion
http://www.sciencemadesimple.net/length.php

Given the fact that virtually all modern medical measurements, including the length of incisions and the diameter of surgical sutures, are commonly presented in metric terms, a conversion chart is a necessity. This site, designed and run by Science Made Simple, Inc., should be retitled "Simply the Best U.S. Standard and Metric Converter Site Ever." Its Metric Conversion Chart is a handy tool for quick reference; for more information, check out any of 14 categories, each of them exhaustive in nature. For example, click "Length/Height" and you get a chart with 49 different measurements starting at *angstrom* and ending at *yard*, with stops in between for such esoteria as *bolts, chains, lines, palms, skeins,* and *spans.*

Surgical Tutor.Org (UK)
http://www.surgical-tutor.org.uk

This British-based site is packed with educational material aimed at medical students preparing for undergraduate and postgraduate surgical examinations.

However, laymen will also appreciate its gallery of famous (British) surgeons, and medically sophisticated readers may want to browse through the collection of radiological studies and pathology slides (tissue samples) that show what a doctor sees when looking at an examination result.

Wound Care Information Network
http://www.medicaledu.com

This site explains in everyday language the nature of wounds (including surgical wounds) and how they heal.

On the home page, click on the picture labeled "Patients" to bring up the offer of a free copy of *Wound Guide for Patients,* a reader-friendly booklet that describes the wound healing process, what to do when a wound does not heal, and where to locate wound care experts. To get a complimentary copy by e-mail, the reader can fill out and submit the simple form with name, e-mail address, type of wound(s), how long the wound has remained unhealed, and what treatment has been used up to now. If the wound fits into a category of particular interest to wound care experts, the reader may also receive information about suitable clinical trials. Naturally, all personal data—collected only for statistical analysis—remains confidential.

Medical/Surgical Language

Online Etymology Dictionary
http://www.etymonline.com

This site, created by Lancaster, Pennsylvania, historian, author, journalist, and lecturer Douglas Harper, employs a long list of sources, including (but not limited to) *The Oxford English Dictionary, Klein's Comprehensive Etymological Dictionary of the English Language,* and Robert L. Chapman's *Dictionary of American Slang,* to track the evolution of common and uncommon words, including many familiar medical terms.

For example, the entry for the word *cosmetic* reads: *Cosmetic 1605, from Gk. kosmetikos 'skilled in adornment,' from kosmein 'to arrange, adorn,' from kosmos 'order.' Fig. sense of 'superficial' is from 1955; cosmetology is from 1855.*

Who Named It
http://www.whonamedit.com

This site is a biographical dictionary of medical eponyms: diseases, conditions, or procedures named for the person who identified or invented them.

From the home page, it is possible to access the eponyms by letter of the alphabet, medical category (i.e., abscess), geographical location (i.e., Argentina, Australia, etc.), or gender, with male entries are in the main list and a separate category for female entries).

As of October 2006, Who Named It listed 7,722 eponyms linked to 3,069 persons, 105 female and 2,964 male. However, the webmasters frankly admit that the list is far from finished. "Many biographical entries are incomplete," they note. "In some cases, we have only the last name, not even knowing that person's sex or nationality. Probably, there are also some errors, both in the eponymic descriptions, bibliography, and biographies." Readers are clearly welcome to add new listings, fill in the gaps and/or correct errors in existing listings by clicking on a Contact button on the home page and proceeding to edit away.

Physician Ratings

The following sites enable a medical consumer in the United States to document and evaluate the credentials, affiliations, and performance for any physician, including plastic surgeons.

Alabama State Medical Board
http://www.albme.org

Alaska Division of Occupational Licensing
http://www.dced.state.ak.us/occ/

Arizona State Medical Board
http://www.azmdboard.org/

Arizona Board of Osteopathic Examiners
http://www.azdo.gov/

Arkansas State Medical Board
http://www.armedicalboard.org/index.asp

Medical Board of California
http://www.medbd.ca.gov/

Colorado State Medical Board
http://www.dora.state.co.us/medical/

Connecticut State DPH - Physician Profile
http://www.dph.state.ct.us/

Delaware State Medical Board
http://www.dpr.delaware.gov/boards/medical
    practice/index.shtml

District of Columbia Medical Board
http://doh.dc.gov/doh/site/default.asp

Florida State Medical Board
http://www.doh.state.fl.us/

Georgia Composite State Medical Board
http://medicalboard.georgia.gov

Hawaii Board of Medical Governors
http://www.hawaii.gov/dcca/areas/pvl/boards/
    medical/

Idaho State Medical Board
http://www.bom.state.id.us/

**Illinois Department of Professional
    Regulation**
http://www.idfpr.com/

Indiana Health Professions Bureau
http://www.in.gov/hpb/

Iowa Board of Medical Examiners
http://medicalboard.iowa.gov/

Kansas State Board of Healing Art
http://www.ksbha.org/

Kentucky Board of Medical Licensure
http://www.state.ky.us/agencies/kbml

**Louisiana State Board of Medical
    Examiners**
http://www.lsbme.louisiana.gov

Maine Board of Licensure in Medicine
http://www.docboard.org/me/me_home.htm

**State of Maine Board of Osteopathic
    Licensure**
http://www.maine.gov/osteo/

Maryland Board of Physicians
http://www.mbp.state.md.us/

**Massachusetts Board of Registration in
    Medicine**
http://www.massmedboard.org/

Michigan Board of Medicine
http://www.michigan.gov/mdch/0,1607,7-132-
    27417_27529_27541-58914--,00 .html

Minnesota State Medical Board
http://www.state.mn.us/portal/mn/jsp/home.
    do?agency=BMP

Mississippi State Medical Board
http://www.msbml.state.ms.us/

**Missouri State Board of Registration for the
    Healing Arts**
http://www.pr.mo.gov/healingarts.asp

Montana Board of Medical Examiners
http://mt.gov/dli/bsd/license/bsd_boards/med_
    board/board_page.asp

**Nebraska Health and Human Services
    Licensure**
http://www.hhs.state.ne.us/

**State of Nevada Board of Medical
    Examiners**
http://www.medboard.nv.gov/

**Nevada State Board of Osteopathic
    Examiners**
http://www.docboard.org/nx/

New Hampshire State Board of Medicine
http://www.state.nh.us/medicine/

**New Jersey State Board of Medical
    Examiners**
http://www.state.nj.us/lps/ca/bme/index.html

New Mexico Board of Medical Examiners
http://www.state.nm.us/nmbme

New Mexico Osteopathic Examiners Board
http://www.rld.state.nm.us/b&c/osteo/

New York State Office of the Professions
http://www.op.nysed.gov/

North Carolina State Medical Board
http://www.ncmedboard.org/

North Dakota State Medical Board
http://www.ndbomex.com/

Ohio State Medical Board
http://www.med.ohio.gov/

Oklahoma Board of Medical Licensure and Supervision
http://www.okmedicalboard.org/

Oregon State Medical Board
http://www.egov.oregon.gov/BME/

Pennsylvania State Bureau of Professional and Occupational Affairs
http://www.dos.state.pa.us/bpoa/site/default.asp

Rhode Island Board of Medical Licensure & Discipline
http://www.health.ri.gov/hsr/bmld/

South Carolina Board of Medical Examiners
http://www.llr.state.sc.us/pol/medical/

South Dakota Board of Medical and Osteopathic Examiners
http://www.state.sd.us/doh/medical/

Tennessee Board of Medical Examiners
http://health.state.tn.us/

Tennessee Board of Osteopathic Examination
http://health.state.tn.us/

Texas State Medical Board
http://www.tmb.state.tx.us/

State of Utah Division of Occupational and Professional Licensing
http://www.dopl.utah.gov/

Vermont Board of Medical Practice
http://www.healthvermont.gov/hc/med_board/bmp.aspx

Vermont Board of Osteopathic Physicians and Surgeons
http://www.vtprofessionals.org/opr1/osteopaths/

Virginia Department of Health Professions
http://www.dhp.virginia.gov/

Washington State Public Health Improvement Partnership
http://www.doh.wa.gov/PHIP/default.htm

West Virginia State Medical Board
http://www.wvdhhr.org/wvbom/

West Virginia Board of Osteopathy
http://www.wvbdosteo.org

Wisconsin Department of Regulation and Licensing
http://drl.wi.gov/index.htm

Wyoming Board of Medicine
http://wyomedboard.state.wy.us/

Health Care Facility Ratings

Accreditation Association for Ambulatory Health Care, Inc.
http://www.aaahc.org

This site offers consumers a guide with which to evaluate any facility that performs outpatient surgery.

The AAAHC accredits ambulatory health care organizations, including (but not limited to) ambulatory and physician office-based surgery centers, managed care organizations, Native American and student health centers to make sure they meet all standards governing patients' rights, quality care, clinical record keeping, dissemination of health information, administration and governance, and facility maintenance.

American Association for Accreditation of Ambulatory Surgery Facilities
http://www.aaaasf.org/consumers.php

This site offers consumers a guide with which to evaluate any facility that performs outpatient surgery.

The AAAASF accredits ambulatory surgery facilities to ensure that they meet local, state, and federal regulations, including fire safety, sanitation, and building codes; follow all pertinent federal laws and regulations such as standards governing hazardous waste and the Americans with Disabilities Act; employ advanced techniques for patient safety during surgery and in the recovery period; permit only qualified surgeons, certified by the American Board of Medical Specialties and with access to an accredited hospital to perform surgery and only board-certified or board-eligible physicians or certified registered nurse anesthetists to administer anesthesic; and certified or registered personnel to maintain the recovery room.

Health Grades
http://www.healthgrades.com/

Health Grades, a health care ratings, information, and advisory services company, ranks more than 5,000 private, state, and city hospitals as one-star (poor), three-star (average), or five-star (excellent), based on their performance in 28 medical procedure and diagnoses in specialties such as cardiac surgery, cardiology, orthopedic surgery, neurosciences, pulmonary/respiratory, vascular surgery, obstetrics, and women's health. The rankings, updated each year, are available free of charge at this site.

Five-star rated hospitals had significantly lower risk-adjusted mortality rates across all three years studied and improved 21 percent more than the U.S. hospital average and 45 percent more than one-star rated hospitals. A typical patient would have, on average, a 65 percent lower chance of dying in a five-star rated hospital compared to a one-star rated hospital, and a 45 percent lower chance of dying in a five-star rated hospital compared to the U.S. hospital average.

Joint Commission on the Accreditation of Healthcare Organizations
http://www.jcaho.org

JCAHO, an independent not-for-profit organization created in 1951, evaluates and accredits health care organizations including hospitals, hospice service, nursing homes, rehabilitation facilities, laboratories, home health care, and medical equipment services. To access the evaluations, select the home page, scroll down to the box on the bottom right labeled "Information for," and click "General Public." When the next page appears, click "Quality Check—Search for Joint Commission accredited organizations," then follow the directions to obtain a complete quality report, including an evaluation of the facility and its individual services, plus its comparative standing in relation to other facilities in the area and across the country. To go directly to this page: http://www. qualitycheck.org/consumer/searchQCR.aspx.

Medicare
http://www.medicare.gov/

In order to participate in Medicare and Medicaid-funded programs, hospitals and other health care facilities must meet government standards of care. To access information about a specific hospital from the home page, scroll down to "Search Tools," click on "Compare Hospitals in Your Area," then follow the prompts as the pages change. Note: When searching for a facility by name, you must have the exact name. For example, Mount Sinai Hospital, a major facility in New York City, is not accessible as "Mt. Sinai."

GLOSSARY

abdomen Section of the body between the chest and the pelvis, often mistakenly called the stomach. The abdomen is divided into nine regions that can be located on a grid of three squares wide by three squares high. The regions of the grid, from right to left, top row: right hypochondriac region, epigastric region, left hypochondriac region. Middle row: right lateral region, umbilical region (over the navel/belly button), left lateral region. Bottom row: right inguinal region, pubic region, left inguinal region.

ablate From the Latin *ab* and *latus,* meaning "to take away." In medicine, to remove a body part or destroy its function, a process called ablation. For example, the use of radiation therapy to ablate the prostate gland in order to prevent the spread of prostate cancer.

abscess An infection in an enclosed space, for example, under the gum at the base of an infected tooth.

acellular Without living cells.

acid In chemistry, a compound that releases a molecular fragment called hydrogen ion (symbol: H+) when dissolved in water; the chemical opposite of a base, a compound that releases an hydroxyl ion (symbol: OH-). Acid substances have a sharp or sour flavor, such as vinegar or lemon juice. Acids are often used as preservatives or, in plastic surgery, as exfoliants, ingredients that smooth the skin by removing the top layer of dead skin cells.

actinic From the Greek *aktis,* meaning "ray." It refers to radiation from the sun.

adhesive Material that enables one surface to stick to another; a glue or paste.

adrenal glands From the Latin *ad,* meaning "near" and *ren,* meaning "kidney." Two glands, one next to or on each kidney; they secrete a variety of hormones including adrenaline (epinephrine), the "fight or flight" hormone, and anti-inflammatory corticosteroids.

adverse effect Uncommon, unexpected, and unusual reaction to a specific medicine, as opposed to a side effect, which is a common, expected, and ordinarily mild reaction. For example, mild drowsiness is a side effect of aspirin; erosion of the stomach lining is an adverse effect.

aerobic From the Latin *aer-,* meaning "air," and the Greek *bios,* meaning "life." Oxygen-dependent, as in aerobic bacteria, bacteria that require oxygen to live.

aesthetic Relating to aesthetics, the branch of philosophy that deals with the nature of art and the standards of artistic judgment. Aesthetic (or esthetic) surgery is a term used to describe medical procedures whose primary aim is to enhance appearance rather than to improve or restore body function.

aesthetician Also esthetician. A person who performs nonmedical services related to appearance; for example, a makeup artist, a hairdresser, or a weight-loss trainer.

afferent From the Latin *afferens,* meaning "bringing to."

agenesis From the Greek *a-,* meaning "without," and *genesis,* meaning "formation." Failure of a fetal body part to develop; as in renal agenesis, a missing kidney in a newborn.

alar From the Latin *ala,* meaning "wing." Winged or wing shape, such as the triangle formed by the nostrils at the base of the nose.

alcohol A synonym for ethyl alcohol, the alcohol used in food and alcoholic beverages. Other common forms of alcohol include *denatured alcohol* (ethyl alcohol plus a chemical that makes the alcohol smell and taste bad); *isopropyl alcohol* (a solution of 90 percent denatured alcohol) is used as an antiseptic; and *rubbing alcohol* (a solution of 70 percent isopropyl alcohol) is used as a skin coolant during a massage.

allo- From the Greek *allos,* meaning "other."

allograft A graft of skin from another individual of the same species; i.e., skin from one human being for another human being or skin from one dog for another dog.

allopathic medicine The predominant form of medicine practiced in the Western world; a discipline that treats illness by inducing a condition opposite to the disease. For example, an allopathic doctor will try to cure a fever by lowering body temperature or to cure an infection by eliminating the infectious agent(s), usually with antibiotics or antiviral drugs.

alopecia From the Greek *alopekia*, meaning "a disease similar to fox [*alopex*] mange." Hair loss.

alpha hydroxy acids (AHA) A group of naturally occurring acidic compounds in food such as citric acid (found in fruits), glycolic acid (found in sugarcane and fruits), lactic acid (found in milk), and malic acid (found in apples).

alternative medicine Techniques used to treat the "whole person" (mind and body); often regarded as an alternative to allopathic medicine, the system of Western medical drugs and treatments. Some alternative medicine therapies are acupuncture, acupressure, biofeedback, chiropractic, herbal medicine, meditation, and yoga. The National Center for Complementary and Alternative Medicine (NCCAM) is the agency of the U.S. government responsible for proving (or disproving) the value of alternative therapies.

aluminum Naturally occurring silver-white metallic element that accounts for about 8 percent of the earth's surface; it is used as a source of energy in a YAG (yttrium-aluminum-garnet) laser and found in health and beauty products such as antacids, astringents, buffered aspirin, and antiperspirants.

ambulatory health care facility Non-hospital setting in which surgery may be performed; also known as a free-standing facility; these facilities should be accredited by the American Association for Accreditation of Ambulatory Surgery Facilities, Accreditation Association for Ambulatory Health Care, Medicare, and by the states in which they are located.

ambulatory surgery Surgery performed on an outpatient basis; the patient comes in, has the surgery, and is released on the same day.

amputation Removal of a body part, most commonly a limb, either by accident as when a finger is caught in machinery or by medical design such as when surgeons opt to remove a leg containing an inoperable bone tumor.

anaerobic From the Latin *an*, meaning "away from," *aer-*, meaning "air," and the Greek *bios*, meaning "life." Non-oxygen dependant, as in anaerobic bacteria, bacteria that can survive in the absence of air.

analgesia From the Greek *an-*, meaning "not," and *algesis*, meaning "pain." Interruption of one or more of the chemical reactions by which the body transmits pain messages from the site of an injury via nerve fibers to the brain; analgesia does not affect consciousness. An *analgesic* is any substance or treatment that relieves pain without causing loss of consciousness.

anastomosis From the Greek *anastomosis*, meaning "opening." A natural or surgically created connection between two tubular structures such as blood vessels.

anomaly A variation from what is generally considered normal; in medicine, an abnormal structure such as extra fingers or toes or a cleft lip or cleft palate.

antero-, anterior Prefix designating "front"; from the Latin *anteus*, meaning "front." In medicine, this prefix is used in compound terms such as the *anterosuperior* (front, upper) quadrant (quarter) of the abdomen.

antibiotic From the Greek *an*, meaning "not," and *bios*, meaning "life." Medical drug that destroys or inhibits the growth of disease-causing organisms. A broad-spectrum antibiotic is one that is effective against the two main classifications of bacteria, thin-skinned Gram-negative bacteria and thick-skinned Gram-positive bacteria organisms. Antibiotic prophylaxis is the practice of giving antibiotics before surgery, including plastic surgery, to reduce the risk of infection afterwards.

anticoagulant Compound such as warfarin (Coumadin™) or vitamin K that reduces the ability of blood platelets to stick together to form a blood clot, thus reducing the risk of a blocked artery.

apex Tip, as in the apex of the nose.

artery From the Latin and Greek *arteria*, meaning "pipe." A blood vessel that carries oxygenated blood from the heart to the tissues and organs of the body, as opposed to a vein, which carries blood from tissue and organs back to the heart. A small artery is called an *arteriole*.

artificial   Not natural; in medicine, a material or device that does not arise from natural cell growth; for example, an artificial hip joint or an artificial limb. Some artificial materials and/or devices such as a metal or plastic replacement joint remain separate and intact inside the body. Others, such as the porous materials used as bone replacements, serve as a base for new cell growth and are ultimately absorbed into the body. Artificial materials and devices are widely used in plastic surgery.

asymmetry   In medicine, a significant difference in size or shape between two parts that are normally assumed to be the same, such as the eyes, ears, or breasts.

atrophy   From the Greek *a*, meaning "without," and *trophe*, meaning "nourishment." Tissue shrinkage or wasting.

augmentation   From the Latin *augmentare*, meaning "to make bigger." In plastic surgery, an enlargement procedure; i.e., "breast augmentation."

auto-   From the Greek *autos*, meaning "self."

autogenous   From the Greek *autos*, meaning "self," and *gen*, meaning "born." In medicine, tissue such as blood or bone cells taken directly from the body of the person for whom it will be used.

autologous   From the Greek *autos*, meaning "self," and *logos*, meaning "place." Term used to describe tissue taken from the patient's own body.

avulsion   From the Latin *avulsio*, meaning "rip, tear." The accidental tearing away of a body part.

axon   From the Greek *axon*, meaning "axis." The part of the nerve cell that sends impulses out from the cell.

bacitracin   An antibiotic used to treat skin infections including mild infection after plastic surgery, commonly used in skin cream that contains two other antibiotics, neomycin and polymyxin B. It is named for its origins *ba*cilli isolated from the blood of an American patient, Margaret *Tracy*, in 1943.

bacteria   From the Greek *bakterion*, meaning "small rod." Member(s) of a family of one-cell microorganisms; some beneficial, others pathogenic (disease causing).

bandage   Material applied to a wound to stop bleeding, to keep out dirt and debris, to prevent drying or to absorb liquid drainage, to hold a dressing in place, or to immobilize a body part, such as a broken arm.

baseline   In medicine, a standard against which to measure future developments, such as a baseline CT-scan or a baseline blood test.

beam   In medicine, a straight line of light or radiation, such as the light from a flashlight or the radiation from an X-ray machine.

bed sore   Decubitus ulcer, pressure ulcer, an injury caused by continuing pressure on skin stretched over a prominent bone, such as the hip bone; occurs in patients who spend long periods of lying in bed without being able to change position frequently.

benign   From the Latin *benignus*, meaning "kind." Mild, as in a benign illness; nonmalignant, as in a benign (noncancerous) tumor.

bi-   From the Latin *bi-*, meaning "two."

bicoronal   From the Latin *bi-*, meaning "two," and *cornu*, meaning "horn." In medicine, an organ or body part with two peaks or projections, such as the mammalian uterus.

bikini incision   Low transverse abdominal incision, surgical incision along the bikini line, the top edge of the pubic hairline; used in gynecological surgery to avoid a visible scar.

bilateral   From the Latin *bi-*, meaning "two," and *latus*, meaning "side." Two-sided, as in bilateral cleft lip, a lip with a cleft on each side.

binder   Bandage used to compress an area so as to reduce post-surgical swelling; for example, after surgery to remove a breast.

biocompatible   Able to interact with a biological system without triggering an adverse reaction; for example, the materials used to create artificial heart-valves and joints, synthetic blood vessels, medical adhesives, sutures, and fill dental defects.

biodegradable   Able to be broken down quickly and safely by biological means, such as bacterial action, and then to be absorbed safely into the environment (i.e., the soil).

biologic adhesive   Material taken from a living organism; for example, the blood protein fibrinogen or chitin, a substance found in the hard outer skeletons of creatures such as beetles and crabs; used in place of sutures to close a wound such as that left by a plastic surgery incision.

biopsy From the Greek *bio-*, meaning "life," and *opsis*, meaning "view." A diagnostic examination of tissue sample.

biosynthesis From the Greek *bio*, meaning "life," *syn*, meaning "together," and *thesis*, meaning "place or arrange." Process by which living cells manufacture complex chemicals from simple constituents via enzyme action; for example, synthesizing proteins from amino acids, the building blocks of proteins.

birth defect Abnormality present at birth.

block Term used to describe anesthesic that numbs a specific area of the body; also known as regional anesthesic.

blood Liquid that transports essential nutrients such as oxygen, vitamins, minerals, hormones, and other biochemicals to every living body cell, while carrying away waste materials such as carbon dioxide.

blood gases Dissolved oxygen (O_2) and carbon dioxide (CO_2) in the blood and dissolved bicarbonate (HCO_3-) in the blood plasma.

blood stream The blood flowing through the blood vessels.

blood vessel Component of the circulatory system; the tube(s) through which blood flows to and from all body organs and tissues.

board-certified Term used to describe a physician who has completed the requirements for becoming a member (diplomate) of one of the 24 specialty boards recognized by the American Board of Medical Specialties.

buttonhole approach Short straight incision; or, occasionally, a synonym for laparoscopic surgery.

calipers Scissorslike instrument with a ruler between the prongs, used to measure the diameter (width) of a round structure such as the inside of a blood vessel.

callus From the Latin *callosus*, meaning "thick skin." On skin tissue, a callosity, thickening of the outer layer of the skin due to repeated rubbing or pressure, as occurs on the bottom or heel of the foot. On bone tissue, a mass of different kinds of tissue, including collagen, that forms at the site of a break in a bone, forming a bridge between the separated ends of the bone, and is ultimately replaced with new bone cells.

calorie From the Latin *calor*, meaning "heat." A unit of energy and/or heat, the amount of energy required to raise one gram of water one degree on the Celsius scale (1.8 degrees on the Fahrenheit scale).

cannula Slim hollow tube to be inserted into a blood vessel or under the skin to remove fluids or deliver medical substances.

carcinoma From the Greek *karkinos*, meaning "cancer," and o*ma*, meaning "tumor." The most common type of cancer; malignant tumor arising from epithelial cells. Examples include some skin cancers, tumors of the lining of the bronchi (tubes leading into the lungs), or tumors of the lining of glands such as the prostate and the breast.

carpus Wrist. From the Latin *carpal*, meaning "of the wrist," as in carpal tunnel syndrome.

catalyst From the Greek *katalysis*, meaning "to dissolve." A substance that facilitates a chemical reaction but is not itself affected by the reaction; for example, platinum, a metal used as a catalyst in the conversion of silicone oil to silicone gel for breast implants. The chemical effect created by a catalyst is called catalysis.

catheter From the Greek *kathiemi*, meaning "to send down." Hollow tube that allows liquid to flow into or out of body cavities or blood vessels; for example, a urinary catheter allows urine to drain directly from a bed-bound patient's bladder into a receptacle; an intravenous catheter is used to administer medication and nutrients directly into a vein.

cauterize From the Greek *kauterion*, meaning "branding iron." To cut or burn body tissues with electric current (electrocautery), or with ultrasound waves, or with a caustic substance such as an acid, or with a cold substance such as liquid nitrogen (cryosurgery), or with heat as in a hot iron poker.

cavity From the Latin *cavus*, meaning "hollow." Any natural or acquired open space in the body such as the nasal cavity (the open space on either side of the nasal septum) or a dental cavity (a hole in the tooth).

cell From the Latin *cella*, "chamber." The smallest unit of a living structure capable of independent life; a nucleus (center) surrounded by protoplasm (cellular fluid) enclosed within a cell membrane.

cement/cementum Heavily mineralized bonelike tissue that anchors ligaments around the root of a tooth.

cephalometrics   From the Greek *kephale*, meaning "head," and *metron*, meaning "measure." System of measurements used to assess the bones of the head and face during imaging studies for oral surgery or orthodontics or to assess facial growth and development in the fetus.

cervico-   From the Latin *cervix*, meaning "neck."

cheilo-   From the Greek *cheilos*, meaning "lip."

chin   The lower jaw (bone) plus the covering layers of fat, muscle, and skin.

chiropractic   A form of drug-free, noninvasive healing that pays special attention to the physiological and biochemical aspects of the body structure (spine, muscles, nerves, blood vessels), sometimes employing specific procedures such as the adjustment and manipulation of the vertebrae (the small, round bones that make up the spine) to cure or alleviate discomfort and illness.

chisel   From the Latin *caedare*, meaning "to cut." Surgical instrument used to chip away excess bone.

chondritis   From the Greek *chondros*, meaning "cartilage," and *-itis*, meaning "inflammation." An inflammation of connective tissue (cartilage).

chromosome   From the Greek *chroma*, meaning "color," and *soma*, meaning "body." Threadlike structures in the cells of all living organisms; composed of DNA (deoxyribonucleic acid), the material that contains an individual's genetic code (inherited characteristics). Human beings normally have 46 chromosomes (23 pairs, one from each parent); each chromosome carries an estimated 20,000 to 30,000 different genes, the basic units of heredity. Many of the congenital defects repaired with plastic surgery are due to damage to one or more chromosomes.

clamp   A device used to hold a tubelike structure closed; for example, to compress a blood vessel so as to reduce bleeding during surgery.

cleft   An opening in a body structure, either normal (such as the cleft between the buttock) or abnormal (as in a cleft lip or palate).

clip   A surgical device used to hold tissue together or close an incision or clamp a blood vessel.

clot   Soft mass of gelled material, as in a blood clot.

collar button abscess   Two-layer infection; one abscess linked to another by a tubelike structure in a manner similar to a collar button or a shirt stud. Also known as shirt stud abscess.

colloid   Thick, gluelike solid, or a liquid or a gas containing suspended microscopic particles.

complexion   From the Latin *complexio*, meaning "combination." Color, texture, and appearance of the facial skin; a predictive guide to the potential success of various cosmetic surgeries such as chemical skin peel.

complication   In medicine, a problem occurs during illness or after a treatment or surgical procedure; for example, the shifting of an implant used to enlarge the breast.

compress   From the Latin *com-*, meaning "together," and *pressus*, meaning "press." This is a dressing used to exert pressure on one spot on the body so as to prevent swelling or stop bleeding from a damaged blood vessel.

congenital   From the Latin *congenitus*, meaning "born with." Existing from birth, as in a congenital defect.

consent form   A written document signed by a patient or his surrogate (e.g., a parent or a guardian), granting doctors permission to treat the patient. Permission may be withdrawn at any time before the procedure or treatment. It is the patient's right to choose whether to consent to or refuse any proposed treatment, including plastic and reconstructive surgery.

contrast material   Substance given orally or by enema or by intravenous injection to highlight areas of the body during an imaging procedure such as a CT-scan, MRI, or X-ray.

corona   From the Greek *korone*, meaning "crown." In anatomy, the top of a structure; i.e., *coronal capitis* (the top of the head), *coronal dentis* (top of a tooth).

corticosteroid   Anti-inflammatory hormone produced naturally on the cortex (outer surface) of the adrenal glands. Cortisone is an anti-inflammatory medicine that mimics the action of natural anti-inflammatory hormones.

cosmeceutical   Cosmetic product that contains an active pharmaceutical ingredient; for example, a cosmetic foundation/base containing a sunscreen.

cosmesis   From the Greek *kosmeo*, meaning "adorning." Any medical procedure that improves appearance.

cosmetic dentistry Dental procedures that improve the appearance and/or restore the structure of the teeth.

cosmetics "Makeup." Products that improve appearance.

counterirritant Chemical or physical agent such as alcohol or heat that mildly irritates the skin, dilating blood vessels just under the skin, increasing the flow of blood, warming the area, and relieving pain caused by inflammation such as a sore muscle or joint.

cranio- From the Greek *kranion*, meaning "skull."

craniofacial This term relates to the skull (cranium) and face, as in *craniofacial cleft* (defect of the face and skull arising from the incomplete fusion of the fetal skull bones during pregnancy), *craniofacial microsomia* (an abnormally small head and face), *craniofacial surgery* (any procedure involving simultaneous operations on the face and head), or *craniofacial syndrome* (a congenital condition such as Apert syndrome which characteristics include defects of the skull and face). In many cases, plastic surgery can repair the defect.

cranioplasty From the Greek *kranion*, meaning "skull," and *plastos*, meaning "formed." Surgery to repair skull damage due to a birth defect or an injury.

cupid's bow The center of the vermillion border, the white line between the reddish mucous membrane of the lip and the facial skin between the upper lip and the nose. The cupid's bow peak is the two highest points on the cupid's bow, on either side of the philtrum, the vertical indentation between the nostrils and the top of the upper lip.

cryo- From the Greek *kryos*, meaning "cold."

curretage Surgery performed with an instrument called a curette, a sharp-edged wire loop or ring attached to a handle, used to scrape a body surface in order to obtain cells for a biopsy or to remove a growth, such as a basal cell skin cancer that has not invaded cartilage or bone.

cutaneous From the Latin *cutis*, meaning "skin." For example, a *cutaneous lesion* is a lesion on the skin.

cyst From the Greek *kystis*, meaning "bladder." A saclike membrane filled with liquid, gas, or solid material; may be found on or in any tissue or organ in the body and named for the material it contains. For example, a cholesterol cyst is a cyst containing fatty tissue including cholesterol; a keratinous cyst is a cyst containing keratin, the most plentiful protein in hair, nails, and skin.

debride From the French *debrisier*, meaning "break apart." To cut away dead tissue, dirt, and debris from a burn or other wound in order to reduce the risk of infection, most commonly before skin transplant to protect a deep burn.

decubitus From the Latin *decumbo*, meaning "lie down." The position of a person lying in bed.

depilation From the Latin *de*, meaning "from," and *pilo*, meaning "hair." Any form of hair removal, whether permanent or temporary. A *depilatory* is any mechanical or chemical agent that breaks, cuts, or dissolves hair or that destroys the hair follicle, thus preventing new hair growth.

derma- From the Greek *derma*, meaning "skin."

dermatology From the Greek *derma*, meaning "skin," and *logos*, meaning "study." The medical study and treatment of diseases of the skin; a dermatologist is a physician specializing in dermatology.

dermoplasty From the Greek *derma*, meaning "skin," and *plassos*, meaning "formed." Use of a skin graft in plastic surgery to correct a congenital defect or to replace skin that has been destroyed by an injury such as a burn, by a disease, or by the treatment for a disease, such as the removal of a tumor.

deviated (nasal) septum An irregularity in the normally straight thin wall of the septum, the bone and mucous membrane that divides the nasal cavity in two.

dexon mesh Synthetic material used during surgery to wrap or support internal organs.

di- Bi-, from the Greek *dis*, meaning "two."

diaphragm From the Greek *diaphragmata*, meaning "partition." The muscular wall that separates the thoracic (chest) cavity from the abdominal cavity.

dilator A surgical instrument used to stretch an open tube such as a blood vessel or the esophagus.

dimple A natural small round indentation in the chin or the cheek or at the base of the spine or a depression resulting from an injury or contraction of scar tissue.

discoloration   Also called hyperpigmentation, this occurs in plastic surgery as a complication following a chemical skin peel, in which dark skin heals lighter than the original color and light skin heals darker. Discoloration may also result if the patient does not apply protective sunblock before going out in the sun.

distal   From the Latin *distalis*, meaning "away." In anatomy, something away from the center of the body or the center of an organ. For example, the farthest part of a limb, such as the hand or foot, or the farthest part of an organ, such as the end of the digestive tract.

dog ear   Excess tissue at the end of a closed wound.

dominant   From the Latin *dominor*, meaning "ruling."

done   As in, "She had her face done"; colloquialism for a tight, unnatural facial appearance resulting from multiple cosmetic surgeries.

donor   A person who gives blood, body tissue, or an organ for a transfusion, transplant, or a skin graft during plastic surgery. The *donor site* is the place on the body from which skin is taken for a skin graft or lifted for a skin flap.

dorsi-, dorso-   From the Latin *dorsalis*, meaning "back."

drain   From the Anglo-Saxon *drehnian*, meaning "draw off." Tube inserted through the skin into a body cavity, commonly after surgery, to allow liquids such as blood or excess spinal fluid to flow out rather than collect under the skin.

dressing   A covering used to protect a wound.

duct   From the Latin *duco*, meaning "lead." A small natural tube leading from a gland or an organ, which allows liquid to flow out from the gland or organ; for example, the tear duct through which liquid flows from a lacrimal (tear) gland in the eyelid.

dys-   From the Greek *dys*, meaning "not, bad"; the opposite of *eu*, meaning "good."

dysostosis   From the Greek *dys*, meaning "bad," *ost*, meaning "bone," and -"*osis*," meaning "condition"; a contraction of dysosteogenesis, from the Greek *dys*, meaning "bad," *ost*, meaning "bone," and *genos*, meaning "birth." Congenital malformation of bone at specific sites in the body.

dysplasia   From the Greek *dys*, meaning "bad," and *plassos*, meaning "mold or form." Abnormal prolifera-tion of cells that disrupts the normal structure of cells and tissues.

dystopia   From the Greek *dys*, meaning "bad," and *topos*, meaning "place"; abnormal position of a body part or organ; for example, bony orbits (the circle of bone surrounding the eyeball) of different sizes and shapes.

ecto-   From the Greek *ektos*, meaning "outside." The opposite of *endo-*, meaning "inside."

-ectomy   From the Greek *ektomia*, meaning "cut out."

edema   From the Greek *oidema*, meaning "swelling." Swelling due to an accumulation of excess fluid. Peripheral edema is excess fluid under the skin of the legs. Pulmonary edema is excess fluid in the air spaces in the lungs. Abdominal or peritoneal edema is fluid collected in the abdomen. Excess fluid throughout the body is called anasarca, from the Greek *ana*, meaning "throughout," and *sark*, meaning "flesh."

efferent   From the Latin *efferens*, meaning "taking out," as in an efferent nerve, a nerve that carries impulses out from the central nervous system (brain and spinal cord) to the body.

elastic cartilage   From the Greek *elastreo*, meaning "to push." Also called yellow cartilage. Tissue containing elastic fibers. Commonly found in expandable structures such as the walls of blood vessels.

elastic fibers   Slender threads in body tissue, woven into a network that forms stretchable membranes of elastin, the primary protein in the connective tissue in expandable body structures such as the walls of blood vessels.

Elastikon™   Brand name for a flexible elastic adhesive tape with tiny openings (pores) that allow air to circulate under the bandage, thus reducing irritation from the adhesive.

elastin   Stretchable protein found in expandable body tissues such as muscles and the walls of blood vessels.

elbow   From the Anglo-Saxon *elnboga*. In anatomy, the joint roughly midway between the shoulder and wrist; in surgery, a J-shape tube or instrument that looks like a bent elbow.

elective surgery   A procedure that is chosen (elected). The Centers for Medicare and Medicaid Services/U.S. Department of Health and Human Services defines elective surgery as surgery that can be scheduled in advance, is not an emergency, and, if delayed, would not result in death or permanent impairment of health.

electrocautery Medical instrument that employs electrical current to burn or cut body tissues. Used in plastic surgery to make an incision or to seal torn blood vessels so as to reduce or stop bleeding.

embolism From the Greek *embolisma*, meaning "something pushed in." An obstruction (blood clot, air bubble, cholesterol plaque) in a blood vessel. In plastic surgery, most commonly a small fat globule released into the vessel during liposuction.

endo- From the Greek *endon*, meaning "within," as in endoabdominal (within the abdomen). The opposite of *exo-, ecto-*, meaning "outside."

energy The potential to do work; in medicine, the potential to affect body tissues such as the energy emitted by an X-ray machine.

epi- From the Greek *epi*, meaning "on or following."

epidermis From the Greek *epi*, meaning "on," and *dermis*, meaning "skin." Collectively, the epithelium, the top layers of skin cells.

Epi-touch™ Brand name laser used to remove hair.

ER Chemical symbol for the element erbium.

erythema From the Greek *erythema*, meaning "flush." Redness due to the temporary pooling of blood in dilated capillaries (tiny blood vessels just under the surface of the skin); for example, a blush or the redness associated with an allergic reaction. In surgery, erythema is a natural consequence of a surgical incision.

eschar From the Greek *eschara*, meaning "scab." Hard covering over a wound or a deep burn.

Ethicon™ Brand name absorbable and nonabsorbable sutures (stitches).

eutectic From the Greek *eu*, meaning "good" (the opposite of *dys-*, meaning "bad"), and *texis*, meaning "melting away." Easily melted.

Eutectic Mixture of Local Anesthetics (EMLA™) Skin cream containing two local anesthetics, lidocaine and prilocaine.

excise From the Latin *excidere*, meaning "cut out." To cut out; for example, to excise a tumor.

excision Removal of a body organ such as the spleen, or a body part such as a bone.

excursion Movement of a body part in one direction and then back to the original position, such as the movement of the bottom jaw from side to side or up and down when chewing.

exfoliant From the Latin *ex*, meaning "off or out," and *folium*, meaning "leaf"; literally, to leaf or flake off. A product or technique that removes the top layer of rough dead skin cells.

exo- From the Greek *exo*, meaning "outside"; the opposite of *endo-*, meaning "inside."

face From the Latin *facere*, meaning "to make," and *facies*, meaning "face." Front part of the head, including the forehead, eyes, nose, cheeks, mouth, and chin, but not the ears.

facial augmentation Surgical transplant of fatty tissue or insertion of synthetic fillers or implants to round or enlarge features such as the cheeks, lip, and chin.

facial features From the Latin *factura*, meaning "making, producing." The distinctive parts of the face (eyes, nose, mouth, ears) that differentiate one individual from another.

facial implant Any prosthesis or filler material surgically inserted to alter the face or any facial feature.

facial reconstruction Any plastic surgery to rebuild or repair a face or facial feature, damaged or missing due to a birth defect, illness, or injury, or, in forensic science, a technique used to reconstruct facial features on a skull in order to identify the skeletal remains of an unknown person.

facial rejuvenation Any plastic surgery technique designed to reverse the signs of facial aging.

factor From the Latin *fascere*, meaning "to make." Any one of several components required for performing a specific activity or producing a specific result; for example, exposure to sunlight is considered a factor in the development of skin cancer.

fascia From the Latin *fascia*, meaning "band, bandage." Layer of fibrous tissue underneath the skin that separates the various layers of tissue in the body; also, a sheet or band of connective tissue enveloping, separating, or binding together muscles, organs, and other soft body structures.

felon　Abscess in the fat pad on the fingertip.

femur　From the Latin *femur*, meaning "thigh." The long bone of the thigh.

fibula　From the Latin *fibula*, meaning "buckle." Calf bone; the smaller, nonweight bearing one of the two bones in the lower leg.

fibroblast　Cell in connective tissue that produces collagen fibers.

fibrous tissue　Body tissue composed of fibroblasts.

filament　From the Latin *filamentum*, meaning "thread." Threadlike structure, such as a muscle fiber or the tail of a spermatozoa (sperm).

fissure　From the Latin *fissure*, meaning "a deep furrow or cleft."

fistula　From the Latin *fistula*, meaning "tube." Abnormal, channel-like opening from one body surface to another; for example, a *salivary fistula*, an opening from the salivary gland to the skin surface.

foam　Solid or semisolid substance containing masses of air bubbles; for example, foam rubber or aerated shaving cream.

follicle　Cup-shape structure in the skin from which a hair grows. From the Latin *folliculus*, meaning "small sac." A closed indentation in the skin, such as the one from which a hair grows.

forceps　From the Latin *forceps*, meaning "tongs." Any instrument used to grasp and remove an object; for example, a bone forceps (for removing pieces of bone) or a capsule forceps (for removing the lens of the eye during cataract surgery).

fore　Front, as in the forehead, the front part of the head, or foreskin, the fold of skin covering the tip (glans) of the penis removed during circumcision.

formaldehyde　Antiseptic and preservative, an ingredient in surgical adhesives; Potent allergic sensitizer (a substance that increases sensitivity to other substances).

fracture　From the Latin *fractura*, meaning "break." A break, as in a bone. In a *compound fracture* the broken bone protrudes through the skin; in a *simple (closed) fracture*, it does not.

freestanding　In medicine, a facility such as a clinic or a nursing home that is independent; not part of a hospital, such as a freestanding surgical facility where plastic surgery is performed.

free tissue transfer　Transfer of a piece of skin lifted entirely off the body.

frown lines　Age-related vertical creases between the eyes and horizontal creases in the forehead.

fungus　From the Latin *fungus*, meaning "mushroom." Microscopic organism such as yeast and mold capable of breaking down complex substances; a few are linked to human fungal infection such as athlete's foot.

fusion　From the Latin *fusio*, meaning "melting, pouring." In medicine, a joining of body structure. A birth defect such as the fusion of two or more bones or membranes that prevents independent movement; for example, polysyndactyly, the fusion or two or more fingers. Plastic surgery is used to repair the defect or mermaid syndrome (fusion of both legs along their entire length).

gangrene　From the Greek *gangraina*, meaning "a devouring sore." Tissue death due to a failure of the blood supply. Gas gangrene is a condition that may occur in wounds infected by bacteria that thrive in a low-oxygen environment, releasing gas and toxins.

gauze　Loosely woven material, commonly cotton, used to cover wounds, including surgical wounds.

gel　A semisolid material such as a jelly.

gender reassignment surgery　Sex reassignment surgery (SRS); plastic surgery to reshape the external anatomy of the body from female to male or male to female as part of the treatment for gender identify disorder, a condition in which a person born with the genitals of one gender feels himself or herself to be a member of the other sex.

gene　A unit on a chromosome that contains DNA, determining a specific hereditary characteristic such as colorblindness or hemophilia.

genitoplasty　Plastic surgery to repair or reconstruct the genitals.

ghost pain　Phantom pain; pain falsely perceived to be originating from an amputated limb.

glucocorticoids　Hormones released by the adrenal glands.

groove Any natural hollow, crevice, depression, or furrow on any internal or external surface of the body.

gyneplasty Gynoplasty, gynoplastica; plastic surgery to repair, reconstruct, or reconfigure the female genitals.

harelip Outmoded term for a cleft lip and/or palate.

harvest Medical term for the process of removing, cleansing, and preserving tissues or cells from a donor for use in transplantation, as in harvesting healthy skin to replace skin destroyed by a severe burn.

hemi- From the Greek *hemisus*, meaning "half."

hemiatrophy From the Greek *hemisus*, meaning "half," and *atrophia*, meaning "wasting away." Shrinking of one half of an organ or body part.

hemoglobin Red protein, pigment in red blood cells that carries oxygen to every tissue in the body.

hemorrhage Bleeding; severe hemorrhage with heavy loss of blood causes shock (dizziness, pallor, weakened pulse, rapid breathing), a potentially fatal condition.

hereditary Describing the transmission of characteristics from one generation to the next through the material in genes and chromosomes.

histology From the Greek *histos*, meaning "web," and *logos*, meaning "knowledge." The study of body tissues; for example, a biopsy is a histological test.

homo- (homeo-) From the Greek *homos*, meaning "same."

homogeneous From the Greek *homos*, meaning "same," and *genos*, meaning "race." Uniform, the same.

hormone From the Greek *hormon*, meaning "impel, set in motion." Chemical substance secreted by a gland, such as estrogen (ovaries), testosterone (testis), adrenaline (adrenal glands), or insulin (pancreas); governs various basic bodily processes such as reproduction, growth, and development.

hump Bulge on the back due most commonly to curves in the spinal bone.

hydr-, hydra-, hydro- From the Greek *hudro-*, meaning "liquid." Prefix meaning moisture, water.

hydration In chemistry, the addition of water. In medicine, techniques such as intravenous fluids designed to maintain the proper fluid balance in the body.

hydroxyapatite (HA) Synthetic material used to rebuild the skull and other boney parts of the body during reconstructive plastic surgery.

hyper- From the Greek *hyper*, meaning "over." Higher amount or degree.

hyperplasia From the Greek *hyper*, meaning "over," and *plasis*, meaning "formation." Abnormal increase in the number of cells in a body tissue/part.

hyperthermia From the Greek *hyper*, meaning "over," and *therme-*, meaning "heat." Fever.

hypertrophy From the Greek *hyper*, meaning "large," and *trophe*, meaning "nutrition, nourishment." Abnormal growth in body cells leading to enlargement of a body tissue/part.

hypo- From the Greek *hypo*, meaning "under." Lesser quantity or degree.

hypoderm- From the Greek *hypo*, meaning "under," and *dermis*, meaning "skin." Under the skin.

hypoplasia From the Greek *hypo*, meaning "under, lesser," and *plasis*, meaning "formation." The incomplete or underdevelopment of a part of the body.

iatrogenic From the Greek *iatros*, meaning "physician," and *gen*, meaning "producing." Something caused by a physician; a response, commonly an adverse reaction, to a prescribed medicine or a medical treatment.

idiopathic From the Greek *idios*, meaning "one's own." Of unknown origin, as an idiopathic disease, an illness for which there is no known cause.

implant Mechanical or cosmetic device inserted into the body; for example, a defibrillator to regulate heartbeat or, in plastic surgery, an implant to reconstruct a breast after cancer surgery or to reshape the face.

incision From the Latin *incisio*, meaning "cut into." Intentional surgical cut through body tissues, most commonly used to describe a cut through the skin.

infection In medicine, presence in the body of disease-causing microorganisms (bacteria, fungi, viruses) that multiply, injure tissues and cells, and trigger inflammation and/or fever and/or tissue death. The normal presence of beneficial microorganisms such as intestinal bacteria that assist in digestion is not considered infection.

inferior   From the Latin *infra*, meaning "below." Below; under.

inflammation   A reaction to an infection, usually involving swelling, heat, and redness at the site. An *inflammatory agent* is a drug or an infectious organism or a process such as irritation that causes inflammation. The *inflammatory response* is the process of inflammation.

infra-   From the Latin *infra*, meaning "below."

inguinal   From the Latin *inguen*, meaning "groin." Of the groin, as in the inguinal region of the abdomen.

injection   From the Latin *injectio*, meaning "throwing in." Introduction of medicine or nutrients under the skin (subcutaneous), into the muscle (intramuscular), into a blood vessel (intravenous/intrarterial), or into a body cavity.

injury   From the Latin *in*, meaning "not," *jus*, meaning "right/law." Damage caused by trauma.

inlay   In dentistry, a device sealed into the tooth cavity as reconstruction for damage resulting from decay or fracture; in plastic surgery, a graft of bone into a cavity in a bone or a skin graft used to fill a defect in the skin.

inpatient surgery   Surgical procedure, performed in a hospital and requiring a patient to remain in the hospital at least overnight.

instrument   In medicine, any tool or implement.

intensity   From the Latin *tensus*, meaning "stretch out." A measure of the strength of energy, as in a high-intensity light.

inter-   From the Latin *inter*, meaning "between."

intergluteal cleft   The space between the buttocks, a.k.a. the natal cleft, the midpoint around which the surgeon aims to create symmetrical shapes during surgery on the buttocks.

interval image   The patient's appearance at one stage in a series of reconstructive procedures such as those required for rebuilding an ear.

intra-   From the Latin *intra*, meaning "inside."

intramuscular   Inside the tissue of a muscle, as in an intramuscular injection, the introduction of a med-

ical substance into muscle tissue via a hollow hypodermic needle.

intraoperative radiation   Technique combining surgery and radiation therapy; immediately after surgical removal of a tumor or part of a tumor, radiation is directed at the area from which the tumor was removed as well as the immediately adjacent areas in an effort to destroy any errant cells.

intraosseous   From the Latin *intra*, meaning "inside," and *os*, meaning "bone." Within a bone, such as an intraosseous implant, an implant, device or filler material inserted during reconstructive surgery into a defect in a bone.

intravenous (IV)   From the Latin *intra*, meaning "within," and *vena*, meaning "vein." Inside a vein, as in an intravenous injection, the introduction of a medical substance such as surgical anesthesic or hydrating fluid directly into a vein via a hollow needle.

involutional   From the Latin *volvo*, meaning "roll up." As in involutional ectropion, an involuntary, age-related folding out of the lower eyelid, or involutional entropion, an involuntary, age-related folding in of the lower eyelid.

ion   From the Greek *ion*, meaning "leaving, going out." An electrically charged atom, group of atoms, or fragment of a molecule.

ionizing radiation   Radiation that damages body tissues by breaking apart cells and separating molecules into electrically charged fragments called ions that can link up with other molecular fragments to form potentially damaging compounds.

irradiation   Exposure to any form of radioactivity, including radiation from any medical diagnostic technique such as a CT-scan (computerized axial tomography) or an X-ray.

irrigate   To clean a wound or body cavity, usually during surgery, by flushing with copious amounts of fluid, generally a saline solution or Ringer's solution. The act of irrigating a wound is called irrigation.

isogenic   From the Greek *iso*, meaning "the same." From the same source.

jacket   In medicine, a stiff bandage such as a cast, used to immobilize the spine; in dentistry, a porcelain or acrylic artificial covering for a tooth.

jaundice From the French *jaune,* meaning "yellow." Yellowing of the skin, mucous membranes, and whites of the eyes due to an accumulation of bilirubin (from the Latin *bilis,* meaning "bile," *ruber,* meaning "red"), a yellow pigment resulting from the degradation of hemoglobin, the red pigment in red blood cells. Ordinarily, as red blood cells die, they are processed and eliminated by the liver. Jaundice occurs when too many red blood cells die at once or when the liver is damaged or cannot process the red blood cells or move bilirubin out of the body.

jelly From the Latin *gelo,* meaning "to freeze." Semisolid compound, such as a red-tinted cosmetic gel to color the face.

joint From the Latin *junctura,* meaning "to join." The point where two or more bones come together. Some joints, such as those between the flat bones of the skull, barely move. In other joints, such as the knee or the elbow, the bones are held together with ligaments in a structure similar to hinges that move in one direction, up and down or side to side. A third type of joint, such as the one between the top two vertebrae (bones in the spine), pivots to allow movement from side to side and up and down.

joule, j Unit of energy; one calorie = 4.2 joules; one joule = 0.23 calories. Named for British physicist James P. Joule (1818–89).

jugular From the Latin *jugulum,* meaning "throat." Relating to the neck or throat, as in the jugular veins, the vessels that carry blood from brain, face, head, and neck toward the heart.

junction, junctio From the Latin *junctura,* meaning "to join." The surface or site where two bones or pieces of cartilage meet, as in a joint.

juxtaposition From the Latin *juxta,* meaning "near," and *posito,* meaning "place." Side-by-side positioning, as in the edges of a wound closing; correct juxtaposition is important to reducing the visibility of a scar after surgery.

keratin The primary protein found in nails, hair, and the top layer of skin cells; the process by which the body deposits keratin in tissues is called *keratinization.*

keratomileusis Surgery to correct vision by altering the shape of the cornea.

labio- From the Latin *labium,* meaning "lip." Used in combinations such as *labiodental* (relating to the lips and teeth).

laceration From the Latin *lacero,* meaning "tear to pieces." A jagged wound.

lacrima From the Latin *lacrima,* meaning "a tear," as in *lacrimal gland* (the glands that produce tears).

lateral From the Latin *latus,* meaning "side." In anatomy, the side of the body or a body part that is farther from the middle or center of the body; for example, the lateral elbow is the side farthest from the opposite elbow.

lattice An open sievelike sheet; in plastic surgery, a meshlike sheet on which skin cells may be grown to produce tissue for a transplant or burn covering.

layer Sheet of one substance lying on top of a sheet of another substance or tissue, for sheet of skin cells.

leakage Escape of fluid from a wound; commonly used to describe the seepage of silicone from a breast implant.

lesion Any change in body tissue, such as a wound or an injury, an infection, or a benign or malignant tumor.

lift Plastic surgery to reshape a facial or body feature; for example, an eye lift or thigh lift.

ligature Thread used to tie off a bleeding blood vessel during surgery.

lipstick sign Term used to describe an indication of a patient's recovery. When a woman begins to apply makeup when recovering from surgery or a serious illness, it signifies a positive attitude or that she is feeling better.

local In the immediate area, as in local excision or local anesthetic.

love handles Slang term for fat deposits at the hip.

lubricant Substance that reduces friction between surfaces; for example, a vaginal lubricant.

lumpectomy Surgical removal of a small tumor; most commonly, the removal of a breast tumor rather than the entire breast.

maceration From the Latin *macerare,* meaning "to soften." Softening due to long-term exposure to liquid.

macro- From the Greek *macros,* meaning "large."

macrognathia   Abnormally large, protruding lower jawbone, often associated with a malfunction of the pituitary gland leading to excess growth; may be corrected with plastic surgery to reduce the size of the lower jaw.

macromastia   Unequal sized breasts, one larger than the other.

macrorhinia   Abnormally large nose.

macula   Macule; flat, pigmented area of skin, less than 10 millimeters across, with a texture similar to the surrounding skin.

mal-   From the Latin *malus*, meaning "bad."

mala-, malar   From the Latin *mala*, meaning "cheekbone." Cheek or cheekbone.

malformation   Deformity; failure of a body structure to develop normally; for example, a cleft palate.

malfunction   Abnormal function of an organ or system; for example, an irregular heartbeat.

malignant   From the Latin *maligno*, meaning "to behave maliciously." Describing a disease that resists treatment, or a tumor that is spreading.

mammo-   From the Latin *mamma*, meaning "breast."

mammoplasty   Breast surgery.

maneuver   From the Latin *manu*, meaning "hand," and *operare*, meaning "to work." Plan or procedure.

margin   From the Latin *margo*, meaning "edge." Border, as in the margin of a cavity (the place where the filling meets the tooth) or the margin of a tumor (the place where the malignant cells give way to healthy tissue).

marionette lines   Fine wrinkles running down from either side of the mouth.

marker   In medicine, a chemical substance or a physical characteristic that identifies a cell, condition, or disease. For example, CA-125 (cancer antigen 125), a protein found at higher levels in ovarian cancer cells than in normal cells, is a marker for ovarian cancer.

matrix   In anatomy, the material between body cells or a framework, as in a matrix in which skin cells are placed to grow into a sheet that can be used as a graft to replace skin lost to an injury such as a burn.

maxillofacial   Referring to the *maxilla* (upper jaw) and the face, as in maxillofacial surgery.

meatoplasty   Reconstruction or repair of the opening to a canal-like body structure; for example, the external ear canal.

meatus   From the Latin *meatus*, meaning "to go." In anatomy, the external opening or a canal, such as the opening of the ear canal or the urethra at the tip of the penis.

medial   From the Latin *medius*, meaning "middle." In anatomy, in or toward the middle of the body or in or toward the center of an organ. For example, the medial side of the elbow is the side closest to the other elbow; the medial layer of a blood vessel is the middle layer of tissue.

medical device   Defined by the Food, Drug and Cosmetic Act as an "article intended to diagnose, cure, treat, prevent, or mitigate a disease or condition, or to affect a function or structure of the body, that does not achieve its primary effect through a chemical action, and is not metabolized."

melanin   From the Greek *melas*, meaning "black." Dark pigment in skin, hair, and retina.

melanoma   From the Greek *melas*, meaning "black," and *-oma*, meaning "tumor." Skin cancer composed of malignant pigmented cells.

membrane   Thin, flexible tissue surrounding body structure; for example, the cell membrane (outer covering of an individual cell) or the membrane lining the mouth.

meso-   From the Greek *mesios*, meaning "middle."

meta-   From the Greek *meta*, meaning "over, above." Beyond, as in meta-analysis, a study consisting of the analysis of many studies.

metabolism   From the Greek *metabole*, meaning "change." The sum of all the chemical and physical changes required for life; anabolism (building up) and catabolism (taking apart) of molecules in body tissues, the conversion of food into energy, and the production of waste in body cells.

micro-   From the Greek *micros*, meaning "small."

micropipette   Extremely small tube for a hypodermic needle.

Micropore™   Brand-name latex-free hypoallergenic paper bandage tape.

mid-   From the Anglo-Saxon *midd*, meaning "middle."

milli- From the Latin *mille,* meaning "1,000." One thousandth, as in a millimeter, one thousandth of a meter.

mixed mesh Titanium-covered plastic mesh (TiMesh®) used as a support in a breast lift.

moustache dressing Dressing that may be placed under the nose after nasal surgery, sinus surgery, tonsillectomy, and/or adenoidectomy, to absorb drainage from the nose.

mucosa From the Latin *mucosus,* meaning "mucous." Tissue lining various body cavities such as the mouth, the stomach, and the vagina; *mucous tissue* (*mucous membranes*) are characterized by the secretion of a clear, sticky liquid called *mucus.*

mucosobuccal fold Fold of mucous membrane extending from the gum at the neck of the teeth and onto the cheek tissue.

Mylar™ Brand-name plastic used in plastic surgery as an implant as in cheek augmentation, or as a supporting structure, for example, in a breast lift.

myo- From the Greek and Latin *mus,* meaning "muscle."

neck The rounded side of the face, from below the eye to the top of the mouth.

necrosis From the Greek *nekrosis,* meaning "death." Death of living cells or tissues.

neo- From the Greek *neos,* meaning "new, young." For example, *neoplasm,* a new growth of tissue.

nerve stimulator Probe use to deliver electrical impulses to body tissues so that the plastic surgeon can locate and avoid damage to underlying nerves, particularly facial nerves during surgery to remove a head and/or neck tumors such as a facial hemangioma.

noble gases Helium, neon, argon, krypton, xenon, and radon; relatively unreactive chemical elements, some of which are used as energy sources for lasers.

node A confined tissue mass; for example, a lymph node. A *nodule* is a small node.

occlusive dressing Any bandage that prevents air and/or bacteria from reaching an open wound, including a surgical wound.

occult From the Latin *occultus,* meaning "hidden."

OMFS Acronym for *o*ral and *m*axillo*f*acial *s*urgery, surgery on the mouth and maxilla (upper jaw).

omo- From the Greek *omos,* meaning "shoulder."

opportunistic infection An infectious illness that does not pose a serious threat to a healthy body but may prove fatal to a person with a compromised immune system.

orbit Circular cavity comprised of parts of the forehead, nose, cheek, and upper jawbones, containing the eyeball and its associated muscles, nerves, and blood vessels.

oro- From the Latin *oris,* meaning "mouth, opening." Referring to the oral cavity, as in orofacial (mouth/face) surgery.

os- From the Latin and Greek *os,* meaning "bone."

oseointegrated prosthesis Artificial body part such as an artificial ear that is implanted into and anchored by the underlying bone.

osteoplastic reconstruction Plastic surgery to repair, reconstruct, or redesign a body part or facial feature using bone grafts; for example, the use of bone grafts to strengthen the framework of the nose during rhinoplasty or rebuilding parts of a missing skull.

oto- From the Greek *ous,* meaning "ear."

packing Process of filling a natural body cavity or wound with absorbent sterile material to slow or stop bleeding; or, the material used to fill the cavity or wound.

pad In medicine, a soft dressing used to relieve pressure or to fill a cavity so that a bandage fits more snugly; in anatomy, a thick piece of body tissue such as the fat pad under the facial skin that rounds out the cheek.

palmar Relating to the palm (from the Latin *palma*) of the hand, as in a palmar injury.

papilla From the Latin *papula,* meaning "pimple." Small, round fingerlike projection, such as one of the tiny bumps on the upper surface of the tongue.

papilloma From the Latin *papula,* meaning "pimple," and the Greek *-oma,* meaning "tumor." Small, round benign tumor composed of epithelial cells; found on the skin or on the surface of a mucous membrane, such as the membrane lining the nose.

papule From the Latin *papula,* meaning "pimple."

para- From the Greek *para-* or *par-,* meaning "next to."

paraffin gauze Wound covering coated with paraffin, a waxy material that prevents the bandage from sticking to an open wound, allowing it to be easily and painlessly removed.

paralysis From the Greek *para*, meaning "around, near," and *lysis*, meaning "cutting, loosening." Generally, a loss of control; in medicine, loss of the ability to move muscles; arising from nerve damage due either to an illness, such as paralytic poliomyelitis, or to an injury, such as a fall that severs the spinal cord, thus preventing the transmission of nerve impulses from brain to muscle.

parenteral From the Greek *para-*, meaning "near," and *enteron*, meaning "intestine." Given by a route other than through the stomach, as in parenteral anesthesia, anesthetics given by injection.

paresthesia From the Greek *para*, meaning "near," and *aesthesis*, meaning "sensation." Unusual, uncomfortable, or annoying sensation such as tingling or burning due to irritation of nerves, sometimes without apparent injury to body tissues.

parietal bone From the Latin *paries*, meaning "wall." Flat bone curved to fit at either side of the top of the skull.

paronychia From the Greek *para-*, meaning "around," and *onyx*, meaning "nail." Infection around the nail on a finger or toe.

paste In general medicine, a semisolid product such as a cream or an ointment, which may contain an active medical ingredient such as an antibiotic or an anti-inflammatory. In plastic surgery, bone paste is a thick filler made from powdered bone and used to fill in a defect in any bone.

patch In medicine, a small, usually round area of skin or mucous membrane with a color or texture different from the surrounding tissue; for example, a mucous patch, a pale yellow, gray, or white spot on the lining of the mouth that may be a sign of syphilis.

pathogen From the Greek *pathos*, meaning "suffering," "disease," *gen*, meaning "made." Anything that causes illness; bacteria, virus, fungi, toxin.

percutaneous From the Latin *per*, meaning "through," and *cutis*, meaning "skin." Through the skin, as a percutaneous medication, a drug that passes through the skin into the body.

peri- From the Greek *peri-*, meaning "around."

periareolar From the Latin *peri-*, meaning "around," and *areaola*, meaning "small area." The area around the nipple.

perineural From the Greek *peri-*, meaning "around," and *neuron*, meaning "nerve." Around the nerve, as in a perineural block, a form of anesthesic that numbs a large area around a specific nerve.

periodontal From the Greek *peri-*, meaning "around," and *odous*, meaning "tooth." Around a tooth, as the soft tissue of the gum and hard bone of the jaws.

peripheral From the Greek *peri-*, meaning "around," and *pherous*, meaning "carry." In anatomy, the parts of the body farthest from the center; i.e., hands and feet or a peripheral nerve, a nerve found around the outer rim of an organ or in the parts of the body, such as hands and feet.

phallo-, phallus From the Greek *phallus*, meaning "penis."

phenol Strong caustic liquid; used as in antiseptic, anesthetic, and exfoliant (rarely) in a deep skin peel.

philtrum From the Greek *philtron*, meaning "love potion." The depression in the center of the upper lip that forms the cupid's bow, the twin-peaked center of the upper lip.

phlebitis From the Greek *phlebs*, meaning "vein," and *-it is*, meaning "inflammation." Inflammation of the walls of a vein, commonly leading to a blood clot (thrombophlebitis, from the Greek *thrombos*, meaning "clot"), accompanied by swelling, stiffness, and pain.

photo- From the Greek *phos*, meaning "light."

photoaging Damaging effects of ultraviolet radiation (sunlight) on skin.

photoallergic reaction A reaction of the immune system such as hives, swelling, or a serious burn due to sensitivity to ultraviolet light (sunlight).

photosensitizer A substance that makes the skin more sensitive to ultra violet light.

pilar From the Latin *pilus*, meaning "hair." Hairy.

pilosabaceous gland From the Latin *pilus*, meaning "hair," *sebum*, meaning "oil." An oil-secreting gland in the skin that contains a hair.

plaque From the French *plaque*, meaning "flat plate." An area of tissue that is different in texture or color from the surrounding skin or mucous membrane; also, commonly a deposit of cholesterol inside an artery.

plaster Adhesive product used to hold the edges of a wound together; or a dressing used to warm the skin (e.g., a mustard plaster) or to apply medicine.

-plasty From the Greek *plastos*, meaning "formed."

plate From the Greek *platys*, meaning "flat." In anatomy, a thin, flat body structure such as the plate (base) under the fingernail; in surgery, a flat piece of metal used to hold the end of a broken bone together.

plexus From the Latin *plexus*, meaning "braid." Site of intertwined nerves and blood or lymph vessels such as the solar plexus, the network of nerves at the back of the stomach that control the organs in the abdomen.

plug A mass of material that fills a body opening; for example, a blackhead, the plug of bacteria and oily matter that blocks the opening to a pore.

polyp From the Greek *poly*, meaning "many," *pous*, meaning "foot." Benign (noncancerous) tumor found in areas lined with mucous membrane; i.e., the inside of the nose, or the colon, or the uterus.

pore From the Greek *poros*, meaning "passage." Opening from the skin into a hair-bearing oil-secreting gland.

povidone iodine Antiseptic; a powder of iodine plus povidone (a synthetic particle polymer used as a vehicle for drugs) mixed with water to produce a water-based antiseptic, disinfectant solution. May irritate the skin and cause burning or itching or, rarely, an allergic reaction.

precancerous Term describing cellular changes that may lead to cancer.

pressure dressing Bandage used to apply pressure to a blood vessel so as to constrict the vessel and stop bleeding; also, bandage used after surgery to reduce fluid accumulation and swelling at the site of the incision.

probe From the Latin *probere*, meaning "to test." In medicine, a thin rod used to examine body cavities and/or wounds; or an instrument such as a laparoscope that enables a surgeon to look into the body through a very small incision, usually no more than an inch in length; or an electrical rod inserted into a liquid or semiliquid substance to determine properties such as temperatures and density.

prosthesis From the Greek *prosthesis*, meaning "addition." Artificial substitute for a body part missing due to a birth defect or destroyed by illness or injury; for example, an artificial eye, or an artificial leg, or a denture.

psoriasis From the Greek *psora*, meaning "scaling." Chronic skin disease, characterized by reddened skin and/or silvery white scale.

ptosis From the Greek *ptosis*, meaning "falling." In medicine, a droop or unnatural relaxation of a specific tissue, such as ptosis of the eyelid.

punch From the Latin *pungo*, meaning "punch." In surgery, tool used to remove a small, circular piece of skin.

pus Thickened, sometimes odorous yellow-white fluid; a sign of infection; composed of phagocytes (white blood cells in the immune system that attack and engulf invading microorganisms), dead microorganisms such as bacteria, and dead and decomposing body tissue at the site.

pyrexia From the Greek *pyr-*, meaning "fire." High temperature; fever.

quadrangular From the Latin *quadrangulus*; meaning "having four corners/angles"; for example, a quadrangular skin flap.

quadrant From the Latin *quadrans*, meaning "quarter, one-fourth." In anatomy, one quarter of an area bounded by a roughly drawn circle such as the upper left quadrant of the abdomen.

quadrate From the Latin *quadratus*, meaning "square"; the term refers to quadrate muscle such as the quadrate muscle of the lower lip, the quadrate muscle of the upper lip, or the quadrate muscle of the thigh.

RAD *R*adiation *a*bsorbed *d*ose; unit of energy absorbed from ionizing radiation.

radial From the Latin *radialis*, meaning "forearm bone." In anatomy, relating to the radius, the shorter of the two bones in the forearm, the one on the outer edge of the arm.

raphe Anatomical term for a ridge or seamlike line between two similar body parts; for example, the line running up the center of the scrotum.

rasp   Surgical instrument with a rough surface used to shave or rub away small amounts of bone.

re-   From the Latin *re,* meaning "again, back, before."

reaction   From the Latin *reacto,* meaning "acting back." Response of a body tissue to a stimulus; for example, skin reddening when exposed to sunlight or nasal stuffiness in response to exposure to allergens.

recessive   From the Latin *recessus,* meaning "pulling away." The opposite of dominant, as in a recessive gene.

reduction   From the Latin *reduco,* meaning "to go back." In plastic surgery, a procedure to reduce the size of an organ or feature, for example, breast reduction or lip reduction.

re-epithelization   Regrowth of skin (epithelial cells) after an injury.

reflex   From the Latin *reflexio,* meaning "bending back." An involuntary response, such as the pupil's contracting when the eye is exposed to light or the leg's flexing when the knee is struck.

regeneration   From the Latin *regene-,* meaning "to reproduce." In medicine, the regrowth of tissue, such as the body's replacement of skin or bone lost to an injury or infection.

region   From the Latin *regio,* meaning "space." A circumscribed or clearly defined area of the body, such as the abdominal region.

reimplantation   Replantation; the surgical reattachment of an organ or body part to its original site; for example, the reimplantation of an accidentally severed finger or finger tip.

rejection   From the Latin *rejectio,* meaning "discard." Immune system response; the body's refusal to integrate foreign tissue, such as a transplanted organ or blood of a type different from the patient's.

rejuvenation surgery   Any plastic surgery procedure such as abdominoplasty, forehead lift, chemical skin peel, dermabrasion, eye lift, face-lift, labioplasty, and/or liposuction designed to reduce signs of facial or body aging.

repositioning   In plastic surgery, a procedure to move organs or tissues as to improve their function; for example, surgery to correct a protruding jaw by moving the bone backward.

resect   From the Latin *sextus,* meaning "cut off." In surgery, to remove part or all of an organ or tissue such as a bone.

resin   Natural substance derived from plants or synthetic substance such as silicone that is solid when cool, pliable when warmed; used in pharmaceutical products as well as lacquers, varnishes, adhesives, and plastics.

resorption   Natural physiological process leading to the loss of body tissue; for example, the resorption of bone in older persons that contributes to the development of osteoporosis.

restoration   From the Latin *restauro,* meaning "to repair." In dentistry, a device such as a bridge, false tooth, or filling used to repair a dental defect or replace missing tooth/teeth.

retractor   Surgical instrument used to hold the edges of an incision apart so as to give the surgeon a clear view of the operating field.

retro-   From the Latin *retro,* meaning "back." Backward; previous.

revascularization   Establishment of a blood supply to body tissue; for example, after the transplant of a piece of skin from one part of the body to another.

rhagades   From the Greek *rhagas,* meaning "tear." Wrinkles and/or cracks in the skin.

rhinocheiloplasty   Procedure involving simultaneous surgeries on the nose and lip.

rhytid   From the Greek *rhytis,* meaning "wrinkle." Commonly, a facial wrinkle. Rhytidectomy, *rhytis + ectome* (cut out), is the scientific term for face-lift, i.e., removing wrinkles.

ridge   In anatomy, an elevation such as the bony ridge above the eyes.

rim   Margin; border; for example, the orbital rim (the edges of the bone surrounding the eye).

ringers solution   Intravenous (IV) solution used to supply water and nutrients to the body, commonly after surgery.

rongeur   From the French *ronger,* meaning "gnaw." Surgical forceps used to chisel away bone.

rubor   From the Latin *rubor,* meaning "red." Redness of the skin or mucous membrane; a sign of infection.

Rule of Nines Diagram of the body that enables physicians to estimate damage due to a burn.

saline From the Latin *salis*, meaning "salt." Salty.

scaffold In surgery, a piece of collagen or absorbable synthetic mesh implanted as a platform on which to grow new body cells.

scapula From the Latin *scapula*, meaning "shoulder." The shoulder blade, a bone with a socket into which the ball-shape head of the humerus (long bone of the arm) fits to create the shoulder joint.

scrub Cosmetic product containing small abrasive particles to smooth the skin by rubbing away the rough dead top cells on the skin.

sensitizer Substance that may produce an allergic reaction after repeated exposure.

sex change Lay term for surgery to alter the external appearance of the body from female to male or male to female.

sex chromosomes These chromosomes determine gender. A female has two X (female) chromosomes; a male, one X and one Y (male chromosome).

shunt Plastic or rubber tube implanted into an organ or tissue to drain off fluids.

sinus From the Latin *sinus*, meaning "curve or hollow." A cavity, such as the sinuses in the skull.

soft tissue Tissues that connect or support body structures and organs; for example, blood vessels, connective tissue (collagen), fatty tissue, muscles, nerves, and synovial tissue (the tissue around joints).

sonogram The picture produce by an ultrasound examination.

speculum Instrument used for widening a body cavity, such as the vagina, during a physical examination.

sponge Gauze-covered materials or nonwoven lint-free fabric used to absorb blood and other fluids during surgery.

stain Dye applied to body cells, tissues, or microorganisms so as to make their structure visible under a microscope.

stenosis Narrowing of any tubular body part such as an artery.

sterile Treated with chemical agents, bombarded with electrons, or exposed to heat, steam, or radiation (ultraviolet light) so as to destroy all microorganisms.

struma From the Latin *strumo-*, meaning "to build." Enlargement of tissue, a tumor.

strut Piece of cartilage, plastic, or metal used to strengthen a body structure, such as the tip of the nose, during surgery.

sub- From the Latin *sub*, meaning "under."

subcutaneous augmentation material (SAM) Biocompatible synthetic device inserted under the skin to alter the shape of an area of the body or face; for example, a cheek implant.

sulcus From the Latin *sulcus*, meaning "furrow." Long, narrow groove, such as the grooves in the surface of the brain or on the surface of the palate.

superinfection A second infection at the same site, usually due to an organism's becoming resistant to the antibiotic used to treat the first infection.

suppuration From the Latin *suppuro-*, meaning "form," and *pur*, meaning "pus."

supra-, super From the Latin *supra*, meaning "on the higher position." Above, or the higher, as *superciliary* (from the Latin *cilium*, meaning "eyelid"), in the area of the eyebrow.

surgery From the Greek *cheir*, meaning "hand," and *ergon*, meaning "work." The branch of medicine that treats with an operation, a procedure that physically cuts, repairs, or manipulates various parts of the body. A *surgeon* is a physician who specializes in surgery.

symmetry From the Greek *sym-* or *syn-*, meaning "together," and *metron*, meaning "measure." Even positioning of parts around a centerline; in anatomy, eyes evenly situated on either side of the face or arms and legs evenly situated on either side of the body.

syngeneic From the Greek *syngeneia*, meaning "family relationship."

system In anatomy, a group of related organs such as the *digestive system*.

telangiectasia Cluster of small blood vessels.

temporo- From the Latin *temporalis*, meaning "temple." In anatomy, the temple or temporal bone, as in temporomandibular (temporal bone/jawbone).

thrombo- From the Greek *thrombus*, meaning "clot." Blood clot.

thyroid eminence Synonym for Adam's apple.

tibia   From the Latin *tibia,* meaning "pipe." The larger of the two bones in the lower leg; the smaller is the fibula.

tissue   In anatomy, tissue is a grouping of similar cells forming material that behaves in a specific way; for example, the basic tissues in the human body are connective tissue, epidermal tissue, muscle tissue, and nerve tissue.

-tomy   From the Greek *tomia,* meaning "incision."

transsexualism   The condition of being born with the genitals of one sex but considering oneself a member of the other.

transverse   Going across. In anatomy, the transverse colon, a section of the intestinal tract lying in a horizontal rather than a vertical position across the mid-body.

trauma   From the Greek *trauma,* meaning "wound, damage." Physical or psychological injury.

unilaminar   One layer, as in a unilaminar skin substitute, artificial skin consisting of a single layer of cells.

vermillion border   Vermillion margin; carmine margin; the pink outer surface of the lips.

vitallium   Alloy (60 percent cobalt, 20 percent chromium, 5 percent molybdenum, plus trace substances) used in dentures, as well as surgical appliances, prostheses, implants, and instruments.

wart   A growth on a body surface caused by a viral infection.

wattle   Sagging skin under the chin, named for its resemblance to the wrinkled piece of skin found under the chin or on the throat of various birds such as the turkey and reptiles such as lizards.

wax   Fatty substance, solid at room temperature, thick syrupy liquid when warmed; similar in appearance to *beeswax,* the natural secretions of a bee. *Mineral wax* is wax extracted from minerals; *Montan wax* is a wax extracted from the mineral lignite.

weeping   In medicine, describes a skin condition characterized by oozing liquid, such as an eczema ("weeping dermatitis").

welt wheal   A raised mark cause by an injury.

wheal   From the Anglo-Saxon *hwele,* meaning "hive." A raised white mark on the skin, a reaction to an allergen, usually one injected to test for allergic sensitivity.

wire   Thin, flexible metal thread or rod, commonly used to hold bones together.

wiring   Surgical technique used to repair or reconstruct broken bones by fixing the ends together with fine wire.

wound   An injury to any part of the body that results in a break in tissue, such as a cut or a surgical incision in the skin or a broken bone.

X-Acto™   Brand-name surgical blade/knife.

xeno-   From the Greek *xenos,* meaning "stranger, foreign." In medicine, material not from a person's own body.

xero-   From the Greek *xeros,* meaning "dry."

xerochilia   From the Greek *xeros,* meaning "dry," and *cheilos,* meaning "lip." Dry lips.

XPS   Abbreviation for extruded polystyrene, a plastic material that may be used by plastic surgeons to prepare models showing the desired results of a proposed reconstructive procedure.

Y bone plate   Y-shape metal bar used to stabilize a fractured bone, or during plastic surgery to reconstruct a boney structure.

yoga   In Western culture, a relaxation technique comprising a variety of postures and body positions together with breathing exercises and meditation. In Eastern culture, yoga is also a set of moral precepts regarding emotional, philosophical, and physical.

yoke bone   Another name for the zygomatic bone (cheekbone).

zero variance   Zero variation; normal; no deviation from the expected norm.

Zest Implant™   Brand-name anchor for a dental implant, invented by and named for Max Zuest (1918–2003), the Swiss-born, Canadian founder of Zest Anchors (devices used to anchor various attachment used in surgery).

Zone *(zona)*   An area or section of the body or of an organ or of an injury; for example, the erogenous zones (areas of the body which produce sexual arousal when stimulated) or the motor zone (the part of the brain that controls movement) or the areas of skin injured by a burn. In plastic surgery, the concept of zones is used to determine treatment for severe burns.

BIBLIOGRAPHY

Books

Braunwald, Eugene, et al. *Harrison's Principles of Internal Medicine,* 15th ed. New York: McGraw-Hill, 2001.

Brown, David L., and Gregory H. Borschel. *Michigan Manual of Plastic Surgery.* Philadelphia: Lippincott, Williams & Wilkins, 2004.

Dorland's Medical Dictionary. Philadelphia: W.B. Saunders, 2000.

Dorland's Plastic Surgery Word Book for Medical Transcriptionists. Philadelphia: W.B. Saunders, 2002.

Magner, Lois N. *A History of Medicine.* New York: Marcel Dekker, 1992.

Stedman's Medical Dictionary, 27th ed. Baltimore: Williams & Wilkins, 2000.

The Visual Dictionary of the Human Body. New York: Dorling Kindersley, 1991.

Weatherford, M. Lisa, ed. *Reconstructive and Cosmetic Surgery Sourcebook.* Detroit: Omnigraphics, 2001.

Webster's New Collegiate Dictionary, 2nd ed. Springfield, Mass.: Merriam-Webster, 1956.

Webster's New International Dictionary, 2nd ed. Springfield, Mass.: Merriam-Webster, 1941.

Weinzweig, Jeffry. *Plastic Surgery Secrets.* Philadelphia: Hanley & Belfus, 1999.

Periodicals/Pamphlets/Reports

The articles listed here are identified by the publication in which they originally appeared; the articles (or an abstract) may also be available on the Internet.

Attin, T., F. Paque, F. Ajam, and A. M. Lennon. "Review of the current status of tooth whitening with the walking bleach technique." *International Endodontal Journal* 36, no. 5 (May 2003): 313–329. Available online. URL: http://www.ncbi.nlm.nih.gov/entrez/query.fcgi?cmd=Retrieve&db=PubMed&list_uids=12752645&dopt=Abstract. Accessed April 20, 2006.

Balakrishnan, C., T. A. Pane, and A. J. Khalil. "Use of groin flap in the closure of through and through defect of a forearm: A case report." *Canadian Journal of Plastic Surgery* 12, no. 1 (Spring 2004): 47–48. Available online. URL: http://www.pulsus.com/Plastics/12_01/bal2_ed.htm. Accessed February 18, 2006.

Berktold, R. E., R. H. Ossoff, G. A. Sisson, and C. F. Wurster. "Chin reconstruction with pectoralis myocutaneous flap." *Otolaryngology Head Neck Surgery* 94, no. 2 (February 1986): 181–186. Available online. URL: http://www.ncbi.nlm.nih.gov/entrez/query.fcgi?cmd=Retrieve&dbPubMed&list_uids=3083332&dopt=Abstract. Accessed May 23, 2006.

Bhatt, Yogesh C., Kinnari Vyas, Dhananjay Nakade, and Manish Zade. "Reconstruction of nasal defects our three years experience." *Indian Journal of Otolaryngology and Head and Neck Surgery* 58, no. 1 (2006): 51–56. Available online. URL: http://www.ijohns.com/article.asp?issn=0019-5421;year=2006;volume=58;issue=1;spage=51;epage=56;aulast=Bhat. Accessed May 24, 2006.

Birkmeyer, J. D., E. V. Finlayson, and C. M. Birkmeyer. "Volume standards for high-risk surgical procedures: Potential benefits of the Leapfrog initiative." *Surgery* 130, no. 3 (September 2001): 415–422. Available online. URL: http://www.ncbi.nlm.nih.gov/entrez/query.fcg...st_uids=115626 2&dopt=Citation. Accessed April 11, 2006.

Birt, B. D. "The 'lip shave' operation for pre-malignant conditions and micro-invasive carcinoma of the lower lip." *Journal of Otolaryngology* 6, no. 5 (October 1977): 407–411. Available online. URL: http://www.ncbi.nlm.nih.gov/entrez/query.fcgi?cmd=Retrieve&db=PubMed&list_uids=926223&dopt=Abstract. Accessed January 30, 2006.

"Body Piercing." *Journal of the American Medical Association* 291, no. 8 (February 25, 2004): 1024. Available online. URL: http://jama.ama-assn.org/cgi/content/full/291/8/1024. Accessed August 29, 2006.

Boque, D. P., A. K. Mundara, M. Thompson, and P. S. Cederna. "Modified technique for nipple-areolar reconstruction: a case series." *Plastic and Reconstructive Surgery* 112, no. 5 (October 2003): 1,274–1,278. Available online. URL: http://www.ncbi.nlm.nih.gov/entrez/query.fcgi?cmd=Retrieve&db=PubMed&list_uids=14504510&dopt=Abstract. Accessed August 1, 2006.

"Botulinum Toxin Helps Facial Scars Heal Better." *Mayo Clinic Proceedings,* August 2006. Available online. URL:

http://www.newswis.com/p/articles/view/522593/. Accessed August 11, 2006.

Buyukunal S. N., and N. Sari. "Serafeddin Sabuncuo-glu, Cerrahiye-i Ilhaniye." *Journal of Pediatric Surgery* 26, no. 10 (February 1986): 1,148–1,151. Available online. URL: http://www.ncbi.nlm.nih.gov/entre/query.fcgi?cmd=Retrieve&db=PubMed&list_uids=1779321&dopt=Citation. Accessed July 10, 2005.

Camber, Rebecca. "Tailor-made skin from 'ink' printer." *Manchester Evening News.* Available online. URL: http://www.manchesteronline.co.uk/news/s/143/143230_tailormade_skin_from_ink_printer.html. Posted January 19, 2005.

Chambers, P. A., C. R. Yavuzer, I. T. Jackson, J. S. Topf, and S. M. Lash. "One-stage correction of complex facial disproportion." *Journal of Craniofacial Surgery* 10, no. 3 (May 1999): 214–221. Available online. URL: http://www.ncbi.nlm.nih.gov/entrez/query.fcgi?cmd=Retrieve&db=PubMed&list_uids=10530230&dopt=Abstract. Accessed June 20, 2006.

Cho, S., S. Y. Lee, J. H. Choi, K. J. Sung, K. C. Moon, and J. K. Koh. "Treatment of 'Cyrano' angioma with pulsed dye laser." *Dermatological Surgery* 27, no. 7 (February 1986): 670–672. Available online. URL: http://www.ncbi.nlm.nih.gov/entrez/query.fcgi?cmd=Retrieve&db=PubMed&list_uids=11442621&dopt=Abstract. Accessed January 15, 2006.

Chuang, D. C., L. H. Colony, and H. C. Chen. "Groin flap design and versatility." *Plastic Reconstructive Surgery* 84, no. 1 (July 1989): 100–107. Available online. URL: http://www.ncbi.nlm.nih.gov/entrez/query.fcgi?cmd=Retrieve&db=PubMed&list_uids=2660172&dopt=Abstract. Accessed February 18, 2006.

Cohen, Michael M., "Cleft lip and palate reconstruction, orofacial clefting: embryonic, pathogenic, epidemiologic, genetic, molecular, and syndromic perspectives." *CME HyperGuide.* N.D. Available online. URL: http://www.cmf.hyperguides.com/default.asp?page=/tutorials/cleft/orofacial_clefting/overview.asp&rID=. Accessed March 28, 2008.

Copcul, Eray, Kubilay Metin, Alper Aktas, Nazan S. Sivrioglu, and Yücel Öztan. "Cervicopectoral flap in head and neck cancer surgery." *World Journal of Surgical Oncology* 1 (2003): 29. Available online. URL: http://www.pubmedcentral.nih.gov/articlerender.fcgi?artid=317373. Accessed August 13, 2005.

Cosmun, B. "The question mark ear: an unappreciated major anomaly of the auricle." *Plastic and Reconstructive Surgery* 73, no. 4 (April 1984): 572–576. Available online. URL: http://www.ncbi.nlm.nih.gov/entrez/query.fcgi?cmd=Retrieve&db=PubMed&list_uids=6709737&dopt=Abstract. Accessed May 26, 2006.

Creighton, Sarah, and Catherine Minto. "Managing intersex (editorial)." *British Medical Journal* 323 (December 1, 2001): 1264–1265. Available online. URL: http://bmj.bmjjournals.com/ci/content/full/323/7324/1264. Accessed October 1, 2006.

Dagregorio, Guy, and Yann Saint-Cast. "Composite Graft Replacement of Digital Tips in Adults." *Orthopedics* 29 (January 2006): 22. Available online. URL: http://www.orthosupersite.com/defaul.asp?page=view&rid=5174. Accessed July 23, 2005.

Dini, Valentina, Marco Romanelli, Alberto Piaggesi, Alessandro Stefani, and Franco Mosca. "Cutaneous Tissue Engineering and Lower Extremity Wounds (Part 2)." *International Journal of Lower Extremity Wounds* 3, no. 2 (June 2004): 80–86. Available online. URL: http://ijl.sagepub.com/cgi/reprint/5/1/27.pdf. Accessed July 26, 2006.

Dogan, T., M. Bayramicli, and A. Numanoglu. "Plastic surgical techniques in the fifteenth century by Serafeddin Sabuncuoglu." *Plastic and Reconstructive Surgery* 99, no. 6 (May 1997): 1,775–1,779. Available online. URL: http://www.ncbi.nlm.nih.gov/entrez/query.fcgi?cmd=Retrieve&db=PubMed&list_uids=9145157&dopt=Citation. Accessed July 10, 2005.

Elliott, L. F., and C. R. Hartrampf, Jr. "The Rubens flap. The deep circumflex iliac artery flap." *Clinical Plastic Surgery* 25, no. 2 (April 1998): 283–291. Available online. URL: http://www.ncbi.nlm.nihgov/entrez/quey.fcgi?cmd=Retrieve&db=PubMed&list_uids=9627786&dopt=Abstract. Accessed May 14, 2006.

Ersek, R. A. "Comparative study of dermabrasion, phenol peel, and acetic acid peel." *Aesthetic Plastic Surgery* 15, no. 3 (Summer 1991): 241–243. Available online. URL: http://www.ncbi.nlm.nih.gov/entrez/query.fcgi?cmd=Retrieve&db=PubMed&list_uids=1897419&dopt=Abstract. Accessed May 15, 2005.

Feldman J. J. "Corset platysmaplasty." *Plastic and Reconstructive Surgery* 85, no. 3 (March 1990): 333–343. Available online. URL: http://www.ncbi.nlm.nh.gov/entrez/query.fcgi?cmd=Retrieve&db=PubMed&list_uids=2304983&dopt=Abstract. Accessed August 12, 2005.

Finlayson, Emily V. A. "Operative Mortality with Elective Surgery in Older Adults." *Effective Clinical Practice* (July/August 2001). Available online. URL: http://www.acponline.org/journals/ecp/julaug01/finlayson.htm. Accessed March 16, 2005.

Freihofer, H. P. "Surgical treatment of the short face syndrome" *Journal of Oral Surgery* 39, no. 11 (November 1981): 907–911.

Friedman, Greg. "Inventing the light fantastic: Ted Maiman and the world's first laser." *OE Reports* 200 (August 2000). Available online. URL: http://www.

spie.org/web/oer/august/aug00/maiman.html. Accessed May 16, 2006.

Friedman, M. "Parietal occipital nape of neck flap. A myocutaneous flap for selected head and neck reconstruction." *Archives of Otolaryngology, Head and Neck Surgery* 112, no. 3 (March 1986): 309–315. Available online. URL: http://www.ncbi.nlm.nih.gov/entrez/query.fcgi?cmd=Retrieve&db=PubMed&list_uids=3942638&dopt=Abstract. Accessed May 15, 2005.

Fuente del Campo, A. "Regional dermolipectomy as treatment for sequelae of massive weight loss." *World Journal of Surgery* 22, no. 9 (September 1998): 974–980. Available online. URL: http://www.ncbi.nlm.nih.gov/entrez/query.fcgi?cmd=Retrieve&db=PubMed&list_uids=9717424&dopt=Abstract. Accessed March 26, 2006.

Fulton, J. E., Jr., A. D. Rahimi, P. Helton, T. Watson, and K. Dahlberg. "Lip rejuvenation." *Dermatology Surgery* 26, no. 5 (May 2000): 470–474. Available online. URL: http://aolsearch.aol.com/ao/search?encquery=58499106e51e72d964cc28e128379046&inocationType=keyword_rollover&ie=UTF-8. Accessed May 6, 2006.

"Gender Reassignment Surgery, Cigna Healthcare Coverage Position." Available online. URL: http://www.cigna.com/health/provider/medical/procedural/coverage_positions/medical/mm_0266_coverage-positioncriteria_gender_reassignment_surgery.pdf. Revised December 15, 2005.

Gmur, Roger U. "Is it safe to combine abdominoplasty with other dermolipectomy procedures to correct skin excess after weight loss?" *Annals of Plastic Surgery* 51, no. 4 (October 2003): 353–357. Available online. URL: http://www.ncbi.nlm.nih/.gov/entrez/query.fcgi?cmd=Retrieve&db=PubMed&list_uids=14520060&dopt=Abstract. Accessed February 12, 2005.

Goodwin, Willard E. "Uncircumcision: a technique for plastic reconstruction of a prepuce after circumcision." *Journal of Urology,* 144 (November 1990): 1203–1205. Available online. URL: http://www.cirp.org/lib rary/restoration/goodwin1/. Accessed February 19, 2005.

Greenwald, A. Seth, Christine Heim, Harri Reddi, Randy Rosier, Harvinder Sandhu, and Donna Toohey. "Profile of orthopaedic accomplishment: Marshall R. Urist, MD." *2004 Annual Meeting Edition of the AAOS (American Academy of Orthopedic Surgeons) Bulletin,* March 11, 2004. Available online. URL: http://www.aaos.org/wordhtml/2004news/c11-4.htm. Accessed February 20, 2005.

Greer, Donald M., Jr., Paul C. Mohl, and Katy A. Sheley. "A technique for foreskin reconstruction and some preliminary results." *The Journal of Sex Research,* 18, no. 4 (November 1982): 324–330. Available online. URL: http://www.cirp.org/library/restoration/greer1/. Accessed February 21, 2005.

Hettiaratchy, Shehan, and Remo Papini. "Initial management of major burns: II—management and resuscitation." *British Medical Journal* 329 (July 10, 2004): 101–103. Available online. URL: http://bmj.mjjourn als.com/cgi/content/full/329/7457/101. Accessed April 18, 2005.

Hage, J. J., F. G. Bouman, and J. J. Bloem. "Construction of the fixed part of the neourethra in female-to-male transsexuals: experience in 53 patients." *Plastic Reconstructive Surgery* 91, no. 5 (April 1993): 904–910. Available online. URL: http://www.ncbi.nlm.nih.gov/entrez/query.fcgi?cmd=Retrieve&db=PubMed&list_uids=8460194&dopt=Abstract. Accessed August 18, 2006.

Kamerer, D. B., B. E. Hirsch, C. H. Snyderman, P. Costantino, and C. D. Friedman. "Hydroxyapatite cement: a new method for achieving watertight closure in transtemporal surgery." *American Journal of Otolaryngology* 15, no. 1 (January 1994): 47–49. Available online. URL: http://www.ncbi.nlm.nih.gov/entrez/query.fcg?cmd=Retrieve&db=PubMed&list_uids=8109630&dopt=Abstract. Accessed February 11, 2006.

Kapoor, Seema, S. B. Mukherjee, Ritu Paul, and Bhavna Dhingra. "OMENS-Plus Syndrome." *Indian Journal of Pediatrics* 78, no. 8 (2005): 707–708. Available online. URL: http://finance.aol.com/usw/quotes/quotesand news?sym=goog&exch=NAS. Accessed June 20, 2006.

Kayhan, F. T., D. Zurakowski, and S. D. Rauch. "Toronto Facial Grading System: interobserver reliability." *Otolaryngology, Head and Neck Surgery* 122, no. 2 (February 2000): 212–215. Available online. URL: http://www.ncbi.nlm.nih.gov/entrez/query.fcgi?cmd=Retrieve&db=PubMed&list_uids=1. Accessed June 7, 2006.

Khouri, R. K. and G. J. Diehl. "Salvage in a case of ring avulsion injury with an immediate second-toe wrap-around flap." *Journal of Hand Surgery (American)* 17, no. 4 (July 1992): 714–718. Available online. URL: http://www.ncbi.nlm.nih.gov/entrez/query.fcgi?cmd=Retrieve&db=\PubMed&list_uids=1629554&dopt=Abstract. Accessed June 7, 2006.

Kitano, M., and M. Taneda. "Subdural patch graft technique for watertight closure of large dural defects in extended transsphenoidal surgery." *Neurosurgery* 54, no. 3 (March 2004): 653–660; discussion 660–661. Available online. URL: http://www.ncbi.nlm.nih.gov/entrez/query.fcgi?cmd=Retrieve&db=PubMed&list_uids=15028140&dopt=Abstract.. Accessed February 11, 2006.

Kligman, Albert H. "Topical treatments for photoaged skin." *Postgraduate Medicine* 102, no. 2 (August 1997). Available online. URL: http://www.postgradmed.com/issues/1997/08_97/kligman.htm. Accessed June 17, 2005.

Lee, W. J., J. S. Chu, S. J. Houng, M. F. Chung, S. M. Wang, and K. M. Chen. "Breast cancer angiogenesis: a quantitative morphologic and Doppler imaging study." *Annals of Surgical Oncology* 2, no. 3 (1995): 246–251. Available online. URL: http://www.annalssurgicaloncology.org/cgi/content/abstract/2/3/246. Accessed February 21, 2005.

Lev, Dorit, Miriam Yanoov, Shlomo Weintraub, and Tally Leman-Sagie. "Progressive neurological deterioration in a child with distal arthrogryposis and whistling face." *Journal of Medical Genetics* 37 (March 2000): 231–233. Available online. URL: http://jmg.bmjjournals.com/cgi/content/full/37/3/231. Accessed February 24, 2005.

Litwin, M. S., M. Relihan, and L. Sillin. "Filtration characteristics of dacron wool (Swank) blood transfusion filters." *Southern Medical Journal* 68, no. 6 (June 1975): 694–698. Available online. URL: http://www.ncbi.nlm.nih.gov/entrez/query.fcg?cmd=Retrieve&db=PubMed&list_uids=124463&dopt=Abstract. Accessed April 18, 2005.

Lockwood, T. "High-lateral-tension abdominoplasty with superficial fascial system suspension." *Plastic and Reconstructive Surgery* 96, no. 3 (September 1995): 603–615. Available online. URL: http://www.ncbi.nlm.nih.gov/entrez/query.fcgi?cmd=Retrieve&db=PubMed&list_uids=7638284&dopt=Abstract. Accessed February 25, 2005.

Mancuso, A., and G. A. Farber. "The abraded punch graft for pitted facial scars." *Journal of Dermatology and Surgical Oncology* 17, no. 1 (January 1991): 32–34. Available online. URL: http://www.ncbi.nlm.nih.gov/entrez/query.fcgi?cmd=Retrieve&db=PubMed&list_uids=1825093&dopt=Abstract. Accessed April 19, 2005.

McCabe, Daniel. "Pain Pioneer Earns Killam Prize." *McGill Reporter,* June 7, 2001. Available online. URL: http://www.mcgill.ca/reporter/33/7/melzack/. Accessed June 9, 2006.

McClintock, Jack. "Bloodsuckers." *Discover* 22, no. 12 (December 2001). Available online. URL: http://www.discover.com/issues/dec-01/features/featblood/. Accessed June 9, 2006.

Meltzer, D. I. "Complications of Body Piercing." *American Family Physician* 72, no. 10 (November 15, 2005): 2029–2039. Available online. URL: http://www.aafp.org/afp/20051115/2029.html. Accessed August 30, 2006.

Miller, P. J., Daniel Grinberg, and Tom D. Wang. "Midline cleft: Treatment of the bifid nose." *Archives of Facial Plastic Surgery* 1, no. 3 (July–September 1999): 200–203. Available online. URL: http://archfaci.ama-assn.org/cgi/content/abstract/1/3/200. Accessed July 11, 2005.

"Minimally Invasive Procedure Restores Sagging Facial Skin without Heavy Lifting." *NewsWise,* July 27, 2006. Available online. URL: http://www.newswise.com/p/articles/view/522212/. Accessed August 23, 2006.

Mole, B. "Lip rejuvenation using chemical abrasion and padding with expanded polytetrafluoroethylene implant." *Aesthetic Plastic Surgery* 20, no. 3 (May–June 1996): 235–242. Available online. URL: http://www.ncbi.nlm.nh.gov/entrez/query.fcgi?cmd=Retrieve&db=PubMed&list_uids=8670390&dopt=Abstract. Accessed May 5, 2006.

Morgan, R. F., L. S. Nichter, H. I. Friedman, and F. C. McCue III. "Rodeo roping thumb injuries." *American Journal of Hand Surgery* 9, no. 2 (March 1984): 178–180. Available online. URL: http://www.ncbi.nlm.nih.nih.gov/entrez/query.fcgi?cmd=Retrieve&db=PubMed&list_uids=6715819&dopt=Abstract. Accessed May 14, 2006.

Most, S., and S. Lee. "Efficacy of an Over-the-counter Lip Enhancer in Lip Augmentation." *Archives of Facial Plastic Surgery* 7, no. 3 (May–June 2005): 203–205. Available online. URL: http://archfaci.ama-assn.org/cgi/content/extract/7/3/203. Accessed February 25, 2006.

Moulin-Romsée C., A. Verdonck, J. Schoenaers, and C. Carels. "Treatment of hemifacial microsomia in a growing child: the importance of co-operation between the orthodontist and the maxillofacial surgeon." *Journal of Orthodontics* 31, no. 3 (September 2004): 190–200. Available online. URL: http://orthod.maneyjournals.org/cgi/content/full/31/3/190. Accessed June 15, 2006.

Muldoon, Matthew F., Steven D. Barger, Janine D. Flory, and Stephen B. Manuck. "Education and debate what are quality of life measurements measuring?" *British Medical Journal,* 326 (February 14, 1998): 542–545. Available online. URL: http://bmj.bmjjournals.com/cgi/content/full/316/7130/542. Accessed March 12, 2005.

Munoz, Sara Schaeffer. "Silicone Again Seeks Approval for Implant Use." *Wall Street Journal,* April 4, 2005.

Namba, K., M. Abe, Y. Narasaki, and K. Harada. "Problems and reconstruction of 'dish face' deformity due to cleft lip and palate." *Annals of Plastic Surgery* 5, no. 1 (July 1980): 7–16. Available online. URL: http://www.ncbi.nlm.nih.gov/entrez/query.fcgi?cmd=Retrieve&db=

PubMed&list_uids=7425498&dopt=Abstract. Accessed March 12, 2005.

Neergard, Lauran. "FDA tightens access to acne drug." Associated Press, August 8, 2005. Available online. URL: http://aolsvc.news.al.com/news/article.adp?id=20050812111309990008. Accessed August 30, 2005.

———. "FDA links anti-wrinkle drugs to deaths," Associated Press, February 8, 2008. Available online. URL: http://www.fda.gov/cder/drug/early-comm/botulinum-toxins.htm. Accessed February 8, 2008.

Newmeyer, W. L., III. "Sterling Bunnell, MD: the founding father." *American Journal of Hand Surgery* 28, no. 1 (January 2003): 161–164. Available online. URL: http://www.ncbi.nlm.nih.gov/entrez/query.fcgi?cmd=Retrieve&db=PubMed&list_uids=12563656&dopt=Abstract. Accessed May 10, 2005.

Patterson, R. "The Le Fort fractures: Rene Le Fort and his work in anatomical pathology." *Canadian Journal of Surgery* 34, no. 2 (April 1991): 183–184. Available online. URL: http://www.ncbi.nlm.nih.gov/entrez/query.fcgi?cmd=Retrieve&db=PubMed&list_uids=2025808&dopt=Abstract. Accessed April 30, 2006.

Pearce, Jeremy. "Bradford Cannon, 98, Surgeon Who Improved Burn Treatment, Dies." *New York Times.* January 15, 2006. Available online. URL: http://www.nytimes.com/2006/01/15/national15cannon.html.

Penn, Jack. "Penile reform." *British Journal of Plastic Surgery* 16 (1963): 287–288. Available online. URL: http://www.cirp.org/library/restoration/penn1/. Accessed April 30, 2006.

Perovic, S. V., and M. L. Djordjevic. "Metoidioplasty: a variant of phalloplasty in female transsexuals." *BJU International* 92, no. 9 (December 2003): 981–985. Available online. URL: http://www.ncbi.nlm.nih.gov/entrez/query.fcgi?cmd=Retrieve&db=PubMed&list_uids=14632860&dopt=Abstract. Accessed May 30, 2006.

Phillips, Vincent M. "Skeletal remains identification by facial reconstruction." *Forensic Science Communications* 3, no. 1 (January 2001): Available online. URL: http://www.fbi.gov/hq/lab/fsc/bakissu/jan2001/phillips.htm. Accessed January 27, 2006.

Ralph, D. J. "Phalloplasty for Female to Male Gender Reassignment." *Endocrine Abstracts* 9 (2005) S46. Available online. URL: http://www.endocrine-abstracts.org/ea/0009/ea0009s46.htm. Accessed January 28, 2006.

Ratkor, Betsy. "New cleft palate surgery gives 'amazing' results." Associated Press, August 31, 2005. Available online. URL: http://aolsvc.news.aol.com/news/article.adp?id=20050830200909990005. Accessed January 27, 2006.

Regnault, P. "Abdominoplasty by the W technique." *Plastic and Reconstructive Surgery* 55, no. 3 (March 1975): 265–274. Available online. URL: http://www.ncbi.nlm.nih.gov/entrez/query.fcgi?cmd=Retrieve&db=PubMed&list_uids=1118485&dopt=Abstract. Accessed August 3, 2005.

Rehman, J., and A. Melman. "Formation of neoclitoris from glans penis by reduction glansplasty with preservation of neurovascular bundle in male-to-female gender surgery: functional and cosmetic outcome." *Journal of Urology* 161, no. 1 (January 1999): 200–206. Available online. URL: http://www.ncbi.nlm.nih.gov/entrez/query.fcgi?cmd=Retrieve&db=PubMed&list_uids=10037398&dopt=Abstract. Accessed February 18, 2006.

Revell, Monica. "Progress in blood supply safety." *FDA Consumer Magazine,* May 1995.

"Rh factor." *The Columbia Electronic Encyclopedia,* 6th ed. New York: Columbia University Press, 2006.

Rose, E. H., M. S. Norris, T. A. Kowalski, A. Lucas, and E. J. Fleegler. "The 'cap' technique: nonmicrosurgical reattachment of fingertip amputations." *American Journal of Hand Surgery* 14, no. 3 (May 1989): 513–518. Available online. URL: http://www.ncbi.nlm.nih.gov/entrez/query.fcgi?cmd=Retrieve&db=PubMed&list_uids=8929250&dopt=Citation. Accessed July 12, 2006.

Rubenstein, Allan E. "Neurofibromatosis." *World Book Online Reference Center,* 2006. Available online. URL: http://www.aolsvc.worldbook.aol.com/wb/Article?id=ar387565. Accessed August 9, 2006.

Sackette, David L., William M. C. Rosenberg, J. A. Muir Gray, R. Brian Haynes, and W. Scott Richardson. "Evidence based medicine: What it is and what it isn't." *British Medical Journal* 312 (January 13, 1996): 71–72. Available online. URL: http://bmj.bmjjournals.com/cgi/content/full/312/7023/71. Accessed August 9, 2006.

Salam, Gohar A., and Janki P. Amin. "The basic Z-plasty." *American Family Physician* 67, no. 11 (June 1, 2003): Available online. URL: http://www.aafp.org/afp/20030601/2329.html. Accessed August 9, 2006.

Samardzic, M. M., L. G. Rasulic, and D. M. Grujicic. "Results of cable graft technique in repair of large nerve trunk lesions." *Acta Neurichir (Vienna)* 140, no. 11 (1998): 1,177–1,182. Available online. URL: http://www.ncbi.nlm.nih.gov/entrez/query.fcgi?cmd=Retrieve&db=PubMed&list_uids=9870065&dopt=Abstract. Accessed June 24, 2006.

Santoni-Rugiu, P., and R. Mazzola. "Leonardo Fioravanti (1517–1588): A barber-surgeon who influenced the development of reconstructive surgery." *Plastic and Reconstructive Surgery* 99, no. 2 (February 1997): 570–575. Available online. URL: http://www.ncbi.

nlm.nih.gov/entrez/query.fcgi?cmd=Retrieve&db=PubMed&list_uids=97182126&dopt=Citation. Accessed June 24, 2006.

Sargent, L. A., R. F. Morgam, and W. B. Davis. "John Staige Davis: Pioneer American plastic surgeon." *Clinical Plastic Surgery* 10, no. 4 (October 1983): 653–656. Available online. URL: http://www.ncbi.nlm.nih.gov/entrez/query.fcgi?cmd=Retrieve&db=PubMed&list_uids=6360481&dopt=Abstract. Accessed May 30, 2005.

Sawaizumi, T., and H. Ito. "Lengthening of the amputation stumps of the distal phalanges using the modified Ilizarov method." *Journal of Hand Surgery* 28, no. 2 (Match 2003): 316–322. Available online. URL: http://www.ncbi.nlm.nih.gov/entrez/query.fcgi?cmd=Retrieve&db=PubMed&list_uids=12671865&dopt=Abstract. Accessed June 24, 2006.

Simhon, D., T. Brosh, M. Halpern, A. Ravid, T. Vasilyev. N. Kariv, A. Katzir, and Z. Nevo. "Closure of skin incisions in rabbits by laser soldering: I: Wound healing pattern." *Laser Surgery Medicine* 35, no. 1 (2004): 1–11. Available online. URL: http://alsearch.aol.com/aol/search?invocationType=topsearchbox.search&query=sutureless+closure+define. Accessed June 30, 2006.

Singh-Ranger, Gurpreet, and Kefah Mokbel. "Capsular contraction following immediate reconstructive surgery for breast cancer—An association with methylene blue dye." *International Seminars in Surgical Oncology* 1, no. 3 (May 2004): Available online. URL: http://www.issoonline.com/content/1/1/3. Accessed June 4, 2006.

Taori, K. B., K. Mitra, N. P. Ghonge, R. O. Ghandi, and T. Mammen. "Sirenomelia Sequence [Mermaid]-Report of Three Cases." *Indian Journal of Radiological Imaging* 12, no. 3 (2002): 399–401. Available online. URL: http://www.ijri.org/articles/archives/2002-12-3/musculo_399.htm. Accessed June 4, 2006.

Thomson, H. G., and M. Lanigan. "The Cyrano nose: a clinical review of hemangiomas of the nasal tip." *Plastic and Reconstructive Surgery* 63, no. 2 (February, 1979): 155–160. Available online. URL: http://www.ncbi.nlm.nih.gov/entrez/query.fcgi?cmd=Retrieve&db=PubMed&list_uids=79116558&dopt=Citation. Accessed August 12, 2005.

Turley, P. K. "Orthodontic management of the short face patient." *Seminars in Orthodontics* 3, no. 1 (March 1997): 73. Available online. URL: http://www.ncbi.nlm.nih.gov/entrez/query.fcgi?cmd=Retrieve&db=PubMed&list_uids=9161276&dopt=Abstract. Accessed July 7, 2006.

Vangelova, Luba. "Botulinum toxin: A poison that can heal." *FDA Consumer,* December 1995.

Vayvada, H., C. Karaca, A. Menderes, and M. Yilmaz. "Question mark ear deformity and a modified surgical correction method: a case report." *Aesthetic Plastic Surgery* 29, no. 4 (July–August 2005): 251–254. Available online. URL: http://www.cbi.nlm.nih.gov/entrez/query.fcgi?cmd=Retrieve&db=PubMed&list_uids=16044239&dopt=Abstract. Accessed May 25, 2006.

Vijay, Gandhi, A. K. Chatterjee, and Sundeep Khurana. "Hemifacial atrophy treated with autologous fat transplantation." *Indian Journal of Dermatology* 50, no. 3 (2005): 150–151. Available online. URL: http://www.eijd.org/article.asp?issn=0019-5154;year=2005;volume=50;issue=3;spage=150;epage=151;aulast=Gandhi. Accessed September 18, 2008.

Vuyk, H. D. "Suture tip plasty." *Rhinology* 33, no. 1 (March 1995): 30–38. Available online. URL: http://www.ncbi.nlm.nih.gov/entrez/query.fcgi?cmd=Retrieve&db=PubMed&list_uids=7784792&dopt=Abstract. Accessed October 24, 2006.

Walker, M. A., C. B. Hurley, and J. W. May Jr. "Radial nerve cross-finger flap differential nerve contribution in thumb reconstruction." *Journal of Hand Surgery* 11, no. 6 (November 1986): 881–887. Available online. URL: http://www.ncbi.nlm.nih.gov/entrez/query.fcgi?cmd=Retrieve&db=PubMed&list_uids=3794249&dopt=Abstract. Accessed May 9, 2006.

Walsh, R. M., M. M. Davies, J. A. McGlashan, and D. A. Bowdler. "The role of the Davis graft technique in the treatment of chronic post-mastoidectomy otorrhoea." *Clinical Otolaryngology* 21, no. 2 (April 1996): 162–167. Available online. URL: http://www.ncbi.nlm.nih.gov/entrez/query.fcgi?cmd=Retrieve&db=PubMed&list_uids=8735404&dopt=Abstract. Accessed May 10, 2006.

Wang, Quincy C., and Brett A. Johnson. "Fingertip injuries." *American Family Physician* 63, no. 10 (May 25, 2001): Available online. URL: http://www.aafp.org/afp/20010515/1961.html. Accessed July 13, 2005.

Wilkins, Robert H. "Edwin Smith Surgical Papyrus." *Journal of Neurosurgery* (March 1964): 240–244. Available online. URL: http://www.neurosurgery.org/cybermuseum/pre20th/epapyrus.html. Accessed July 13, 2006.

Wood, V. E., and J. Biondi. "Treatment of the windblown hand." *American Journal of Hand Surgery* 15 (May 1990): 431–438. Available online. URL: http://www.ncbi.nlm.nih.gov/entrez/query.fcgi?cmd=Retrieve&db=PubMed&list_uids=2348061&dopt=Abstract. Accessed February 12, 2006.

Wright, Chris. "Grow jobs: Why penis enlargement is poised to become the next big thing." *The Boston Phoenix,* January 20–27, 2000. Available online. URL: http://www.bostonphoenix.com/archive/features/00/01/20/

PENIS_ENLARGEMENT.html. Accessed February 1, 2006.

Zuber, Thomas J. "Dermal Electrosurgical Shave Excision." *American Family Physician* 65, no. 9 (May 1, 2002): Available online. URL: http://www.af.org/afp/20020501/contents.html. Accessed February 10, 2006.

Zucchero, Theresa, et al. "Interferon Regulatory Factor 6 (IRF6) Gene Variants and the Risk of Isolated Cleft Lip or Palate." *New England Journal of Medicine* 351, no. 8 (August 19, 2004): 769–780. Available online. URL: http://content.nejm.org/cgi/contentshort/351/8/769. Accessed March 1, 2005.

Internet

The articles listed here are available only on the Internet. Not all Web addresses require "www."

Albright, Ann L., and Judith S. Stern. "Adipose tissue." *Encyclopedia of Sports Medicine and Science.* Available online. URL: http://www.sportsci.org/encyc/adipose/adipose.html. Accessed January 6, 2006.

American Academy of Dermatology. "Acne scarring." Available online. URL: http://www.skincarephysicians.com/acnenet/scarring.html. Accessed January 6, 2006.

———. "Soft tissue fillers." Available online. URL: http://www.aad.org/public/Publications/pamphlets/SoftTissueFillers.htm. Accessed July 13, 2006.

———. "Statement on layered closure." Available online. URL: http://www.aad.org/professionals/pramanage/practicemgmtinfo/LayeredClosure.htm. Accessed April 21, 2006.

American Academy of Family Physicians. "Botulinum toxin injections: A treatment for muscle spasms." familydoctor.org. Available online. URL: http://familydoctor.org/017.xml. Accessed January 6, 2006.

———. "Hirsutism (excess hair)." familydoctor.org. Available online. URL: http://familydoctor.org/210.xml. Accessed August 18, 2008.

———. "Warts." familydoctor.org. Available online. URL: http://familydoctor.org/105.xml. Updated July 2005.

———. "Warts." familydoctor.org. Available online. URL: http://familydoctor.org/209.xml. Updated April 2004.

American Academy of Ophthalmology. "Botulinum toxin (BOTOX®) for treating facial wrinkles." Medem.com. Available online. URL: http://www.medem.com/medlb/article_detaillb.cfm?article_ID=ZZZ7QNLURDD&sub_cat=2019. Accessed January 27, 2006.

American Academy of Orthopaedic Surgeons. "Limb lengthening." Available online. URL: http://Orthoinfo.aaos.org/fact/thr_rport.cfm?Thread_ID=310&topcategory=About%20Orthopaedics. Accessed January 8, 2006.

American Academy of Periodontology. "Periodontal (gum) disease." Available online. URL: http://www/perop.org/consumer/2a/html. Accessed October 28, 2006.

———. "Soft tissue grafts." Available online. URL: http://www.perio.org/consumer/grafts.htm. Accessed July 13, 2006.

American Association for Clinical Chemistry. "Blood gases." LabTestsOnLine. Available online. URL: http://www.labtestsonline.org/understanding/analytes/blood_gases/test.html. Accessed September 18, 2008.

American Cancer Society. "Breast reconstruction after mastectomy." Available online. URL: http://www.cancer.org/docroot/CRI/content/CRI_2_6X_Breast_Reconstruction_AfterMastecto my_5.asp. Revised August 23, 2004.

American College of Mohs Micrographic Surgery and Cutaneous Oncology (ACMMSCO). "About Mohs micrographic surgery." Available online. URL: http://www.mohscollege.org/AboutMMS.html. Accessed June 12, 2006.

American Melanoma Foundation. Available online. URL: http://www.melanomafoundation.org/facts/Facts.htm. Accessed October 24, 2006.

American Psychiatric Association. "Let's talk facts about: Depression." Available online. URL: http://www.psych.org/disasterpsych/fs/depression.cfm. Accessed January 8, 2006.

American Psychological Association. "Depression and how psychotherapy and other treatments can help people recover." Available online. URL: http://www.apa.org/pubinfo/depression.html. Accessed January 7, 2006.

American Sleep Apnea Association. "Considering surgery for snoring?" Available online. URL: http://www.sleepapnea.org/resources/pubssnoring.html. Accessed April 18, 2006.

American Society for Aesthetic Plastic Surgery. "Cosmetic plastic surgery statistics." Available online. URL: http://www.cosmeticplasticsurgerystatistics.com/statistics.html#2004-HIGHLIGHTS. Accessed May 21, 2006.

———. "Lip augmentation." Available online. URL: http://surgery.org/public/procedures-lipaug.php. Accessed April 20, 2006.

American Society of Plastic Surgeons. "Abdominoplasty/tummy tuck." Available online. URL: http://www.plasticsurgery.org/public_education/procedures/Abdominoplasty.cfm. Accessed August 15, 2005.

————. "Blepheroplasty." Available online. URL: http://www.plasticsurgery.org/public_education/procedures/Blepharoplasty.cfm. Accessed January 5, 2006.

————. "Breast reconstruction following breast removal." Available online. URL: http://www.plasticsurgery.org/public_education/procedures/BreastReconstruction.cfm. Accessed January 6, 2006.

————. "Breast reduction." Available online. URL: http://www.plasticsurgery.org/public_education/procedures/ReductionMammaplasty.cfm. Accessed January 6, 2006.

————. "Camouflage cosmetics, makeup techniques." Available online. URL: http://www.plasticsurgery.org/public_education/procedures/CamouflageCosmetics.cfm. Accessed January 6, 2006.

————. "Dermabrasion, skin refinishing." Available online. URL: http://www.plasticsurgery.org/public_education/procedures/Dermabrasion.cfm. Accessed July 3, 2006.

————. "Endoscopic plastic surgery." Available online. URL: http://www.plasticsurgery.org/news_room/Terms-and-Definitions.cfm. Accessed January 7, 2006.

————. "Facelift alternatives rid patients of neck 'wattle' without the downtime of surgery." Available online. URL: http://www.plasticsurgery.org/news_room/press_releases/Facelift-alternatives.cfm. Accessed January 7, 2006.

————. "Hair replacement." Available online. URL: http://www.plasticsurgery.org/public_education/procedures/HairReplacement.cfm. Accessed February 27, 2006.

————. "Hand surgery." Available online. URL: http://www.plasticsurgery.org/public_education/procedures/HandSurgery.cfm. Accessed September 29, 2006.

————. "Injectible fillers." Available online. URL: http://plasticsurgery.org/public_education/procedures/InjectableFillers.cfm. Accessed January 8, 2006.

————. "Jaw, cheek and chin surgery." Available online. URL: http://www.plasticsurgery.org/public_education/procedures/FacialImplants.cfm. Accessed January 8, 2006.

————. "Male breast reduction." Available online. URL: http://www.plasticsurgery.org/public_education/procedures/Gynecomastia.cfm. Accessed January 8, 2006.

————. "Mastopexy: breast lift." Available online. URL: http://www.plasticsurgery.org/public_education/procedures/Mastopexy.cfm. Accessed January 8, 2006.

————. "Pyschological aspects: Your self-image and plastic surgery." Available online. URL: http://www.plasticsurgery.org/public_education/procedures/psychological_aspects.cfm. Accessed January 6, 2006.

————. "Rhinoplasty: surgery on the nose." Available online. URL: http://www.plasticsurgery.org/public_education/procedures/Rhinoplasty.cfm. Accessed May 22, 2006.

————. "Scar revisions: surgical treatments for scars." Available online. URL: http://www.plasticsurgery.org/public_education/procedures/ScarRevision.cfm. Accessed June 29, 2006.

————. "Sclerotherapy/spider veins." Available online. URL: http://www.plasticsurgery.org/public_education procedures/Sclerotherapy.cfm. Accessed July 26, 2006.

————. "Smoking and elective plastic surgery: some surgeons say 'No' to specific procedures, PRS article reveals." Available online. URL: http://plasticsurgery.org/news_room/press_releases/Smoking-and-Elective-Plastic-Surgery.cfm. Accessed July 18, 2006.

————. "Tissue expansion: creating new skin from old." Available online. URL: http://www.plasticsurgery.org/public_education/procedures/TissueExpansion.cfm. Accessed August 30, 2006.

————. "2004 reconstructive surgery procedures." Available online. URL: http://www.plasticsurgery.org/public_education/loader.cfm?url=/commonspot/security/getfile.cfm&PageID=16160. Accessed May 21, 2006.

American Urological Association. "Vaginal anomalies: vaginal agenesis." UrologyHealth.org. Available online. URL: http://www.urologyhealth.org/pediatric/index.cfm?cat=01&topic=150. Accessed August 3, 2006.

Answers.com. "Blood Type." Available online. URL: http://www.answers.com/topic/blood-type. Accessed January 5, 2006.

Armeniapedia, the Armeniam Encyclopedia. "Varaztad Kazanjian." Available online. URL: http://www.armeniapedia.org/index.php?title=Varaztad_Kazanjian. Modified April 17, 2005.

Bashour, Mounir, and Mirelle Benchimol. "Myopia, radial keratotomy." Available online. URL: http://www.emedicine.com/oph/topic669.htm. Updated June 10, 2005.

"Belly button reshaping (umbilicoplasty)." CosmeticSurgeryAustralia. Available online. URL: http://www.cosmeticsurgeryaustralia.com.au/umbilicoplasty.htm. Accessed July 26, 2006.

Berman, Brian, and Sonia Kapoor. "Keloid and hypertrophic scar." eMedicine. Available online. URL: http://www.emedicine.com/der/topic205.htm. Updated March 3, 2005.

Biavati, Michael J., and Benjamin Bassachis. "Cleft palate." eMedicine. Available online. URL: http://www.emedicine.com/ent/topic136.htm. Updated April 21, 2003.

Biavati, Michael J., and Joseph L. Leech. "Ear reconstruction." eMedicine. Available online. URL: http://www.emedicine.com/ent/topic79.htm. Updated November 13, 2002.

"Bio-eye hydroxyapatite orbital implants." Available online. URL: http://www.ioi.com/Accessed June 26, 2006.

Brannon, Heather. "What causes wrinkles." About.Inc. Available online. URL: http://dermatology.about.com/cs/beauty/a/wrinklecause_2.htm. Accessed January 7, 2006.

"A brief history of the 'Habsburg Chin.'" Antiquesatoz.com. Available online. URL: http://www.antiquesatoz.com/habsburg/habsburg-jaw.htm. Accessed February 24, 2006.

British Association of Oral and Maxillofacial Surgeons. "Craniofacial surgery." Available online. URL: http://www.baoms.org.uk/ce/ce_canfac.html. Accessed August 21, 2006.

Brown, Clarence William Jr. "Cherry hemangioma." eMedicine. Available online. URL: http://www.emedicine.com/DERM/topic73.htm. Updated May 24, 2005.

Buford, Gregory A., and Armand R. Lucas. "Rhinoplasty, supratip deformity." eMedicine. Available online. URL: http://www.emedicine.com/plastic/topic83.htm. Updated March 15, 2005.

Calvert, J. B. "Rare earths." Available online. URL: http://www.du.edu/~jcalvert/phs/rare.htm. Accessed May 15, 2006.

Camer, Richard H. "Skin resurfacing." HealthAtoZ.com. Available online. URL: http://www.healthatoz.com/healthatoz/Atoz/ency/skin_resurfacing.jsp. Accessed January 9, 2006.

Cancer Research (UK). "Bone scan." CancerHelp.com. Available online. URL: http://www.cancerhelp.org.uk/help/default.asp?page=151. Updated March 23, 2005.

Center for Nonverbal Studies. "Blank face." Available online. URL: http://members.aol.com/nonverbal2/blank.htm. Accessed January 7, 2006.

Center for Nonverbal Studies. "Facial expressions." Available online. URL: http://members.aol.com/nonverbal3/facialx.htm. Accessed January 7, 2006.

Chakrabarty, S. P. "The Ilizarov technique." Vardaan Hospital (India). Available online. URL: http://www.vardaan.net/ilizarov.htm. Accessed January 6, 2006.

Chen, Amy Y. "Facial reanimation of the chronically paralyzed face." Baylor College of Medicine, Bobby R. Alford Department of Otorhinolaryngology and Communicative Sciences. Available online. URL: http://www.bcm.edu/oto/grand/92994.html. Accessed January 6, 2006.

Children's Hospital (Boston). "Constriction band syndrome (amniotic band syndrome)." Available online. URL: http://www.childrenshospital.org/az/Site1156/mainpageS1156P0.html. Accessed January 6, 2006.

———. "Macrodactyly." Available online. URL: http://www.childrenshospital.org/az/Site1093/mainpageS1093P0.html. Accessed May 31, 2006.

Circumcision Information and Resources Pages (CIRP). "Foreskin restoration for circumcised men." Available online. URL: http://www.cir.org/pages/restore.html. Revised February 8, 2003.

Clark, J. Madison, and Tom D. Wang. "Skin flap, design." eMedicine. Available online. URL: http://www.emedicine.com/ent/topic14.htm. Updated October 31, 2003.

Cleveland Clinic. "Collagen replacement therapy." Available online. URL: http://www.clevelandclinic.org/dermatology/patient/collagen.htm. Posted November 11, 2002.

———. "Pain management evaluation and treatment." Available online. URL: http://www.clevelandclinic.org/painmanagement/eval_treat/. Updated September 6, 2005.

Coaschini, Michael, and Steven L. Bernard. "History of plastic surgery." eMedicine. Available online. URL: http://www.emedicine.com/plastic/topic433.htm. Updated January 18, 2005.

Columbia University, College of Physicians and Surgeons, Department of Otolaryngology. "Head and neck surgery, eyelash transplant." Available online. URL: http://www.entcolumbia.org/eyelash.htm. Accessed October 24, 2006.

"Common and minor complications." Liposuction.com. Available online. URL: http://www.liposuction.com/safety/common_minor.php. Accessed January 6, 2006.

"Compression Garments FAQs." BeautySurg.com. Available online. URL: http://www.beautysurg.com/index.html. Accessed July 21, 2006.

Conway, Lynn. "Vaginoplasty: male to female sex reassignment surgery." Available online. URL: http://ai.eecs.umich.edu/people/conway/TS/SRS.html. Updated October 14, 2005.

Cordes, Stephanie. "Reanimation of the paralyzed face." Available online. URL: http://www.utmb.edu/otoref/Grnds/Reanimation-9811/reanimation.html. Posted November 11, 1998.

"Cosmetic procedures: laser tattoo removal." WebMD. Available online. URL: http://www.webmd.com/content/article/76/90242.htm. Accessed August 29, 2006.

"Cosmetic surgery safer under local anesthetic." MacLeans.Ca. Available online. URL: http://www.macleans.

ca/topstories/health/article.jsp?content=20050420_103620_3628. Posted April 20, 2005.

"Craniostenosis." drkoop.com. Available online. URL: http://drkoop.com/encyclopedia/93/30.html. Accessed January 6, 2006.

"Definition of Bell, Charles." MedicineNet.com. Available online. URL: http://www.medterms.com/script/main/art.asp?articlekey=39326. Accessed June 10, 2006.

"Definition of 'body surface area.'" MedicineNet.com. Available online. URL: http://www.medterms.com/script/main/art.asp?articlekey=39851. Accessed September 17, 2006.

DeLaria, Giacomo A. "Gangrene." Available online. URL: http://www.aolsvc.worldbook.aol.com/wb/Article?id=ar216460&st=Gangrene. Accessed January 7, 2006.

"Dental health: dental bonding." WebMD.com. Available online. URL: http://webmd.com/oral-health/guide/dental-bonding. Reviewed March 7, 2007.

"Dental health: veneers." WebMD.com. Available online. URL: http://webmd.com/content/article/66/79605.htm?z=4208_00000_9001_to_08. Edited May 2005.

Department of Physics and Astronomy, Georgia State University. "Ruby Laser." HyperPhysics.com. Available online. URL: http://hyperphysics.phyastr.gsu.edu/hbase/optmod/lassol.html. Accessed May 16, 2006.

"Dermatologists use antigen shots to alleviate warts without scarring." Newswise.com. Available online. URL: http://www.newswise.com/articles/view/513144/?sc=mwtr. Updated July 14, 2005.

"Diagnostic laparoscopy." MedlinePlus.com. Available online. URL: http://www.nm.nih.gov/medlineplus/ency/article/003918.htm. Updated July 14, 2006.

Duke University Medical Center. "Cheek augmentation." Available online. URL: http://www.dukehealth.org/ServicesAndLocations/Services/Aesthetics/Procedures/Enhancements/CheekAugmentation. Accessed January 6, 2006.

"Electrolysis." Hairfacts.com. Available online. URL: http://www.hairfacts.com/methods/electro/electrolysis.html. Revised December 30, 2001.

"Electrolysis guide." TransGenderCare. Available online. URL: http://www.transgendercare.com/electrolysis/methods/epilators.htm. Accessed February 16, 2006.

Englewood Hospital and Medical Center. "Techniques to make bloodless surgery possible." Available online. URL: http://www.bloodlessmed.com/Pags/BS_methods.htm. Accessed January 9, 2006.

Esan, Temitope, and Adeyemi Oluniyi Olusile. "Hemifacial atrophy: a case report and review of literature." *The Internet Journal of Dental Science* 1, no. 1 (2004). Available online. URL: http://www.spub.com/ostia/index.php?xmlFilePath=journals/ijds/vol1n1/hemifacial.xml. Accessed March 4, 2006.

Ethicon, Inc. "Skin replacement." Available online. URL: http://www.skinhealing.com/3_3_burntreatments.shtml. Accessed January 9, 2006.

Facial Plastic Surgery Network. "Lip reduction." Available online. URL: http://www.facialplasticsurgery.net/lip_reduction.htm. Updated November 3, 2003.

Fardo, Dean, and Gregory A. Buford. "Facelift, skin only." eMedicine. Available online. URL: http://www.emedicine.com/plastic/topic49.htm. Accessed July 2, 2006.

Fishman, Scott M. "Fifth Vital Sign." Painfoundation.org. Available online. URL: http://www.painfoundation.org/page.asp?file=QandA/FifthVitalSign.htm. Posted January 2004.

Food and Drug Administration, Center for Devices and Radiological Health, *FDA Breast Implant Consumer Handbook* (2004). Available online. URL: http://www.fda.gov/cdrh/breastimplants/handbook2004/specificissues.html. Updated June 8, 2004.

"Frequently asked questions about buccal fat pad extraction." Facial Plastic Surgery Network. Available online. URL: http://www.facialplasticsurgery.net/buccal_fat_faq.htm#1. Accessed January 7, 2006.

Gabriel, Barbara A. "A Hippocratic oath for our time." AAMC Reporter, September 2001. Available online. URL: http://www.aamc.org/newsroom/reporter/sept2001/hippocraticoath.htm. Accessed March 20, 2006.

Gatti, John M., and Andrew J. Kirsch. "Hypospadias." eMedicine. Available online.URL: http://www.emedicine.com/PED/topic1136.htm. Accessed May 28, 2006.

"Gender identity disorder, disorder information sheet." PsycheNet-UK. Available online. URL: http://www.psychnet-uk.com/dsm_iv/gender_identity_disorder.htm. Accessed January 7, 2006.

"George Crile." WhoNamedIt.com. Available online. URL: http://www.whonamedit.com/doctor.cfm/1959.html. Accessed January 7, 2006.

Gibson, F. Brian. "Facial reanimation and rehabilitation." Available online. URL: http://www.utmb.edu/oto/Grand_Rounds_Earlier.dir/Face_Reanimation_1990.txt. Posted December 19, 1990.

Goodheart, Herbert P., and Hendrik I. Uyttendaele. "Hirsutism." eMedicine. Available online. URL: http://www.emedicine.com/DERM/topic472.htm. Updated February 24, 2006.

Gore Medical Products. "Where Thoracic Surgery Is Going." Available online. URL: http://www.goremedical.com/English/index.htm. Accessed January 6, 2006.

Gosselin, Benoit J. "Malignant Tumors of the Mobile Tongue." EMedicine. Available online. URL: http://www.emedicine.com/ENT/topic256.htm. Updated May 4, 2006.

"The Gram Stain." Microbiology @ Leicester. Available online. URL: http://www.micro.msb.le.ac.uk/Video/Gram.html. Accessed February 18, 2006.

Greenwald, A. Seth, Christine Heim, Harri Reddi, Randy Rosier, Harvinder Sandhu, and Donna Toohey. "Profile of orthopaedic accomplishment: Marshall R. Urist, MD." 2004 Annual Meeting Edition of the AAOS (American Academy of Orthopedic Surgeons) Bulletin, March 11, 2004. Available online. URL: http://www.aaos.org/wordhtml/2004news/c11-4.htm. Posted March 11, 2004.

Haines, Cynthia, ed. "Breast augmentation." WebMD. Available online. URL: http://aolsvc.health.webmd.aol.com/content/article/76/90226.htm. Accessed January 4, 2006.

———. "Cosmetic procedures: hair removal." WebMD. Available online. URL: http://www.webmd.com/content/article/76/90229.htm. Accessed January 5, 2006.

"Hammer, Claw, and Mallet Toes." Available online. URL: http://aolsvc.health.webmd.aol.com/hw/foot_problems/hw143429.asp?src=AOLConditionWidget. Updated July 19, 2005.

Hannibal, Matthew, and Daniel Roger. "Gamekeeper's thumb." eMedicine. Available online. URL: http://www.emedicine.com/orthoped/topic112.htm. January 5, 2006.

"Hemangioma." AllRefer.com. Available online. URL: http://health.allrefer.com/health/hemangioma-info.html. January 4, 2006.

"Hemangioma." MedlinePlus, U.S. National Library of Medicine. Available online. URL: http://www.nlm.nih.gov/medlineplus/ency/article/001459.htm. Updated October 29, 2004.

Henry, Kimberly A., and Penny S. Heckaman. "Permanent tattoo for lips, eyebrows and eyeliner." WebMD. Available online. URL: http://www.webmd.com/content/article/85/98423.htm. Accessed May 6, 2006.

"Hippocratic Oath." Available online. URL: http://www.bbc.co.uk/dna/h2g2/A1103798. Accessed September 18, 2008.

Hom, David B. "Incision Placement." eMedicine. Available online. URL: http://www.emedicine.com/ent/topic34.htm. Updated July 5, 2005.

Huang, Conway. "Scalp reconstruction." eMedicine. Available online. URL: http://www.emedicine.com/derm/topic906.htm. Updated October 28, 2004.

"Hyperelastic skin." AllRefer.com. Available online. URL: http://health.allrefer.com/health/hyperelastic-skin-info.html. Accessed September 18, 2008.

"Intense pulsed light therapy." DermNetNZ. Available online. URL: http://www.der mnetnz.org/procedures/ipl.html. Accessed July 4, 2006.

International Hyperhidrosis Society. "Botulism toxin injection." Available online. URL: http://www.sweathelp.org/English/PFF_Treatment_Injections.asp. Accessed January 4, 2006.

"Intersex." MedlinePlus. Available online. URL: http://www.nlm.nih.gov/medlineplus/ency/article/001669.htm. Updated October 15, 2007.

Ipsen. "Ipsen product list." Available online. URL: http://www.ipsen.com/?page-products. Accessed September 18, 2008.

Jansen, David A., and Jennifer McGee. "Flaps, muscle and musculocutaneous flaps." eMedicine. Available online. URL: http://www.emedicine.com/plastic/topic472.htm. Accessed June 5, 2006.

Jiang, S. Brian. "MOHS surgery." eMedicine. Available online. URL: http://www.emedicine.com/ent/topic29.htm. Accessed June 11, 2006.

"Johan Friedrich Dieffenbach." WhoNamedIt. Available online. URL: http://www.whonamedit.com/doctor.cfm/1959.html. Accessed January 8, 2006.

Johnson, Carla K. "Tongue piercing linked to severe facial pain." Available online. URL: http://articles.news.aol.com/news/_a/tongue-piercing-linked-to-severefacial/20061017160409990005?cid=2194. Accessed August 21, 2008.

"Key gene controls skin colour." BBCNews, December 16, 2005. Available online. URL: http://news.bbc.co.uk/2/hi/health/4531966.stm. Accessed July 15, 2006.

Khosh, Maurice M. "Upper eyelid reconstruction." eMedicine. Available online. URL: http://www.emedicine.com/ent/topic83.htm. Updated November 18, 2003.

Kilpatrick, Jefferson K., and Keith A. LaFerriere. "Rhytidectomy, deep plane facelift." eMedicine. Available online. URL: http://www.emedicine.com/ent/topic131.htm. Updated July 11, 2003.

Kremkau, Frederick W. "Ultrasound." Available online. URL: http://www.aolsvc.worldbook.aol.com/wb/Article?id=ar573860. Accessed July 24, 2006.

Kuwahara, Raymond T. "Chemical peels." eMedicine. Available online. URL: http://www.emedicine.com/derm/topic533.htm. Updated August 5, 2005.

Lai, Stephen Y., and Daniel G. Becker. "Sutures and needles." eMedicine. Available online. URL: http://www.emedicine.com/ent/topic38.htm. Accessed July 11, 2006.

Langford, F. P. Johns. "Nasal reconstruction following soft tissue resection." eMedicine. Available online. URL: http://www.emedicine.com/ent/topic655.htm. Updated October 3, 2005.

"Laser history." About.Inc. Available online. URL: http://inventors.about.com/library/inventors/bllaser.htm. Accessed May 27, 2006.

"Laser-assisted uvulopalatoplasty." WebMD. Available online. URL: http://www.webmd.com/hw/health_guide_atoz/aa75802.asp. Updated August 3, 2005.

"Leg length discrepency." Orthoseek.com. Available online. URL: http://www.orthoseek.com/articles/leg-length.html. Accessed May 6, 2006.

Lehnert, Paul. "Laser surgery for warts." Yahoo! Health. Available online. URL: http://health.yahoo.com/ency/healthwise/hw61559. Updated November 17, 2004.

"Liposuction techniques." Liposuction.com. Available online. URL: http://www.liposuction.com/lipoinfo/lipo_techniques.php. Accessed January 8, 2006.

Loftus, Jean M. "Wrinkles." InfoPlasticSurgery.com. Available online. URL: http://www.infoplasticsurgery.com/facial/wrinkletreatment/index.html. Accessed January 27, 2006.

Louis Calder Memorial Library. "Dr. Ralph Millard." Available online. URL: http://calder.me d.miami.edu/Ralph_Millard/index.html. Accessed January 7, 2006.

Lustig, J., H. Librus, and A. Neder. "Bipedicled myomucosal flap for reconstruction of the lip after vermilionectomy." Available online. URL: http://www.ncbi.nlm.nih.gov/entrez/query.fcgi?cmd=Retrieve&db=PubMed&list_uids=8065722&dopt=Abstract. Accessed August 7, 2006.

"Lymph system." MedlinePlus, U.S. National Library of Medicine. Available online. URL: http://www.nlm.nih.gov/medlineplus/ency/article/002247.htm. Updated October 23, 2004.

"May 2001—Machines, methods and mechanics of human hair removal." Consumerbeware.com. Available online. URL: http://www.consumerbeware.com/cbs0501.htm. Accessed February 12, 2006.

March of Dimes. "Cleft lip and cleft palate." Available online. URL: http://www.marchofdimes.com/professionals/681_1210.asp. Accessed August 21, 2008.

Meals, Roy A. "De Quervain tenosynovitis." EMedicine. Available online. URL: http://www.emedicine.com/orthoped/topic482.htm. Accessed September 18, 2008.

Mercandetti, Michael, and Adam J. Cohen. "Facelift, SMAS plication." eMedicine. Available online. URL: http://www.emedicine.com/plastic/topic50.htm. Accessed July 2, 2006.

———. "Implants, soft tissue, Gore-Tex." WebMD. Available online. URL: http://www.emedicine.com/ent/topic376.htm. Updated August 2, 2005.

———. "Wound healing, healing and repair." eMedicine. Available online. URL: http://www.emedicine.com/plastic/topic411.htm. Updated August 1, 2006.

Microtitia-Congenital Ear Institute. "Microtia overview." Available online. URL: http://www.microtia.net/Webpages.asp?WPID=3. Accessed January 8, 2006.

Midha, Rajiv. "Peripheral nerve repair and grafting techniques: a review." Available online. URL: http://ots.utoronto.ca/users/howardg/nerverepair.html.

Nahabedian, Maurice Y. "Flaps, free tissue transfer." eMedicine. Available online. URL: http://www.emedicine.com/plastic/topic473.htm. Updated June 26, 2005.

National Blood Data Resource Center. "FAQs." Available online. URL: http://www.aabb.org/About_the_AABB/Nbdrc/faqs.htm. Accessed January 7, 2006.

National Center for Complementary and Alternative Medicine. "Get the facts: acupuncture." Available online. URL: http://nccam.nih.gov/health/acupuncture/. Accessed June 16, 2006.

National Institute for Clinical Excellence (U.K.). "Interventional procedures consultation document-transilluminated powered phlebectomy for varicose veins." Available online. URL: http://www.nice.org.uk/page.aspx?o=83862. Accessed January 8, 2006.

National Institute of Allergy and Infectious Diseases. "The immune system." Available online. URL: http://www.niaid.nih.gov/final/immun/immun.htm. Updated September 25, 2003.

National Institute of Arthritis and Musculoskeletal and Skin Diseases. "Acne." Available online. URL: http://www.niams.nih.gov/hi/topics/acne/acne.htm. Posted October 2001.

National Institute of Neurological Disorders and Stroke. "Chiari malformation information page." Available online. URL: http://www.ninds.nih.gov/disorders/chiari/chiari.htm. Updated February 9, 2005.

National Kidney and Transplant Division of Urology (Philippines). "Oath and law of Hippocrates." Available online. URL: http://members.tripod.com/nktiuro/hippocra.htm. Accessed March 21, 2006.

National Necrotizing Fasciitis Foundation. "Necrotizing fasciitis." Available online. URL: http://www.nnff.org/nnff_factsheet.htm. Accessed June 18, 2008.

———. "Chloasma." Available online. URL: http://dermnetnz.org/colour/melasma.html. Updated June 14, 2005.

New Zealand Dermatological Society. "Fat grafting." Available online. URL: http://dermnetnz.org/procedures/fat-implants.html. Updated May 29, 2005.

———. "Myxoma syndrome." Available online. URL: http://www.dermnetnz.org/systemic/myxoma.html. Updated April 4, 2006.

———. "Thermage." Available online. URL: http://www.dermnetnz.org/procedures/thermage.html. Accessed August 24, 2006.

Nova Online. "Hippocratic oath: classic version." Available online. URL: http://www.pbs.org/wgbh/nova/doctors/oath_classical.html. Accessed March 20, 2006.

"Odor reducing dressings." Family Practice Notebook. Available online. URL: http://www.fpnotebook.com/SUR105.htm. Accessed January 6, 2006.

Oklulicz, Jason F., and Sergius Jozwiak. "Lentigo." eMedicine. Available online. URL: http://www.emedicine.com/DERM/topic221.htm. Updated July 14, 2005.

"Orbital reconstruction/ocular prosthetics (false eyes)." EyeMDLink.com. Available online. URL: http://www.eyemdlink.com/EyeProcedure.asp?EyeProcedureID=35. Accessed June 26, 2006.

Oregon Health and Science University. "Ice packs vs. warm compresses for pain." Available online. URL: http://www.ohsuhealth.com/htaz/ortho/treatmen/ice_packs_vs_warm_compresses_for_pain.cfm. Accessed January 7, 2006.

———. "Cardiovascular diseases: vital signs." Available online. URL: http://www.ohsuhealth.com/htaz/cardiac/vital_signs.cfm. Accessed July 28, 2006.

"Over-the-counter facial stimulators do little to enhance aging skin." Newswise.com. Available online. URL: http://www.newswise.com/articles/view/517384/?sc=mwtr. Posted January 18, 2006.

"Over-the-counter lip enhancers fail to deliver promises." Newswise. Available online. URL: http://www.newswise.com/articles/view/511875/?sc=mwtr. Posted May 16, 2005.

Palo Alto Medical Foundation. "Thigh/buttock lift." Available online. URL: http://www.pamf.org/cosmeticsurgery/procedures/thighbutt_lift.html. Accessed January 9, 2006.

"Penile implants for erection problems." WebMD. Available online. URL: http://my.webmd.com/hw/impotence/hw111556.asp. Updated April 1, 2005.

Persoff, Myron M. "Uses of the postoperatively adjustable implant in aesthetic breast surgery." eMedicine. Available online. URL: http://www.emedicine.com/plastic/topic507.htm. Updated June 24, 2005.

"Phantom pain." MayoClinic.com. Available online. URL: http://www.mayoclinic.com/invoke.cfm?=DS00444. Posted November 9, 2005.

"Platinum in breast implants." CNN.com. Available online. URL: http://www.cnn.com/aol/story/2004/08/26/cnn_HEALTH_breast.implants.ap.html. Posted August 26, 2004.

"Port wine stain." MedlinePlus, U.S. National Library of Medicine. Available online. URL: http://www.nlm.nih.gov/medlineplus/ency/article/001475.htm. Updated July 22, 2005.

Potted Biography. "Who was Ilizarov." Available online. URL: http://www.ilizarov.org.uk/biog.htm. Accessed January 6, 2006.

Prasad, Srinivasa, and Dushyant Sahani. "Cavernous hemangioma, liver." eMedicine. Available online. URL: http://www.emedicine.com/radio/topic136.htm. Updated May 16, 2003.

Radiological Society of North America. "Computed tomography (CT)-body." Radiology Info. Available online. URL: http://www.radiologyinfo.org/content/ct_of_the_body.htm. Accessed August 25, 2005.

———. "General nuclear medicine." Radiology Info. Available online. URL: http://www.radiologyinfo.org/en/info.cfm?pg=gennuclear&bhcp=1. Accessed August 9, 2006.

———. "MRI imaging-body." Radiology Info. Available online. URL: http://www.radiologyinfo.org/content/mr_of_the_body.htm. Accessed June 5, 2006.

Radio National: The Health Report with Norman Swan. "Fat cells in our bodies." Available online. URL: http://www.abc.net.au/rn/tals/8.30/helthrpt/stories/s20847.htm. Posted March 29, 1999.

"Results with newer bladeless LASIK equivalent to standard microkeratome LASIK." Newswise. Available online. URL: http://www.newswise.com/p/articles/view/520056/. Accessed May 3, 2006.

Revis, Don R., and Michael B. Seagel. "Skin, grafts." eMedicine. Available online. URL: http://www.emedicine.com/plastic/topic392.htm. Updated November 5, 2003.

———. "Skin resurfacing: chemical peels." eMedicine. Available online. URL: http://www.emedicine.com/ent/topic625.htm. Updated October 27, 2005.

Robinson, Michael E. "Mallet finger." eMedicine. Available online. URL: http://www.emedicine.com/sports/topic72.htm. Updated November 23, 2005.

Rosenberg, Lawrence, and Jorge de la Torre. "Wound healing, growth factors." eMedicine. Available online. URL: http://www.emedicine.com/plastic/topic457.htm. Updated February 17, 2006.

Royal Children's Hospital(UK). "Burn diagram." Clinical Practice Guidelines. Available online. URL: http://rwh.org.au/clinicalguide/cpg.cfm?doc_id=5250. Accessed July 5, 2006.

Schmucker, Tracy M., and Roy Hampton, Sr. "Xanthelasma." eMedicine. Available online. URL: http://www.emedicine.com/oph/topic610.htm. Updated November 17, 2004.

Schwade, Nathan C. "Wound adhesives, 2-octylcyanoacrylate." eMedicine. Available online. URL: http://www.emedicine.com/ent/topic375.htm. Updated June 6, 2005.

Sclafani, Anthony P., and Michael Fozo. "Rotation flaps." eMedicine. Available online. URL: http://www.emedicine.com/ent/topic654.htm. Accessed May 16, 2006.

"Septoplasty." MedLinePLus. Available online. URL: http://www.nlm.nih.gov/medlineplus/ency/article/003012.htm. Updated January 30, 2008.

Sheldon, Nina. "SMAS refinement offers superior cheek elevation." Cosmetic Surgery Times, March 1, 2005. Available online. URL: http://www.cosmeticsurgery times.com/cosmeticsurgerytimes/article/articleDetail.jsp?id=147515. Accessed September 18, 2008.

Shenaq, Saleh M., and Aldona J. Spiegel. "Hand, brachial plexus surgery." eMedicine. Available online. URL: http://www.emedicine.com/plastic/topic450.htm. Updated October 7, 2002.

Sheridan, Robert L. "Burns, rehabilitation and reconstruction." eMedicine. Available online. URL: http://www.emedicine.com/plastic/topic155.htm. Updated July 22, 2005.

Sheth, Raj D. "Café au lait spots." eMedicine. Available online. URL: http://www.emedicine.com/ped/topic2754.htm. Updated October 31, 2002.

"Short-Form McGill pain questionnaire: I. pain rating index (PRI)." Available online. URL: http://www.med.umich.edu/obgyn/repro-endo/Lebovicresearch/Pain Survey.pdf. Accessed June 9, 2006.

"Skin, abnormally dark or light." MedlinePlus, U.S. National Library of Medicine. Available online. URL: http://www.nlm.nih.gov/medlineplus/ency/article/003242.htm. Updated July 22, 2005.

Skin Cancer Foundation. "Actinic keratosis: what you should know about this common precancer." Available online. URL: http://www.skincancer.org/ak/index.php. Accessed April 7, 2006.

"Skin cancer: melanoma." WebMd. Available online. URL: http://aolsvc.health.webmd.aol.com/hw/cancer/hw206764.asp?pagenumber=3. Updated January 28, 2005.

Smith, Jeffrey B., and Sidney B. Smith. "Cutaneous manifestations of smoking." eMedicine. Available online. URL: http://www.emedicine.com/derm/topic629.htm. Accessed July 18, 2006.

"Special plastic surgery needed for soaring obese population." Newswise, June 21, 2006. Available online. URL: http://www.newswise.com/articles/view/521416/?sc=mwtr. Accessed June 22, 2006.

Stavile, Karen L., and Richard Sinert. "Metabolic acidosis." eMedicine. Available online. URL: http://www.emedicine.com/emerg/topic312.htm. Updated September 22, 2005.

"Stem cell research hints at better looking cosmetic, reconstructive surgery." Newswise, February 16, 2005. Available online. URL: http://www.newswise.com/articles/view/509895/?sc=mwtr. Accessed July 17, 2006.

Stevens, Rusty, Karen Calhoun, and Francis B. Quinn. "Facial analysis." Department of Otolaryngology, UTMB, Galveston, Texas. Available online. URL: http://www.utmb.edu/otoref/grnds/facial2.html. Accessed April 13, 2006.

Streeten, David H. P. "General organization of the autonomic nervous system." Available online. URL: http://www.ndrf.org/ans.htm#FunctionsoftheAutonomicNervousSystem. Modified February 7, 2002.

"Surgeon who pioneered burn treatment dies." AP Wire. Available online. URL: http://www.bradenton.com/mld/bradenton/living/health/13509208.htm. Posted December 29, 2005.

Surgical-Tutor.org. UK. "Wound dressings." Available online. URL: http://surgical-tutor.org.uk/default-home.htm?core/preop2/dressings.htm%7Eright. Updated December 27, 2005.

"Surgical treatment of erectile dysfunction." EMedicine. Available online. URL: http://www.emedicinehealth.com/articles/44788-4.asp. Accessed January 9. 2006.

Taylor, Ben, and Ardeshir Bayat. "Basic plastic surgery techniques and principles: Choosing the right suture material." studentBMJ. Available online. URL: http://www.studentbmj.com/issues/03/05/education/140.php. Accessed July 14, 2006.

"Teeth whitening." iEnhance.com. Available online. URL: http://www.ienhance.com/cosmeticdentist/teeth whitening.asp. Accessed January 8, 2006.

Tennessee Craniofacial Center. "Maxillary fractures." Available online. URL: http://www.craniofacialcenter.com/book/Trauma/Trauma_3.htm. Accessed May 4, 2006.

Terhune, Margaret. "Materials for wound closure." eMedicine. Available online. URL: http://www.emedicine.com/derm/topic825.htm. Updated December 21, 2005.

"Tongue splitting: forking the tongue." InfoPLasticSurgery.com. Available online. URL: http://www.infoplasticsurgery.com/facial/tonguesplitting.html. Accessed August 30, 2006.

Tsue, Terry, and Douglas A. Girod. "Free tissue transfer, osteocutaneous radial forearm flap." eMedicine. Available online. URL: http://www.emedicine.com/ent/topic720.htm. Updated July 15, 2005.

United Crystals Company. "Potassium titanyl phosphate." Available online. URL: http://www.unitedcrystals.com/KTPProp.html. Accessed January 9, 2006.

U.S. Food and Drug Administration. "Breast implants: saline-filled breast implant surgery: making an informed decision (Mentor Corporation)." Available online. URL: http://www.fda.gov/cdrh/breastimplants/labeling/mentor_patient_labeling_5900.html. Accessed June 27, 2006.

———. "The darker side of tanning." Available online. URL: http://www.fda.gov/cdrh/consumer/tanning.html. Accessed August 22, 2006.

————. "FDA clears medicinal leeches for marketing." Available online. URL: http://altmedicine.about.com/gi/dynamic/offsite.htm?zi=1/XJ&sdn=altmedicine&zu=http%3A%2F%2Fwww.fda.gov%2Fbbs%2Ftopics%2Fanswers%2F2004%2FANS01294.html. Accessed April 12, 2006.

————. "Lasik eye surgery." Available online. URL: http://www.fda.gov/cdrh/lasik/. Updated March 9, 2005.

————. "Premier ink shades associated with adverse reactions." Available online. URL: http://www.cfsan.fda.gov/~dms/cos-tat2.html.

————. "Tattoos and permanent makeup." Available online. URL: http://www.cfsan.fda.gov/~dms/cos-204.html. Accessed September 18, 2008.

U.S. Department of Labor, Bureau of Labor Statistics. "Chiropractors." Available online. URL: http://stats.bls.gov/oco/ocos071.htm. Modified December 20, 2005.

University of California, San Diego. "A practical guide to clinical medicine." Available online. URL: http://medicine.ucsd.edu/clinicalmed/vital.htm. Accessed July 28, 2006.

University of Maastricht. "A randomised controlled trial comparing vacuum assisted closure (V.A.C.(r)) with modern wound dressings." Available online. URL: http://www.clinicaltrials.gov/ct/show/NCT00243620. Accessed August 2, 2006.

University of Michigan Health System, Plastic Surgery. "Osteoarthritis." Available online. URL: http://www.med.umich.edu/surgery/plastic/clinical/hand/osteoarthritis/index.shtml. Accessed October 26, 2006.

————. "Rheumatoid arthritis." Available online. URL: http://www.med.umich.edu/surgery/plastic/clinical/hand/rheumatoid/index.shtml. Accessed October 26, 2006.

University of Virginia Health System. "Micropenis." Available online. URL: http://www.healthsystem.virginia.edu/uvahealth/peds_urology/mcrpenis.cfm. Accessed June 13, 2006.

Vaughn, Glen. "Fingertip injuries." eMedicine. Available online. URL: http://www.emedicine.com/emerg/topic179.htm. Updated April 26, 2005.

"Varicose veins." MayoClinic.com. Available online. URL: http://www.mayoclinic.com/health/varicose-veins/DS00256. Accessed July 24, 2006.

"Varicose veins." WebMD. Available online. URL: http://aolsvc.health.webmd.aol.com/hw/skin_and_beauty/hw113840.asp?pagenumber=4. Accessed August 1, 2006.

"Varicose vein therapy." MedlinePlus. Available online. URL: http://www.nlm.nih.gov/medlineplus/ency/article/002952.htm. Updated March 1, 2005.

Vartanian, A. John, and Steven H. Dayan. "Nonablative facial skin tightening." eMedicine. Available online. URL: http://www.emedicine.com/ent/topic769.htm. Accessed August 9, 2006.

Vartanian, A. John, and J. Regan Thomas. "Rhinoplasty, Saddle Nose." eMedicine. Available online. URL: http://www.emedicine.com/Ent/topic121.htm. Accessed September 18, 2008.

"Vein ligation and stripping." WebMD. Available online. URL: http://aolsvc.health.webmd.aol.com/hw/health_guide_atoz/hw113736.asp. Updated August 25, 2004.

"Vital signs." Medline Plus. Available online. URL: http://www.nlm.nih.gov/medlineplus/ency/article/002341.htm. Accessed July 28, 2006.

Wang, Peter, and Vipul R. Dev. "Lip reduction." eMedicine. Available online. URL: http://www.emedicine.com/plastic/topic66.htm. Accessed June 1, 2006.

Weiss, Robert, and Albert-Adrien Ramelet. "Varicose veins treated with ambulatory phlebectomy." eMedicine. Available online. URL: http://www.emedicine.com/derm/topic748.htm. Updated November 25, 2004.

Whitaker, Elizabeth. "Facelift, composite." eMedicine. Available online. URL: http://www.emedicine.com/plastic/topic44.htm. Accessed July 2, 2006.

Wilhelmi, Bradon J., and Michael Neumeister. "Hand, finger nail and tip injuries." eMedicine. Available online. URL: http://www.emedicine.com/plastic/topic309.htm. Updated January 8, 2002.

Woodbury, Kerri M., and Keither Robertson. "Flaps, fasciocutaneous flaps." eMedicine. Available online. URL: http://www.emedicine.com/plastic/topic243.htm. Updated November 6, 2003.

Wound Care Information Network. "Hydrogel sheets." Available online. URL: http://www.medicaledu.com/hydrogellsheet.htm. Accessed March 1, 2006.

Yang, Jun Yi, and Timothy Damron. "Histology of bone." eMedicine. Available online. URL: http://www.emedicine.com/orthoped/topic403.htm. Updated August 19, 2002.

Yaseen, Samir, and Christie Thomas. "Metabolic alkalosis." eMedicine. Available online. URL: http://www.emedicine.com/med/topic1459.htm. Updated August 2, 2002.

Yugoslav Society for Plastic, Reconstructive and Aesthetic Surgery. "History of plastic, reconstructive and aesthetic surgery in Yugoslavia." Available online. URL: http://www.yupras.co.yu/history.htm. Accessed March 27, 2006.

Zabawski, Edward J., Jr., and Clay J. Cockerell. "Halo nevus." eMedicine. Available online. URL: http://www.emedicine.com/DERM/topic174.htm. Updated May 18, 2005.

INDEX